Mother Food

For Breastfeeding Mothers

Foods and herbs that promote milk
production and a mother's health

With sections on colic,
allergy, depression, weightloss,
and low milk supply

Hilary Jacobson

"Mother Food" has been compiled as an informational guide for mothers and their health care providers.

Neither the publisher nor the author can assume medical or legal responsibility if the contents of this book are taken as a prescription.

Treatment of lactation difficulties and health issues should be supervised by a lactation specialist in conjunction with a licensed health care provider.

You and your healthcare-provider take full responsibility for the use that you make of this book. – Hilary Jacobson

Mother Food © 2004 by Hilary Jacobson.

Imprint: Mother Food Books Series / Rosalind Press

All rights reserved. No part of this publication may be used or reproduced without written permission by the author.

Jacobson, Hillary A. (Ann), 1956 –

Mother Food: lactogenic food and herbs for milk production and for a mother's and her baby's health.

Includes bibliographical references, endnotes, and index.

ISBN 978-0-9795995-0-7

First Printing June 2004

Cover: Cathi Stevenson   http://www.bookcoverexpress.com

*dedicated in hope and trust
to the health and the future
of our children*

Contents

Measures ... Caffeine (coffee, tea, soda, chocolate) ... Limit or Stop Smoking ... Alcohol—Set Your Limit

Balance Your Use of Caffeine ... A Resource for Sugar Addicts ... Mothers With Eating Disorders or Abuse Issues during Birth ... Foods that Strengthen the Center and Support Milk Supply ... Two TCM Herbal Remedies

Acknowledgments

I would like to thank my family for their patience, my friends for their support—and to give a *big hug* to my children, whose joy of breastfeeding remains an inspiration.

I would like to thank three professional women for their assistance in my exploration of milk supply issues, Christiane Husi, the founder of the school for holistic breastfeeding support in Switzerland, Beverly Morgan, IBCLC, author of "Reading Your Baby's Body Language" and "Breastfeeding's Number One Question: How Do I Know My Baby is Getting Enough Milk?", and Susan Chick, childbirth educator, doula, and founder of the email forum for "Mothers Overcoming Breastfeeding Issues," (MOBI).

I wish to acknowledge my debt of gratitude to the mothers and professionals who contributed their knowledge, insights, and recipes to this book. Though too many to name individually, your experience and wisdom are present on all these pages.

I would like to express my appreciation to the IBCLCs Patricia Gima, for her insights on fats and minerals and their impact on milk supply, to Sheila Humphrey and Cheryl Renfree for their insightful conversation, and to acknowledge Lisa Marasco, whose innovative research has given comfort to countless women who have low milk supply. A special thanks to John M. Riddle, Ph.D., for the identification of plants from Dioscorides' ancient herbal, and to James Akre, for his enthusiasm that extends to all-things-breastfeeding. On cold, rainy days, his encouragement helped me not give up on writing this book.

Finally, to the kind and courageous mothers at MOBI, my heartfelt gratitude for allowing me to learn with you.

Hilary Jacobson

Foreword

Throughout time there have been changing views toward breastmilk and its relationship to a mother's diet. In the 30 years that I have been involved in breastfeeding, I have seen what we once believed to be true shift to another perspective. Whereas we know that many cultures traditionally have a list of foods and herbs to avoid or add to the diet of a breastfeeding woman, during the last several decades in Western cultures, breastfeeding experts placed the notion of 'lactation foods' in the 'myths category.' Now this is changing.

When I became involved in breastfeeding in 1973, mothers were told to eat wholesome food. Supplements were limited to brewers yeast to make more milk and prenatal vitamins to assure a balanced diet. The list of foods to avoid in the United States had shrunk considerably, with drugs, cigarettes, and alcohol being on the short list. As there was no proof that other suspected foods were a problem for *all* mothers and babies, it seemed prudent not to deprive all mothers of potentially healthy and enjoyable foods. Over time however, foods were informally added back to the 'avoid list' as women noticed, for example, that their children were unsettled or colicky after they had caffeine or cow's milk. This food avoidance was mother to mother wisdom.

In 1991, the Institute of Medicine's Subcommittee on Nutrition During Lactation, the Committee on Nutritional Status During Pregnancy and Lactation, the Food and Nutrition Board, the Institute of Medicine, and the National Academy of Science published their findings on "Nutrition During Lactation." In answering the question "Does Maternal Nutritional Status Influence Milk Composition?" they made a number of generalizations. The report stated that many major minerals, such as calcium, phosphorus, magnesium, sodium and potassium in human milk are not affected by diet. However, there was a link between a mother's diet and the composition of mother's milk in other cases.

1) The proportions of different fatty acids in human milk vary according to maternal dietary intake.

2) Maternal intakes of selenium and iodine are positively related to their concentrations in human milk.

3) The vitamin content of human milk is dependent upon the mother's current vitamin intake and her vitamin stores, but the

strength of the relationship varies with the vitamin. Chronically low maternal intake of vitamins may result in milk that contains low amounts of these essential nutrients.

As the connection between maternal diet and the composition of the mother's milk was strengthened, people began looking at the connection between allergy, sensitization and fussiness in an infant that is related to a mother's diet.

Research done mostly in Europe has been uncovering connections between the ratios of fatty acids in a mother's milk and her baby's tendency to develop certain allergies. Furthermore, a recent study from T. Dunder in Finland, *"Diet, serum fatty acids, and atopic diseases in childhood"*[17] concluded that children who develop atopic disease usually come from a home where margarine instead of butter is used. This makes sense from the point of view of fatty acid metabolism and allergy.

Many experts are now convinced that babies are presensitized in the womb to proteins that later act as allergens in a mother's milk. This has lead to new guidelines for mothers in families with a history of allergy, including that they avoid one of the most potentially dangerous allergens during pregnancy and breastfeeding: the peanut.

Science is now leading where women's wisdom once prevailed. Still, many mothers make assumptions about foods that limit their diet unnecessarily. They try to find a universal list of foods to avoid rather than keying in to foods more specific to themselves and their babies. When the role of foods in a mother's diet is understood, mothers can discover their unique intolerances and avoid them, enhancing health for both mother and baby. Mrs. Jacobson's book takes us in this direction.

Studies have also shown that certain foods and chemical substances, including nicotine, some antihistamines, estrogen, vitamin B6, garlic, beer and several herbs may enhance or hamper milk production. While this has changed our understanding of milk production, the old assumption—that every mother makes an adequate amount of milk for her baby(s)—has been slower to change. Mothers who have difficulties maintaining or producing enough milk are often told that they have just not tried the right strategies, causing these mothers to feel abandoned by the breastfeeding community.

The notion that milk volume could be influenced by adding herbs or lactation enhancing foods was not widely embraced in Westernized

Introduction

In 1985, after the birth of my first child, I had low milk supply. The inability to produce enough milk to nourish my baby led to profound feelings of failure as a mother. Nothing I did seemed to help increase my milk supply. Weeks passed. Then, one day, I chanced to drink a Swiss soda that is made from whey and flavored with herbal extracts*. Suddenly I had so much milk that my baby could not keep up with the flow. How was this possible?

With each of my four children, I learned more about foods and herbs that increased my meager milk supply. If I did not eat these foods and take these herbs, within two days my milk supply dwindled to a trickle. I recognized that I was unusual, an exception to the rule, but I nonetheless began to wonder why we in the West say that what we eat has no effect on milk supply, whereas around the world, mothers have elaborate traditions of *mother food.*

To learn more I consulted the University Library of Basel in Switzerland, where I live, and corresponded with researchers and authors. I also spoke to persons from different countries to learn how mothers in their cultures support their milk supply.

Understanding the mystery of foods and their relationship to milk supply was like putting together a puzzle. I was exhilarated each time I discovered a new piece. However, none of my friends or colleagues shared my enthusiasm for this subject, and I felt very alone. Finally, in 1996, I was able to go online. There I met a community of mothers dealing with low milk supply. I felt like I'd come home.

At about this time it occurred to me that these foods and herbs might have had special importance in early human history—a time when the survival of babies depended solely on breastmilk. I decided to look for clues in mythology. The late scholar Robert Graves called myths "ancient newspapers." He said that myths used symbolic language to describe stone-age culture. Well, I soon discovered that these foods and herbs were associated with a dozen mother-goddesses the world over. But what could this mean? The answer seemed

---

* It is called *Rivella* and is used in Swiss maternity wards to help mothers build their milk supply (though I did not know this at the time that I tried it). My midwife believes that it increases milk flow.

obvious: stone-age women saw milk-enhancing herbs and foods as the gifts of a mother-goddess, provided to support their milk production.

Mother-goddesses were worshipped as the protectors of crops. To my amazement, I realized that the list of milk-enhancing foods is identical to the list of crops that were cultivated earliest by Neolithic peoples. It was *women* who cultivated these staple food crops, and botanists have long wondered what prompted our foremothers to prefer the foods that they did. To me, the answer seemed clear: they cultivated food that supported their milk supply.

What was good enough for my foremothers was good enough for me. Indeed, with the help of these foods and herbs I exclusively breastfed my third and fourth children for more than a year (they did not accept solid foods though I did offer). Both were plump babies— the type you'd expect to see on an advertisement for formula. And of my four children, these are the two who have no allergies.

Back when I had these experiences, breastfeeding experts did not understand why some mothers had low milk supply. Today, thankfully, physiological causes for low milk supply are being explored. Research is also providing explanations for the influence that foods and herbs have on milk production.

Many experts, however, are still hesitant to talk about herbs and food. They fear that mothers could believe that breastfeeding success depends on herbs and diet, rather than on a mother's responding to her baby's cues of hunger, and on her baby's ability to latch on to the areola and to remove milk. Another fear is that mothers might become upset or depressed by what they perceive as dietary restrictions.

It is my hope that in the long run, helping mothers to understand the impact that food and herbs can have on their breastfeeding experience will increase both the number of breastfeeding mothers and the length of time that they breastfeed. Knowledge that enhances a skill leads to greater confidence and empowerment. And these are major factors in breastfeeding success.

I also believe that this information is beneficial to the fundamental health of mothers and their families. Historically, human beings have been eating a whole-foods diet up to a few generations ago. This diet included a wealth of nutrients that benefited both a mother's health and the composition of her breastmilk. For instance, a study done in England from 1991 showed a *significant and sustained increase* in the fat content of breastmilk, *if* mothers supplemented with fish oil. The milk of mothers in the control group, who were not taking this supplement, saw a *decrease* in the fat content of their milk over the same period. This indicates that the diet of early humanity, which typically included plenty of fish, would have provided babies with higher-caloric milk for a longer time, as well as with milk that contained higher levels of omega-3 fatty acids. These same fatty acids have been shown to prevent depression and foggy-mindedness in mothers after birth and to improve the overall development of babies.

We have known for decades that the kinds of fats that a mother takes will influence the fatty acid content of her milk. Specific fatty acids promote the neural development of babies, or increase the immunity-strengthening properties of breastmilk. Trans-fatty acids, however, found in processed vegetable oils and processed foods, decrease these same properties. Surely all mothers want to know how to make their milk richer in 'good' fatty acids.

In addition, low milk supply is an issue for many more mothers than is commonly thought. For instance, even successfully nursing mothers may see a slump in their milk production at around 3–4 months, or later. Many mothers, once they have their period, see a dip in their milk supply two weeks before menstruation. And, when returning to work, mothers may have problems keeping up their supply while pumping. Finally, some mothers who exclusively breastfeed can only meet their baby's needs by breastfeeding almost constantly, day and night.

These issues can often be addressed through diet and herbs. For instance, mothers report that they pump more milk in the office on days when they drink herbal teas, have oatmeal for breakfast, or hummus for lunch. Mothers who exclusively pump can also use these foods and herbs to help support their supply.

Clearly, information that helps mothers to sustain their milk supply when they pump at work, during "milk-slumps," during illness, before their period, during a baby's growth spurt, or during a nursing strike can help mothers have a more positive experience of breastfeeding.

Mothers who have an overly-high milk supply may also benefit. They can learn which foods and herbs to avoid while bringing their supply down to the needs of their baby.

Finally, some babies learn how to suppress their mother's milk production. They may suppress milk production if they cannot keep up with the milk flow, for instance, but also if the mother's milk contains chemicals or tastes that they do not like, or if the mother takes foods that trigger a baby's allergies, or colic, or heartburn. In learning how to identify and eliminate a baby's problem foods from her diet, mothers can prevent this baby-caused reduction in milk supply from reoccurring.

This book looks at the impact that food and herbs can have on a mother's physical and emotional health, on her milk supply, on her baby's digestion or indigestion, and on allergic reactions. There is also a section on toxins, and on toxins in the home environment. These subjects tie into the prevention of neurological, behavioral, and learning problems later on in the child's life.

I have also explored questions that many mothers pose about diet. For instance, mothers frequently ask how they can overcome sugar or soft drink cravings and develop better eating habits while losing weight. I address food cravings and food addictions, based on the work of DesMaisons and others. Since weightgain is often related to blood sugar issues, some discussion is devoted to this as well.

Mothers frequently report that they don't have enough time to eat or cook. I address this by providing a selection of simple, milk-enhancing *mother food* recipes. I have also included basic whole-foods cooking instructions. I hope this will help young mothers pick up cooking techniques that, up until four generations ago, were an integral part of the culture of motherhood.

I have included a discussion of the ways that lactogenic foods and herbs were perceived in ancient Greece, India, and China. I find this subject fascinating and I hope it will interest my readers as well. Otherwise—there's no harm in skipping these chapters.

Before continuing, I would like to state that the information in this book is for educational purposes only and is not intended to replace the diagnosis and treatment of your health care provider or lactation expert. I cannot be held liable for any ill effects that may be incurred through the remedies or treatments described here.

I would also like to say that there is no instant cure for low milk supply. Some mothers see a drastic improvement when taking a combination of foods and herbs, while others, even with expert guidance, frequent pumping, and the use of medication, do not. For these mothers, it may be helpful to know that you are not alone: other mothers experience breastfeeding grief and understand what you are going through. Most of these mothers say that in doing everything possible to make breastfeeding work, and by giving their baby whatever breastmilk they do have, they have fewer regrets later on.

In this book, recommendations and warnings for herbs are based on their safety rating from the US and Germany. The bibliography lists sources on allergy and herbal medicine; source references are listed in the endnotes section; and indexes are divided into *Herbs*, *Foods*, and a general *Subject* Index.

When writing this book, it was difficult to decide what to include and what not. I was relieved to realize that I could save certain subjects for articles published on my website. Please check my website for more information: www.mother-food.com.

This book is being published through the venue of digital demand printing. The advantage is that the author has full control over content, and that it can be revised at any time. This book is easily ordered online, but will only become available in bookstores, healthfood stores and libraries if mothers inform their local resources of their interest in "Mother Food" and request its availability. If you find that this book is helpful to you, please spread the word in your community so that other mothers can benefit.

"Mother Food" will hopefully be read by people of many cultural backgrounds living in many countries. I hope that mothers and fathers will be inspired to talk to the "old folk" in their family or community about the traditions they followed to support milk production, and that you will write me and share what you learn. Documentation through photos, dvd, video or cassette recordings are welcome. Soon our oldest generation will have passed on, and with them, their knowledge of *mother food* traditions. Let's preserve what we can.

With all my heart – wishing radiant health to parents, their children, and to their children's children.

Hilary Jacobson   (June 2004)

Part One

About Mother Food

CHAPTER ONE

Tools To Build and Sustain Milk Supply

"From the beginning of time, mothers have used various herbs to increase their milk supply." — Jack Newman, MD, "The Ultimate Breastfeeding Book of Answers."

This chapter outlines ways that mothers can prepare before birth to prevent breastfeeding problems, and it looks at measures to prevent these problems from escalating if they do occur. It also looks at the choices available to mothers who have extraordinary problems. The history of milk-enhancing foods and herbs at the beginning of this chapter ties into the theme of *tools to build milk supply*. These tools include pumps, feeding devices, supply-enhancing food and herbs, getting enough to eat and drink, and having contact with a lactation specialist and a community of supportive mothers.

It is beyond the scope of this book to present breastfeeding basics in detail. I refer the reader to a range of excellent breastfeeding books, for instance by J. Newman, K. Huggins, M. Renfrew, B. Morgan, and J. Tamaro, among others.

Galactagogue - Lactogenic

Pharmacists call a food, herb, mineral, or medication that increases milk production a *galactagogue*. This chewy word stems from the ancient Greek language, in which *galacta* means "milk" and *gogos* means "leading." A galactagogue *leads milk from the breast*.

The ancients had a special relationship to breastfeeding. They thought that a breastfeeding goddess created the galaxy! (Note the nod to *milk* in the word "*gala*xy.") She tried to feed her baby, but missed his mouth. Endless sprays of droplets flew across the sky, where they coagulated into the stars and planets. The *Milky Way* was born. Today, all we recall of this creation myth is that the moon is made of cheese.

Galactagogues, too, have ancient roots in human culture. One of the historically oldest goddesses was called *Demeter*. The Greeks worshipped her as the great "mother of grain." In the Greek language, *de* means "grain" and *meter* means "mother," but perhaps *De-meter* also means the "grain of mothers." The grain referred to here is barley, a hardy grain, and the oldest and most sacred grain in Greece. We know that the Greeks used barley as a galactagogue. We also know that a special sugar in barley, *beta-glucan*, increases levels of *prolactin*, the hormone that regulates milk production. Barley is a confirmed *mother food*.

Most people today have never heard of galactagogues. This is not surprising. Up until the 1990s, people thought that galactagogues work through the placebo effect. Then the breastfeeding expert, Kathleen Huggins, had significant milk supply difficulties, and was able to increase her milk production by taking fenugreek seed. After that, breastfeeding experts observed countless mothers whose low milk production improved, often dramatically, with food and herbs.

Now breastfeeding experts frequently recommend galactagogues, in combination with other measures, for problems with low milk supply. Unfortunately, scientists in the US have not yet studied the effect of herbal galactagogues *on women* (studies have been done on rats and other animals[1]). Safety is therefore a concern, though the herbs recommended in this book have no record of toxicity. You can read more about these herbs in *A Lactogenic Herbal* in Part Four.

  *

In this book, the word "lactogenic" is used to describe a food, herb or medication that enhances milk production. "Anti-lactogenic" describes a food, herb, or medication that reduces milk production. "Lactogenic diet" refers both to a choice of foods and to a manner of eating that support breastfeeding, and also a mother's and her baby's best health.

Milk-Medicinals: Ancient Tools of Motherhood

Long before cattle, sheep, and goats were domesticated, and their milk used as food, our foremothers naturally preferred foods and herbs that supported their milk production. This was a time when breastmilk alone sustained the lives of infants and ensured our survival as a species. Mothers noticed that certain plants had a supportive effect on their milk supply. These were cultivated as our earliest crops, for instance, barley, carrot, corn, fennel, fenugreek, garlic, lettuce, onion, peanut*, sesame, sweet potato, and yam. Many were revered as the sacred plants of women, for instance the lotus, fig, date, coconut, elder flower, and almond.

Lactogenic grains, such as barley and millet, were fermented into *grain-drinks* and taken by mothers to increase their milk production. Grains were also the holy plants of ancient mother-goddesses. In the earliest days of human culture, Neolithic mother-goddesses were portrayed with breasts that were large and laden with milk. Later, they were shown breastfeeding a baby. Clearly, early cultures viewed the breastfeeding relationship as synonymous with divine, motherly love—and these earliest grains were sacred, at least in part because they supported milk production.

The prevalence of *mother foods* in early cultures appears to reflect women's timeless concern with milk production. We are not alone. Animals, too, prefer certain plants when they nurse, or so say rural peoples from around the world. Women observed their nursing animal's preferences and learned from them.

Ancient medical texts contain a plethora of galactagogues, suggesting that a mother's ability to breastfeed was highly regarded both by medical doctors and by philosophers (they were originally one and the same). In the first century B.C., a doctor in India named Caraka† wrote a comprehensive book of herbalism based on older works. He wrote that herbs have fifty therapeutic effects, two of which are beneficial to nursing mothers—*to increase milk supply* and *to clean the milk.* Caraka cleansed a mother's milk *by using herbs to*

---

* Peanuts are not advised as a galactagogue due to their being dangerously allergenic for about 1% of all babies. In Asia and Africa, cooked green peanuts are used to build milk supply. It is possible that in this form they are less allergenic.

† Some historians place Caraka one to six centuries earlier, and some believe he was not one man, but a school of doctors.

cultures over the last several decades. Even the old standby, brewers yeast, had been discredited as something of a myth. Mrs. Jacobson is among the first to focus on foods as well as herbs from around the world that promote lactation. Luckily for us, people such as Mrs. Jacobson have continued to research lactation foods, so the wisdom of the ages has not been lost. Her years of personal research to bolster her own low milk supply can now benefit today's mothers, not only women with low milk supply, but all breastfeeding mothers.

Mrs. Jacobson has learned that mothers in other cultures stress herbs that support digestion and boost the immune system, that soothe the mood and strengthen the nerves, and also foods that have hormonal components that apparently steady the chemistry of lactation. In other words, she has found that these food-traditions support the health of the mother and baby on many basic and beneficial levels.

The last decade has seen a resurgence of interest in galactagogues (foods that increase milk supply or milk flow). The herb of choice for promoting milk supply, fenugreek, opened the door of interest to other herbs and foods. The climate is now right for *"Mother Food."* Sit back, enjoy a cup of herbal tea, and take this world tour of lactation foods.

Beverly Morgan IBCLC

Georgetown, Texas, USA
Author of the audiobooks series *Breastfeeding Basics and Beyond*

improve her digestion. Today, with so many babies suffering from colic and allergies, perhaps we could learn from this ancient doctor.

In the 1st century AD, a Greek doctor, Dioscorides, compiled a huge treatise on herbal medicine. In the preface, he stated that he was putting the knowledge of the 'ancients' to paper—referring to doctors and midwives who lived centuries before his time. It is noteworthy that John M. Riddle, Ph.D., a renowned medical historian, showed that Dioscorides was correct in the herbs that he prescribed for abortion. Riddle discovered identical remedies in Egyptian herbals that were centuries older than Dioscorides' book. *Just how old are the remedies that Dioscorides records?* It is possible that these remedies were passed down from mother to daughter in an unbroken chain for hundreds if not thousands of years.

Dioscorides provides 30 remedies for breastfeeding mothers, three of which are foods. He has remedies for increasing milk, for the milk-ejection reflex, to improve milk-flow, even for keeping milk fresh in the breast (this one is for wet-nurses who were unable to regularly empty their breasts), for treating engorgement, milk clots, mastitis, for extinguishing milk production, and for re-lactating.

Dioscorides carefully differentiates between herbs that promote the milk-ejection reflex ("bring the milk down") and those that increase milk supply ("make milk more abundant"). The women of his day clearly knew that whereas some mothers produced on the low side, others had problems "letting down."

Medical historians who read ancient languages will find many more references to galactagogues in Chinese and Egyptian herbals. However, the *high art* of galactagogues will remain a mystery. Anthropologists in the 19th and early 20th centuries, writing from Africa and the Americas, noted that elderly women could fully re-lactate, within a few days, by using special, potent herbal remedies. (If a mother became ill or died, her own mother or aunt would re-lactate and feed her baby.) Sadly, these powerful remedies were not revealed to the anthropologists. They were closely guarded as sacred tribal knowledge—knowledge that is probably now lost.

Still, traditions do live on. Some are even created anew. We, too, can avail ourselves of lactogenic foods and herbs, and invent our own traditions. For instance, we can have oatmeal for breakfast, snack on almonds throughout the day, enjoy chickpea spread (hummus) with our meals, press garlic into salad sauce, or use lactogenic spices in our meals (they make a great spaghetti sauce).

The Benefits of a Lactogenic Diet

A lactogenic diet addresses maternal health in a broad way. During the postpartum, mothers have increased vulnerability to blood sugar highs and lows, to mood swings, to hypothyroidism, and to fatigue. By addressing these problem areas through their diets, mothers may experience less postpartum exhaustion and depression, enabling us to enjoy motherhood more.

Digestion is a central theme for many breastfeeding mothers. If a mother's digestion is poor, and if she has a *permeable* intestine, due to antibiotics or other causes, partially digested food molecules will enter her bloodstream and then her milk. These can cause digestive discomfort in her baby and lead to fussiness, to crying, perhaps to food sensitivity or allergies—even to refusal to breastfeed in some cases. The good news is that breastfeeding provides mothers with time to improve their digestion, and it is a unique opportunity to recognize and recover from so-called *problem foods*. (These subjects are discussed in detail in Chapters Four and Five.) The benefit for her baby is a perfect food. Her baby is no longer fussy, and she is healthier, too. She has more energy with which to enjoy and care for her happier baby.

A lactogenic diet contains foods that enrich the fat content of breastmilk, and fats are crucial to the development of young children. This is discussed in Chapter Three.

Lactogenic food and herbs help stabilize a mother's milk supply during illness (her own or her baby's), during her baby's growth spurts (they help her body respond more quickly to the higher demand for milk), if she returns to work, if her baby goes on a nursing strike, and also when her baby begins to eat solid food. Mothers who naturally have an abundant milk supply will want to choose foods that benefit their digestion and enrich their milk, but avoid foods and herbs that create an over-supply.

About Low Milk Supply

Milk production is based on the law of *supply and demand*. A baby drinks according to his hunger, and the mother's body responds to that demand with an appropriate amount of milk. In order for this law to function, a baby must be able to remove milk from his mother's breasts, and he must be allowed to breastfeed as often as he would like. During the first few weeks, some babies may drink every hour or two around the clock.

Most cases of low milk supply result when the baby is unable to efficiently remove milk due to poor positioning on the breast and a shallow latch that does not encompass the areola. A visit with a lactation specialist can help mothers and babies improve their position and latch. Also, if the mother does not follow her baby's cues of hunger, but rather feeds her baby according to a fixed schedule, her supply will probably not be appropriate to meet her baby's needs.

Less common factors for low milk supply include: a baby's nipple preference (when a baby receives a bottle and develops a preference for it); immature suck (in spite of good latch, the baby cannot effectively remove milk); a mismatched size of a baby's mouth to his mother's nipple or areola; a baby's tight or short frenulum preventing good suck (the frenulum is the strap of skin between the tongue and the floor of the mouth); the baby refusing the breast for any myriad of reasons; a baby actively suppressing his mother's supply by under-drinking, for instance because he can't deal with the strong flow, or because he has indigestion or heart burn.

Painful conditions of the breast can cause a mother to avoid or limit breastfeeding. When the pain resolves, the mother's milk supply will rebound. Rarely, physiological factors are involved in low milk supply: large blood loss during birth can damage the pituitary gland; tiny pieces of the placenta in the womb generate pregnancy-hormones that inhibit the onset of lactation; thyroid imbalances hinder milk production; other hormonal imbalances may be involved; and a mother may have insufficient glandular tissue in the breast. (For more discussion on low milk supply, see Chapter Thirteen.) The good news is that these problems can almost always be resolved with time, guidance, and in some cases, specific therapy or training for the baby.

Building Milk Supply

If you suspect that you have low milk supply, talk to your local La Leche League (LLL), or see a lactation specialist for a diagnosis of your breastfeeding situation. Until you know what the problem is, you cannot know which strategy will help. The specialist will adjust your baby's latch and position, and observe your baby's suck. She may teach you special suck training techniques, or refer your baby to a specific physical or occupational therapist. She may also advise that you borrow, rent, or buy a pump. Pumps that work most reliably to build supply are so-called *hospital grade pumps*, the Medela Classic™ or a Lact-E® by Ameda-Hollister. While these are more expensive, they are generally more effective than smaller pumps, which are adequate for pumping at work. Each mother is individual, however, and some mothers successfully build their supply using smaller pumps. One hand pump, the Avent® Isis™, is handy and effective for many women—occasionally leading to better results than a hospital grade pump. Mothers often find it helpful to use the gentle, massaging Isis™ flange insert in hospital grade pumps.

For some mothers, finding the right pump can be tedious trial and error work. Different mothers, different breasts, respond to different pumps and flanges. Ask your local lactation expert or hospital for advice. You can also find information at online support groups, such as at http://groups.yahoo.com/group/pumpmoms.

Some mothers prefer to hand-express their milk, rather than using a pump, and for some, hand-expression is more effective. This gentle procedure is best taught person to person: ask your local La Leche League leader or lactation specialist to show you how. An excellent description of hand-expression is found in the book, *Bestfeeding*.

Sometimes, pumping is not necessary. The LLL suggests that mothers take their babies into bed with them to cuddle and rest for twenty-four hours, allowing the baby to feed at his leisure. This intense cuddle-time increases milk supply very well for most mothers.

For a very few mothers, however, no amount of resting with her baby or pumping will result in a significant increase in milk supply. For these mothers, taking lactogenic foods, herbs, and sometimes medication, can help their bodies gradually build an abundant supply of milk. Some of these mothers see a greater increase in their milk supply through galactagogues than through pumping

<u>*Let-Down Strategies*</u>

Milk-Ejection Reflex –Learning to Let-Down

Let-down difficulties are another possible cause of low milk supply. Mothers who find it difficult to let-down when feeding their baby may find it doubly hard to let-down while pumping. Here are some tips that can help.

- **Nap or relax**. Lay down a few moments before pumping, and let all your worries go. Feel your body fall heavily into the bed or floor. An optimal length of time to nap or relax is 25 – 30 minutes, but even as little as 5 minutes helps.

- **Gravity**. Lean over, so that your breasts hang downward. Swing your upper body and your breasts gently from side to side. Gravity promotes milk flow. Some mothers support themselves above their baby—lying on his back on the bed or floor—so that her breast hangs to the baby's mouth.

- **Breathing**. Breathe softly and deeply through the nose to stimulate a let-down (rhythmic breathing stimulates the pituitary to produce oxytocin).

- **Compress**. A compress of warm, moist towels on the breasts before pumping can help the milk flow.

- **Breast massage**. Stroke your breast from the chest wall to the areola. Gently explore your breast with your fingertips until you find the milk glands, and massage these, one cluster, or hard, tender area, at a time. Move your fingertips in small circles above the pea-sized glands, pushing your fingertips gently downward into your breast. This massage stimulates that cluster to release its milk. The area will then become soft, and you may even feel the milk flowing down the milk duct to the areola.

- **Breast compression**. With your breast-supporting hand in the 'C-position,' and the fingers and thumb well back from the areola, press the breast gently but firmly toward the wall of the chest. This effectively compresses, or presses out, the milk. Breast compression should not hurt! Pressing too hard could damage your glandular tissue.

- **Drink**. Drink a large glass of water or other beverage before or while nursing or pumping. The let-down reflex makes some mothers extremely thirsty. Some say that drinking helps their milk flow more freely. Getting enough fluid will also help prevent plugged milk ducts.

- **Rescue Remedy**. Take a dropperful of the Bach flowers "Rescue Remedy" before pumping. This remedy eases anxiety, and some mothers find that it makes all the difference.

- **Visualization**. Imagine a peaceful scene, or a scene of particular beauty, or meaning, to you. Breathe deeply, and visualize your milk flowing. Keep a photo of your baby close to your pump.

- **Receive a massage**. While breastfeeding or pumping, have someone stand behind you and massage your shoulders and the area between your shoulder blades with her thumbs.

- **Double stimulation**. Mothers with let-down difficulties may find that pumping both breasts at once, or pumping one breast while breastfeeding their baby on the other, helps with the let-down and increases the flow. Some mothers become expert at this balancing act, supporting the baby with pillows on one side, and attaching the pump to the other breast, perhaps using a special holding bra, so that they have a hand free to hold a book or glass to drink.

- **Oxytocin nose-spray**. If deep breathing and other techniques are not sufficient, an oxytocin nose-spray enables some mothers to finally experience a let-down. Ask your doctor for a prescription, and have it compounded by a pharmacist. Do not use the nose-spray more than a few times, however, as this can reduce the body's sensitivity to its own oxytocin and impair the let-down!

Pumping Strategies

Frequency of Pumping

Pumping frequently with a hospital grade pump—every two hours around the clock—is the most common recommendation for building milk supply. Usually, two or three days of frequent pumping suffice to increase milk production. To ensure that the breast is completely emptied, remember to perform breast compression while pumping, and pump five minutes after the milk stops flowing. Pump for a minimum of 15 – 20 minutes.

Less frequent pumping—every three to four hours—but pumping for a longer time, produces better results for a minority of mothers. If possible, continue to pump until you have another let-down.

It is generally recommended that mothers pump every two or three hours throughout the night as well. Some mothers see a marked increase in their supply if they pump in the early morning hours, when prolactin production is naturally highest. Other mothers, however, find that getting a stretch of 4 – 5 hours of sleep is better for building their supply.

If you drink plenty of liquid before going to bed, you will automatically wake up about five hours later to empty your bladder. While still half asleep you can feed the baby (if she wakes up and is hungry), and/or pump, put the milk in the fridge or freezer, rinse out the tubes and flanges, and go back to bed. (Yes, this does become automatic routine with time!)

No Milk at the Pump

Some women do not pump very much milk—less than an ounce, sometimes only a few drops. This does not mean that the mother has no milk—though it *can* mean this. It is more likely that this pump is not right for this mother, or that she is not able to let-down while pumping. Hand expressing may be the solution for some mothers, and a different pump and flange could produce better results for others. Most mothers are eventually able to let-down while pumping (see suggestions above).

A few mothers, however, never do produce well through pumping or hand expression, try what they might. This still does not mean that they have no milk. Women are not *designed* to let-down for anything but a baby. Do not be discouraged if you only get a few drops at the pump. This does not necessarily mean that you have too little milk, or that your baby is getting too little milk at your breast.

To Pump or Not to Pump – Limiting Stress

Mothers occasionally find that their milk supply increases when they *stop* pumping, even when they stop using foods and herbs altogether. When they stop *obsessing* over breastfeeding and just relax, their milk production picks up naturally.

It is also possible that, coincidentally, these mother's babies develop a more efficient suck just at the time when they stop pumping. Many mothers go through 2 – 4 months of pumping before their baby becomes an efficient drinker. Then they suddenly find themselves with a competent breastfeeding baby and a full supply.

If you are feeling exhausted by pumping, the decision to reduce, or to stop pumping, although very difficult and sometimes painful, could be right for you. Topping off milk with formula is a decision that some mothers are forced to make—either because they cannot produce enough milk, or because they do not have the time or energy to pump. Most mothers want to do everything they can to succeed at breastfeeding, and the decision to stop pumping, and to supplement with more formula, is painful. I hope that you will find what is best for you and your baby.

Lactation Aid: Using a Supplemental Feeding Device

> *"My son was born at 35 weeks gestation and spent his first week in the NICU. Fortunately, I was prepared to try a lactation aid to keep him at the breast instead of going to bottles right away like we had before. It worked! He will take a bottle now when necessary, but he's fully breastfed."*

A lactation aid is, very simply, a container for expressed milk or formula, with a long tube attached to deliver this fluid to your breast. Two kinds of lactation aids are available commercially: the Medela supplemental nursing system™ (SNS) and the Lact-Aid®. Before purchasing a lactation aid, you may wish to discuss your choice with your lactation consultant or research their pros and cons online.

Lactation aids serve many purposes. If a baby has problems nursing after birth, or if a mother's milk production is delayed, having a lactation aid at hand will make it unnecessary for the hospital staff to give your baby a bottle. By using the lactation aid, you avoid *nipple confusion*, a possible cause of later breastfeeding problems.

If a young baby has a weak suck, or if the mother's milk does not initially flow quickly enough to keep the baby happy, a lactation aid will help keep the baby at the breast, rewarding his early efforts with a reliable flow of milk. If a mother wishes to train her baby's suck using the finger feeding technique, she can use the Lact-Aid® with her expressed milk or formula.

If a mother adopts a baby, a lactation aid will keep her baby on her breast while she is building her supply. If a mother has low milk supply, a lactation aid will enable her to breastfeed long term. As one mother put it, "There is more to breastfeeding than milk. If you can't breastfeed, you can still breastbond."

In most cases, mothers use lactation aids for only a short time. Low-supply mothers who use a lactation aid long term discover tricks that make it convenient. For instance, they hold the tube in place by slipping it beneath the upper part of their nursing bra, or discover practical ways to use butterfly strips or hairstyling tape, or to hold the tube lightly with their fingers. They discover the best place to situate the bottle or sack so that the milk flows steadily but not too quickly, so that their baby still has to work for her milk[*].

By starting with a wider tube and working up to a more narrow tube, and by gradually placing the bottle or sack lower than the baby, so that the baby has to suck more strongly to bring up the milk against the force of gravity, mothers train their babies to suck more efficiently. Mothers can also press the tube shut for a while and then release it to imitate a let-down, or different rates of milk flow in the breast, or close off the second tube, creating a vacuum effect, so that the baby will have to work harder and develop a more efficient suck.

> *"I had to learn that there is more to breastfeeding than providing milk. Even if I can never provide all of my baby's nourishment, I am going to offer my breast to him for as long as he wants it."*

Weaning From a Lactation Aid

Weaning a baby from a lactation aid can be easy if you have strong milk production. Low-supply mothers on the other hand often wean gradually. It can take an act of courage for a low-supply mother to believe that her supply will fully respond to her baby's sucking and

---

[*] Jimmie Lynne Avery provides free consultation regarding the use of the Lact-Aid in building supply. She can be reached through the contact address on the website: http://www.lact-aid.com

that she will have enough milk without supplementing with a lactation aid. If this is your situation, it is recommended that you increase your use of lactogenic herbs and foods, and give yourself time and space to concentrate on this transition—your baby may wish to drink more frequently for a few days to stimulate the extra milk she needs.

Even if you continue to rely on the lactation aid, the time will come when she takes solid foods and no longer gets the bulk of her nourishment from your breast. At that time, low-supply mothers can breastfeed without a lactation aid, even if they produce very little milk. This kind of extended breastfeeding offers mothers and children very special time together. (You will not want to miss it!)

Medication for Milk Supply

Medication is sometimes prescribed to increase milk supply. One such medication, metoclopramide, with the brand name Reglan®, is manufactured in the US. Commonly used for stomach ailments, Reglan has the "side effect" of increasing prolactin, the hormone of milk production. Unfortunately, Reglan® frequently causes fatigue and depression, especially if used longer than two weeks, but sometimes after only a few days. If you take Reglan®, *keep an eye on your energy level and your mood, and stop if necessary.*

Another stomach medication, domperidone, sold as Motilium™, has the same milk-enhancing effect, but rarely causes fatigue and depression because only small amounts cross the blood-brain barrier. Domperidone is not manufactured in the US. In Switzerland, where I live, and in many countries, domperidone is sold over the counter. Formally, mothers in the US ordered it from Mexico, Canada, England, or New Zealand, or they had it compounded in pharmacies.

In June 2004, after a decade of widespread use, and no reports of more than rare, minor side effects in mothers, the FDA ruled against breastfeeding mothers using domperidone. This ruling was based on incidents decades old, when extremely high dosages of domperidone were given intravenously to severely ill patients, causing heart complications and contributing to fatality.

The FDA did not consult experts in the lactation community before making this ruling. They could, for instance, have consulted the leading international expert in medication and breastfeeding, Thomas W. Hale, Ph.D., Professor of Pediatrics. In his book, *Medications and Mother's Milk: A Manual of Lactational Pharmacology*, Hale lists Domperidone as an L2(SAFER), pediatric concerns: none reported.

Mothers in the US with insufficient glandular tissue (IGT) and low milk supply have been grateful for the availability of domperidone. Many have better success with domperidone than with Reglan®. However, medication, while improving supply in most mothers with IGT, does not always lead to a full supply. For many mothers, it is still necessary to pump, and to take herbs and foods. For some mothers, herbs, foods, and healthy fats have a better effect than medication. Finally, while most mothers can wean off galactagogues while maintaining their improved milk supply, some mothers find that they have to continue taking these galactagogues on a long-term basis, to maintain a steady and sufficient level of milk production.

> Jack Newman, M.D., endorses domperidone in his book, *The Ultimate Breastfeeding Book of Answers*. To get up-to-date information on the breastfeeding medication, do an internet search on "Jack Newman" and "domperidone."

Domperidone proves the 'intestine theory,' as do herbs

One of the anecdotal benefits of domperidone is that babies suffering from colic or heartburn often improve when their mothers take it. Since domperidone is taken to treat heartburn, nausea, and constipation, as well as to generally improve digestion, it seems likely that when a mother takes domperidone, her meals are better digested and fewer 'irritants' enter her milk. The result is a happier baby. For more information, read Chapter Five, on colic.

This digestive benefit is shared by lactogenic herbs, such as dill seed, fenugreek, and marshmallow, among many others: they increase a mother's milk supply but they also improve her digestion, and lead to a happier baby with less colic and heartburn[*].

---

[*] This is what Caraka, the ancient doctor from India mentioned earlier, may have meant by "cleansing the milk."

Prepare Before Birth

Mothers who have "been there" recommend that new mothers prepare for any eventuality by renting a hospital grade pump and buying or making a lactation aid (see pages 11-12) before birth. That way, a mother will not have to resort to formula and a bottle in an emergency.

The Avent Isis—a hand pump with gentle flange inserts that massage the areola—works as well for many low-supply women, and only costs about one month's rent, or $40 - 50. Still, hospital grade pumps are reliable and user-friendly (you may become tired using a hand-pump). If money is a problem, consider that pump rental is cheaper than formula in the long run. You may wish to buy a pump if it is clear that you have chronic low supply, or if you plan to pump at work.

Prepare to Prevent Pain

We tend to think of breastfeeding as a joy-only activity. Especially in the beginning, however, new mothers may experience excruciating conditions that make breastfeeding or pumping difficult. Pain is one of the most common causes behind mothers stopping breastfeeding— so be prepared! (It *does* get better.)

Some worst-case scenarios include severe engorgement, bad latch and torn nipples, plugged-ducts, mastitis and thrush. Intervention can bring relief and stop the problem or problems from escalating further.

There is only space to scratch the surface of these issues here. Fortunately, most breastfeeding books discuss this in detail. "The Nursing Mother's Herbal" by Sheila Humphrey discusses both medical and alternative therapies in detail.

It cannot be stressed enough that mothers should read and learn about prevention and treatment of these common problems before birth (you will not have much time afterwards).

- To avoid **extreme, painful engorgement** when the milk arrives, nurse often (and/or pump) during the first few days after birth before and after the milk comes in. Frequent feeding or emptying prevents extreme engorgement.

- **Cabbage leaves**, chilled, and softened by rolling in the hand and applied to the breast as a poultice for about twenty minutes, relieve swelling. This method may be repeated as often as necessary until the breasts are slacker.

- **Bra**: make sure your bra is large enough and loose—or go braless if possible. A tight bra can lead to plugged ducts, mastitis, and even low milk supply.

- **Drink plenty of water** to help **prevent plugged milk ducts**, which are more frequent during the early weeks of breastfeeding.

- **Latch**: avoid painful, cracked nipples by having your baby's latch diagnosed soon after birth. Pain that persists beyond the first few moments of breastfeeding is a sign that the latch or suck is not right.

- **Cracked nipples:** Spread a drop of colostrum or breastmilk onto your nipple, and air-dry before applying Lansinoh® or PurLan™ cream to the wounded area only. Soothies® are another option, both to prevent cracking and to promote healing. If the wound seems infected, use calendula tincture: dilute a teaspoon into a cup of boiled water, allow it to cool to room temperature, and wash the nipple with this dilution after feeding.

- **Breast infection** or **inflammation,** may be either an inflammation of tissues (similar to having a swollen, tender ankle), or a bacterial infection (mastitis). Follow the suggestions in this book to boost your immune system. Most important, get regular meals and rest up as much as possible. These routines of day-to-day life support your immune system as well.

- **Echinacea,** an herb that increases the immune response, can be taken orally to ward off breast infection at the first sign of redness, swelling, tenderness, or a distinctly warm area on the breast. Preventatively, it may be less helpful.

- Because **thrush** (yeast infection of the nipple and breast) is increasingly common (due to the overuse of antibiotics and to *diets rich in refined white flour and sugar*), it is wise to act preventatively. Good results have been observed when mothers take grapefruit seed extract before and after birth, and preparations of probiotic lactobacilli (healthfood store), or probiotic yogurt.

- If you have a history of yeast infections, be on the safe side and have **medication for thrush** at hand to use at the first sign of red, itchy, painful nipples, or shooting pain from the nipple to the wall of the chest. Gentian violet tincture is available over the counter. Though messy to use, it often solves the problem after only one application. The baby's mouth is treated as well when he drinks from your purple-stained breast. Read more about medication to treat thrush on Dr. Jack Newman's webpages.

More Preparation

Galactagogues

A kitchen cabinet full of lactogenic foods and spices, plus lactation tea, herbal supplements, and/or tincture, can help ensure that a mother's milk production becomes well established during the first few weeks after birth. Read in Chapter Twenty to learn which herbs are appropriate after birth, and which are better avoided.

Contact Your Breastfeeding Expert

Contact a local lactation consultant, preferably an *internationally board certified lactation consultant* (IBCLC). Give her a call before birth and let her know about any breastfeeding concerns you may have.

An IBCLC has the equivalent to a Master's degree in breastfeeding. She has seen hundreds of mothers, many with complex problems. Unfortunately, it is possible that the IBCLC in your area may not be available, or may not have time, just when you need her. In this case, your local La Leche League (LLL) may be able to help you, or be able to recommend other competent lactation experts.

An IBCLC may not be covered by your health insurance. Mothers who had breastfeeding problems with their first baby have told me that they put money aside during their second pregnancy to cover several visits with an IBCLC if necessary: it still costs less than formula in the end, and it is an investment in their baby's health.

When Breastfeeding Seems Impossible

Support and Guidance

When mothers encounter breastfeeding problems, life suddenly becomes more difficult, and sometimes more frightening, than they ever thought possible. In this situation, the support of friends and family, the comfort of a mother's support group such as La Leche League, or of an on-line support group, such as parentsplace.com, pumpmoms.org, or MOBI, and the professional guidance of a pediatrician and an IBCLC, are of utmost importance to the success of breastfeeding.

Feeling Up To the Task

Mothers can feel overwhelmed by breastfeeding difficulties—crying, fussy baby, apparent low milk supply, torn nipples, thrush, etc. Weaning may seem like the only sane solution, but mothers often regret this choice later on. If you are thinking of weaning your baby, please take a moment to consider the following.

You probably know that babies benefit from the brain-nourishing and immune-strengthening substances found only mother's milk—though this may be hard to believe if your baby is fretful at the breast. Ironically, it is the fussy, fretful baby who needs these substances the most, and it is precisely the fussy baby who tends to become sensitive to formula with time. The search for formula that is tolerated by your baby can be just as exhausting as the struggle to breastfeed. It can end with a mother having to purchase expensive hypoallergenic formula, or by her trying to re-lactate, in the hopes of having a food that her baby tolerates.

There are many tools available to help mothers and babies overcome breastfeeding difficulties—as insurmountable as these may seem now. Breastfeeding books offer excellent advice, and LLL-Leaders and lactation consultants provide support and individual guidance.

The sections in this book that focus on colic and food allergy, and the sections that focus on depression and exhaustion may also help, as these issues commonly accompany and compound breastfeeding problems.

Finding Specialized Help or Therapy

Cranio-sacral therapy, Occupational therapy, Speech Language Pathologists, Chiropractic

Therapy often turns breastfeeding around. For instance, if a baby is feeling physical trauma from birth, such as a kink in her neck, shoulders, or spine, it can be difficult to find a comfortable feeding position. Tenderness in the muscles surrounding her skull may cause her to feel pain when her head is touched or held. Many such babies become better feeders after gentle therapy from a *cranio-sacral therapist*. Chiropractics can also specialize in treating infants, and Speech Language Pathologists can help develop better suck.

Many breastfeeding experts today, such as Beverly Morgan, who wrote the foreword to this book, would like to see cranio-sacral therapy become routine for both mothers and babies after birth. In India, mothers and babies traditionally receive several sessions of massage after birth—working out their kinks and tension. This treatment doubtless contributes to their high rate of breastfeeding success.

A baby's inability to stimulate milk production may sometimes signal *"sensory integration dysfunction,"* or *developmental delays*. These babies are frequently high-need. Their sucking difficulties may be compounded by colic, by an inability to accept cuddling, by crying all the time, or GERD. An occupational therapist can recognize these issues, and a few therapy sessions may bring resolution to a baby's feeding problems. Talk to your doctor or IBCLC about therapy available in your area. Whatever form of therapy you choose, always ask if the therapist you are consulting has extensive experience treating infants.

High Palate

Sometimes, babies are born with the roof of their mouths, the "palate," arched so highly that they cannot create an adequate latch. These babies need *feeding help*, such as finger feeding, or a lactation aid at the breast. Their mothers will need to pump to replace the stimulation for milk production that they are not receiving from their baby's suck. Therapy (see above) may help, and the guidance of a lactation specialist is invaluable. Fortunately, most high-palate babies do learn to suckle well eventually.

She Refuses to Take the Breast

Occasionally, a baby will refuse to breastfeed for no apparent reason, either from the get-go or within the first few days after birth. These babies should be seen by an IBCLC for a diagnosis. If your IBCLC is as perplexed as you are, you may have a breast-refusing baby. But why would a baby refuse the breast?

Sometimes breast refusal is a reaction to having been physically forced to drink at the breast by a well-meaning nurse or lactation consultant. Some babies do not like being forced and may then refuse to take the breast. Some babies have what is called an *oral defensiveness* to objects that extend into the mouth. An IBCLC will usually be able to help a baby overcome oral defensiveness. However, specialized treatment by an occupational therapist may be necessary. Some babies may be sensitive to a mother's perfume, cosmetics or deodorant, and avoid the breast to avoid close contact to these odors. Fungal infection in the baby's mouth may also cause him to clamp up. Sensitivities to food the mother is eating may play a role as well.

You may have to consult several IBCLCs and therapists until you find one whose experience includes your issues, and who can provide the correct diagnosis and therapy or strategy. You may have luck, and your very first consultation will yield results. Most babies do overcome their issues, though it may require time and patience. If, in the meantime, a mother keeps up her supply, she will then be able to breastfeed.

Sadly, it is not always possible to resolve this problem. Some babies continue to refuse the breast, and a mother may never know the cause. If you are in this heartbreaking situation, realize that it does not mean you are a bad mother or that your relationship to your child is less valuable.

If you choose, you may still feed your baby your pumped or hand-expressed breastmilk. Such mothers are called *Express Pumpers*. Many succeed in providing breastmilk for their baby for the same duration that they had planned to breastfeed. In any case, and regardless of what you choose, *try to focus on the joy of mothering* as you find ways to move on.

Defend Your Choice

No one has the right to criticize a mother who decides to express-pump, to formula-feed, or only partly feed her baby breastmilk. Mothers who cherish breastfeeding are always willing to go an extra mile to make it work *if they possibly can.* These mothers may deeply regret the loss of their breastfeeding relationship. They may be experiencing *breastfeeding grief.* They may be fighting depression. They deserve all our support and encouragement as they focus on bonding with their baby in other ways and moving on with their lives.

I would like to share some advice offered by a very wise mother: focus on the fact that it is the *good mother* in you that is making these terribly hard decisions. Do not let anyone make you feel you are a bad mother for doing what you recognize is necessary for you and your family.

Medical professionals, however, should never tell mothers who are experiencing problems that they might just as well formula-feed. *Mothers want solutions, not an easy fix.* Professionals should rather refer the mother to a breastfeeding support group and to an IBCLC. Countless mothers stop breastfeeding every day because healthcare providers do not refer them to persons who are qualified to provide the guidance that they need.

Re-lactation

Mothers who have already weaned their babies, and who wish to re-lactate and possibly breastfeed, are often not encouraged by their family, doctors, and sometimes even by their breastfeeding experts who may wish to spare the mother stress and disappointment. Many mothers wish, retrospectively, that they had not listened to the nay-sayers and had at least tried. Pumping for a few days every two hours around the clock, increasing the use of lactogenic herbs and foods, and feeding at the breast, initially with a supplemental feeding device, will kick-start lactation. That said, not every mother can build a full milk supply, and not every mother can re-lactate. Still, every bit of milk is beneficial to a baby, and bonding at the breast is desirable if at all possible. Getting a baby back onto the breast can be difficult, but frequently it can be achieved through cultivating close, cuddly times with your baby (co-bathing, co-sleeping) with lots of skin-to-skin contact, and by offering the breast in a non-stressful manner.

Take Life Day to Day

Mothers who build their milk supply through difficult times do so by living day to day. Mothers encourage other mothers by saying, "If you do have to quit, you can quit tomorrow. Just try to get through today. Be kind to yourself and forgiving. You are doing something far more difficult than most people can imagine."

After a while, caring for your baby and building your milk supply becomes a routined way of life—though thankfully, a temporary one: breastfeeding, supplementing, washing the feeding device, diapering, pumping, cleaning the flanges and tubes, and having perhaps only twenty minutes to rest before your baby is hungry again is certainly more than trying!

The good news is that the reward does make up for the effort. Eventually, most mothers find themselves able to breastfeed without pumping or supplementing with formula. As one mother put it, "The slogan shouldn't be: 'All women can nurse.' The slogan should be: 'It's worth it.'"

Acknowledge and Accept

If breastfeeding simply does not work out, for whatever reason, and if you are not able to *breastbond* with a lactation aid or by comfort feeding, it may be healing to consider that motherhood is much larger than what happens at the breast. Motherhood is the bond of love and the commitment of care between you and your baby.

Most mothers do the best they knew at the time they were having breastfeeding problems. We cannot do more than that. Acknowledge to yourself that whatever happened, the very fact that you care shows that you are a good mother.

Grieving

When mothers grieve the loss of a breastfeeding relationship, they do not always find understanding from family and friends. It may be helpful to find a community of mothers going through similar issues. Online breastfeeding communities, such as "Breastfeeding-Grief" at yahoogroups, provide this opportunity. Know that you are not alone. Whereas some mothers move quickly through breastfeeding grief, others mourn for a long time, even years later. If you find that you need professional help, look for a compassionate therapist.

CHAPTER TWO

Basics of a Lactogenic Diet

"The mother's food should be warm....

"Even if we include some amount of raw vegetables such as carrot, most vegetables should be cooked, to protect the baby from bloating and gas. It has been found that root-vegetables are particularly lactogenic, especially red beet, black-root, then cauliflower prepared with mustard and caraway seeds. Otherwise, be careful with cauliflower due to flatulence! If the produce is bio-dynamically grown and properly spiced, it is surprising how well it may be tolerated.

"Grains should be soaked to make their nutrients accessible, and carefully prepared. Rice, oats and millet appear to have the best effect on lactation. Spices include bitter leaves such as thyme, basil, marjoram and chervil; also the umbel seeds, caraway, anise, fennel. Sprinkle fresh, hacked nettle over the meal. But avoid parsley—it dries up the milk." — U. Renzenbrink, M.D., 1979, translation from German to English by the author[2].

This chapter explores dietary and lifestyle factors that contribute to building and sustaining milk supply, including weightloss; calorie and fluid intake; warm or cold food, cooked or raw food; and it also introduces basic concepts on how the mother's diet can impact her baby's digestion.

Make Time to Eat

For many years, breastfeeding mothers were advised to get an additional 500 calories each day. Now, experts agree that while a normal intake of calories is usually sufficient, mothers should not skip meals: three full meals a day, with healthy snacks in between, will safeguard a mother's milk supply and her health.

The reality is, however, that many breastfeeding mothers do not eat regular meals and snacks. It is not uncommon for mothers to eat practically nothing at all, or to eat mainly leftovers and yogurt straight from the fridge, or a microwaved meal now and then (note: microwaving damages some nutrients).

These mothers often believe that their diet is sufficient. They may have heard that *starving women can still produce adequate milk*, or that *what we eat is not important to milk quality or quantity,* and to their minds, this seems to justify a poor diet or under-eating.

Yes, it's true that undernourished women *do* manage to produce milk under extreme conditions (severe undernourishment pushes the body into survival mode, when prolactin is naturally higher), but when women in the US reduce their caloric intake, or skip lots of meals and snacks, their milk supply usually drops.

The first rule of a lactogenic diet is therefore to eat meals and snacks at regular intervals throughout the day. Most important: never miss breakfast. Consider this: when we miss meals or snacks, our bodies produce an abundance of *stress hormones*. Stress hormones inhibit the milk-ejection reflex. They can also lead to irritability, exhaustion, and panic attacks. In pregnancy, going without regular meals has been linked to premature delivery[3]—due to the effect of stress hormones from hunger.

If you hardly have time to eat, discuss this matter with your lactation specialist or healthcare provider. Work out a few recipes for quick meals and snacks, using wholesome, nutrient-rich foods, and eat at least one warm meal a day. If you don't have time to get adequate nutrition through food, look into vitamin and mineral supplements, vegetable juices, "green drinks", and nutritious herbal teas or herbal supplements.

"When my milk supply went up, I was hungry all the time."

"I find that eating more calories increases my supply."

Eat To Satisfaction

When we eat to satisfaction—and this usually means eating a good amount of food—a wave of happy contentment fills the body. This feeling of emotionally fullness, of satiety, is evoked by oxytocin, one of the hormones of lactation. Oxytocin is responsible for the milk-ejection reflex, and also for the digestion of a large meal. And oxytocin makes us feel emotionally wonderful.

It's no coincidence that oxytocin triggers the milk ejection reflex and *also* triggers more enzymatic activity in the intestines. Nature uses this trick to ensure that breastfeeding women digest their food better. Some researchers suspect that the opposite may also be true: that oxytocin, sent out to digest a large meal, may help mothers breastfeed[4] by signaling to the brain that it is safe to produce milk, i.e., that the mother can spare the calories.

Enjoy at least one large, satisfying meal a day—preferably sitting down at a table with someone you love—to get that extra dose of oxytocin.

Drink to Thirst

Over-Drinking

Mothers are advised to drink to thirst while breastfeeding. Studies have shown that when mothers drink somewhat above or below their thirst, their supply is not affected. But if *mothers drink far above their thirst* they see a drop in their milk supply[5].

Lactation consultants often get calls from women who say that they have insufficient milk, in spite of drinking *four or more quarts* of fluid every day. These mothers are over-drinking. When the mother drinks less, her milk supply recovers.

The same thing has been observed when mothers receive IV infusions before birth, causing their legs and arms to swell. The sharp increase in bodily fluids suppresses milk production. These women may then formula feed in the mistaken belief that they have no milk, when in fact the problem is only temporary and they should pump and put their baby to the breast anyway (with the help of a lactation aid if necessary). As soon as the excess fluid has been worked out of her body—it can take up to a week for the kidneys to work out extra fluids—milk production will pick up.

Under-Drinking

The opposite also occurs. Although mothers are advised to drink to thirst, we often plain forget. We ignore feelings of thirst, or we mistake thirst for hunger and take a bite to eat rather than a cup of something to drink.

Usually, under-drinking will not impact a mother's supply (the body will reduce urine output rather than reduce milk production). Some mothers however do see their supply drop if they do not drink enough fluid, and some also say that drinking throughout the day improves their milk supply.

Understanding Thirst

Water plays a crucial role in the body's health. It transports water-soluble vitamins to cells, it participates in the metabolism of cells, and it transports toxins out of the body through urine and perspiration.

In the US, mothers are advised to drink to thirst, or approximately 8 cups a day. The amount anyone drinks depends on their body size, weight, and the weather. Hot weather, or very dry, cold weather, makes us thirstier. Don't wait until you are thirsty to drink. Carry a bottle of water or herbal tea around the house with you, and take a sip every now and then.

The color of morning urine can indicate whether your fluid intake is sufficient—though its color can be altered by food or supplements, for instance, vitamin B complex will darken its color, and eating beet root will turn urine pink. Usually, a light yellow, nearly transparent color indicates that you are drinking sufficient amounts. Dark-yellow color, or urine with an intensive smell, signals that the body needs more fluid. Colorless urine signals that you are drinking too much.

If you are the type who forgets to drink, you may wish to check off 8 – 12 cups a day on a pad of paper. Take into account that black and green tea, coffee, nettle, and dandelion tea deplete the body of fluids because they activate the kidneys (though recent research suggests that this effect is less if you drink these beverages frequently). Keep an eye on possible extra thirst if you drink these beverages.

Experiment with fluids to find out what works best for you. In my case, drinking an additional 4 cups before bedtime enhanced my milk production throughout the night and the next day. But that's just what worked *for me*.

- Filtered water is best. The Brita water filter is not too expensive.
- Constant thirst can be a symptom of EFA deficiency. See the section, *Get Your Fats Right, in Chapter Three.*

Note: If you have low milk supply or are at risk for mastitis, do not drink iced beverages. In general, avoiding cold foods and drinks and dressing warmly is said to help prevent mastitis[*].

Tips for Losing Those Extra Pounds

Throughout this book you will find tips on how to balance your blood sugar, which will help you lose weight because you will no longer binge eat. Actually, most breastfeeding mothers, if they eat healthfully, will gradually lose weight and reach their pre-pregnancy during the latter half of the first year after birth. However, some mothers maintain their weight, and others actually gain weight while breastfeeding. You won't know which group you belong to until it happens. And since you have little influence over this, it's best to focus on caring for your baby and maintaining your milk supply. This is particularly true for women with low milk supply, as eating more calories may help boost their supply.

Two common dietary habits that contribute to weightgain:

- Frequently taking high concentrations of sugar, such as fruit juice, dried fruit[†], soda, candy, cookies, pastry, chocolate, and also white flour products, such as white bread or pasta. Artificial sweeteners also lead to weightgain because they stimulate hunger that may lead to compulsive eating later in the day.
- Large meals or large snacks taken late in the evening lead to weightgain, because the body does not have time to work off the calories.

---

[*] This advice is taken from Ayurvedic, Anthroposphic and Traditional Chinese Medicine.

[†] Dried fruit and trail mix are a good snack for most mothers, but women who easily gain weight may have to be careful about their intake of even these healthy sources of concentrated sugar.

The following concerns weight loss:

- Eat a hearty breakfast. Not eating breakfast frequently leads to a higher intake of starchy foods and calories later in the day.

- Quick weight loss leads to a flood of fat-soluble toxins and trans-fatty acids entering a mother's milk—a good reason to lose weight slowly.

- Exercise. Mothers often pick up their exercise routine soon after birth in the hopes of losing weight. While moderate exercise helps mothers feel better overall and may also increase milk supply, exercising without calorie restriction usually doesn't lead to weightloss in the postpartum[6]. Since calorie restriction often leads to a drop in supply, it is not advisable. Mothers who exercise *very strenuously* in the postpartum may see their baby fussy or unhappy following their next feeding, due to lactic acid in their milk.

- Low level exercise is sufficient to lose weight gradually: a long walk a few times a week, slow dancing, or gentle weight-lifting will gradually shift the body's metabolic rate toward weightloss. Exercise experts are now suggesting that we aim for half of the level we think we can manage, and gradually build up from there.

- Drink enough. We commonly mistake thirst for hunger, and take a bite to eat rather than a cup to drink. Drinking a glass of water or cup of tea ten minutes before a meal will reduce the tendency to overeat. Drinking a glass of water or tea after a meal will dilute the digestive fluids, and according to Asian medicine, will promote weightgain.

- Get enough of the right kinds of fats. Supplements of essential fatty acids will reduce cravings for fatty foods such as chocolate and ice cream (see 'Get your Fats Right').

- When you deem it is time to really work towards weight loss, reduce your total intake of fat but be sure you continue to get a balanced assortment of fats, including EFAs.

- In traditional yoga, mothers do not return to their yoga routine for up to six weeks after birth; it is thought that the mother should remain 'soft,' both emotionally and physically, in order to be more responsive to her baby. Indeed, this is an unique time in which we can emotionally 'mesh' with our new partner in life; if concentrating on body-building takes away from that 'meshing' in this crucial period of time, it should be postponed a few weeks.

- Balance your blood sugar. Blood sugar highs and lows lead to cravings for sweet food and coffee, both of which are not compatible with a long term weightloss program. For more information, see the section on balancing blood sugar on pages 99-100 and on insulin resistance on page 104.
- Overcome food cravings. See *Overcoming Food Cravings,* pages 107-117.

A Nightly Review of the Day's Food

Mothers frequently say that they are too preoccupied with their baby to pay much attention to what they eat and drink during the day. My solution—and I found it helped stabilize my milk supply—was to evaluate, sometime during the evening, what I had had to eat and drink that day.

It's really very simple. Ask yourself whether you had food from each food category (fat, carbohydrates, vegetables (green and yellow), fruit, and protein), and whether you drank enough during the day.

If not, take something from the missing category. It doesn't have to be much. You ate no vegetable? Eat a carrot. You had too few carbohydrates? Eat a piece of whole-grain bread, with a layer of butter or 1/2 teaspoon of flaxseed oil if you didn't get enough fat that day. Drink as much as you forgot to drink during the day. You should aim for at least two quarts of fluid a day (see section on drinking above).

Balance Hot and Cold Food

Asian systems of medicine say that a mother's body should be in balance between *hot* and *cold*. The thought behind this is that mothers after birth are more *cold* than usual. 'Cold' here means that major organs and glands are slightly underfunctioning (what we call convalescence, during which time a mother 'warms up,' or regains her strength and vitality). This cold state is countered by taking *warming* foods that are cooked with *warming* herbs. There are even special recipes that are said to nourish a mother's vitality. For instance, in China, mothers are given chicken soup, once a week, that has been simmered for several hours along with the blood-tonic herb, dong quai.

Traditional Chinese Medicine (TCM) and Ayurvedic wisdom from India recommend that cooked, *warming* foods should form the basis of a mother's diet. The heat of cooking breaks open the cellular walls of food so that its nutrients can be extracted more easily. It is in these walls that minerals are stored. Doctors from India or China typically ask, "What is the point of eating raw vegetables if you can't absorb their nutrients?"

- In the early postpartum months, it's a good idea to eat warm food at least once a day, and to drink warm beverages. Breastfeeding mothers who have low milk supply and who eat mainly raw foods may see an increase in their milk supply by eating warm, cooked foods.

- Also, mothers with low milk supply, who eat mainly cold foods, such as yogurt from the fridge or cold sandwiches, may see their supply improve when they begin eating warm foods.

- Foods and spices that add heat to the body, such as meat and curry, should be taken in larger amounts during winter; cooling foods, such as oil, fresh fruit and salad-type vegetables such as cucumber and tomato should be taken in larger amounts during summer. Grains and legumes are only slightly warming and should form the basis of our diet at all seasons—according to these traditions.

- Warming lactogenic herbs such as Nigella sativa and the umbel seeds should not be taken every day—unless the mother frequently feels cold or exhausted, in which case they can help restore her energy.

- **Fenugreek** and **nettle** are considered to be thermally 'neutral' and so are among the herbs that can be used every day[7].

From a 'Western' point of view, cooked foods are comfort foods. Warmth helps us to relax. It imparts a sense of satiety and safety—and this affects our brain chemistry in a good way. Warm breakfasts such as oatmeal (porridge) support milk production as countless mothers testify. Warm rice, millet, polenta, and warm veggie dishes or vegetable soups are all used to support milk production around the world. Even a piping warm plate of spaghetti or pizza support milk production—especially if they are spiced with basil and marjoram, and covered with a drizzle of olive oil.

Vegetables that are crunchy and compact, such as broccoli, carrot, beet, turnip, and cauliflower should preferably be cooked with carminative herbs such as caraway, cumin and mustard seed to make them more digestible; vegetables that are easily chewed such as lettuce are less likely to cause digestive problems when eaten raw— though some sensitive mothers do have difficulties even with soft vegetables.

Diet is a highly personal matter. The information here is to be taken as suggestions with which mothers can experiment.

Vary Your Diet – Prevent Colic and Food Sensitivity

Eat a *varied* diet—even before conception. A varied diet will ensure that a mother is well nourished. It will introduce her baby to different tastes, both in the womb and through her milk, so that he eats a wider range of food later on. A varied diet has an additional plus: *it reduces the risk for food sensitivities and allergies in yourself and your baby.*

- Getting a varied diet may be even more important than usually thought, as some allergists, such as Dr. Doris Rapp, believe children's developmental problems can be linked to a baby's food sensitivities that develop during pregnancy.
- The foods that you crave or eat *every day* during pregnancy and while breastfeeding will be the most likely 'culprits,' should your baby have food sensitivities.
- Eating a varied diet may be difficult, especially if a mother has food cravings or feels repelled by fresh food. Read the sections on overcoming food cravings and addictions for suggestions.
- Two foods in particular to avoid overeating are dairy and wheat, as these are the most common culprits behind colic. Corn, soy, fish, nuts and citric fruit are also common triggers, as are sugar and caffeine.
- Take the list of lactogenic foods with you when you go shopping (see pages 119-122), and make sure you have a variety of fresh or frozen whole foods in your kitchen for days when you have no time to cook.

Breastmilk - The Best It Can Be

A mother's breastmilk uniquely meets her baby's individual nutritive and immunological needs, so that the title of this chapter, suggesting that breastmilk can be more or less best, seems over the top. Yet, experts are beginning to suggest that there can be very slight degrees of *bestness* to breastmilk. One factor involves the fats found in breastmilk—whether fats are available at good levels that boost a child's immunity and overall development, or if trans-fatty acids are available instead. The good news is that mothers can influence the kinds of fats found in their milk though the kinds of fats that they eat.

Chapter Three takes a close look at the fats we eat. Because fatty acids are a complicated matter to talk about, Chapter Three contains technical language. If you do not wish to read the technical parts, you can look at pages 52-55 for a summary of suggestions.

Chapter Three also looks briefly at choline (so-called *brain-food*), and at birth control, medication, caffeine, cigarette smoking, and at alcoholic beverages, i.e., at some of the many ways that what we eat, drink, or otherwise ingest can ever so slightly impact the bestness of breastmilk.

Carefulness and Responsibility

The Navaho people have a fascinating philosophy. They hold that breastfeeding mothers cannot just eat what they want, or do what they want, because it will affect their milk. A breastfeeding mother is told to eat 'old' foods: corn, vegetables, herbs, and meat. These foods are said to support her supply and also to keep her milk healthy for her child.

Here is the really intriguing part: Navaho tradition has it that when a mother is *careful* about what she eats and does, the child *will drink in this quality of carefulness* along with her milk. He will get a *taste of responsibility*. This is the reason, they say, that a breastfed child is more willing to listen to the elders of the tribe than a bottle-fed child, and why he is more likely to become a responsible member of his culture. This means that for a Navaho mother, being careful about her diet while breastfeeding is an expression of love and concern on many levels[8].

American mothers frequently have a hard time eating old, traditional foods. In fact, many of us don't know what old foods are. To illustrate this point, I'd like to share an episode from *Only in America*, by Harry Golden. In this book, Golden describes his life in New York as a boy in the early 20th century, and the joy he felt on discovering venders of snack foods on street corners. One of the names painted on a wooden stand was "Cracker Jack".

Caramel-covered popcorn is a good example of America's old foods. People arriving here, usually poor, were grateful to enjoy inexpensive, sweet foods—and even more happy to sell them. In order to make a profit these foods had to taste rich while being cheap to produce—and this is still a good description of the food that Americans typically prefer. That's why, quite frankly, most of us no longer are in touch with the wholesome foods that helped our great-grandmothers produce milk. That healthy sense was forfeited in childhood when we accepted sweet and fatty foods as a staple ingredient of happiness. No, eating a whole-foods diet is not easy for most of us.

Compounding the situation is the fact that most women in the US (and increasingly in Europe) have had an eating disorder at some point, and almost all of us are uptight about carrying extra weight. Along the same line, we may feel uptight about eating enough calories and especially enough fat to produce milk well.

To top it off, almost all of us have learned to think of many unhealthy foods as being perfectly healthy, and of healthy foods as being bad for us (examples are scattered throughout Part One of this book). Finally, we have learned to judge the value of food based on its cost and on how quickly it can be prepared and served. Traditional foods are inexpensive, but their preparation requires know-how. They aren't pre-cooked.

The result is that although we know we should eat more healthily, especially during pregnancy and breastfeeding, the transition is difficult, and not all women do manage to change their eating habits. In fact, many continue to eat in ways that they know are outright unhealthy. This goes to show how strongly food ties into our emotions and lifestyle—indeed, many of us believe that eating habits are beyond our control.

I would like this book to support women in making a transition to a healthier diet. By choosing foods that support your milk supply, you integrate healthier foods into your diet. By learning to keep an eye on your body's responses to the foods you eat, you can learn which foods are harming and which are helping you. The good news is that in taking the time to build this awareness, you lay a foundation for better health throughout your life to come.

Get Your Fats Right

Pregnant and breastfeeding mothers need to know about fats—not about avoiding them, but rather how to use them correctly. The wrong kinds of fats increase a baby's risk of allergies and illness, but the right fats will help him be healthier and smarter.

Many people still do not realize that fats can help or harm a person's immune system, affect their mental health, and even increase or lower their intelligence. Although these insights on fats have become the centerpiece of recent studies and books, most people still have not heard the news[*].

Because fats are so important, the following section is one of the largest in this book. It is also one of the most complex. I have tried to reduce medical terminology as much as possible and to provide concise, clear explanations. Still, the material is not easy to grasp, especially the first time around[†].

Fats and The Diseases They Cause – Or Do They?

Most people believe that a low-fat diet is healthy, that saturated fat (butter, animal fat, and coconut oil) should be avoided at all costs, and that other fats should also be kept to an absolute minimum.

---

[*] See Dr. Leo Galland's "Superimmunity for Kids" for help integrating healthful fats into your diet and the diet of your family. This is one of the few health books written with pregnant and breastfeeding mothers in mind. It contains crucial information for formula-feeding mothers as well.

[†] **Check my website, www.mother-food.com, for updates on fatty acids.**

The goal is to protect ourselves from disease, especially from heart disease, cancer, and overweight, by avoiding fat. The consensus is that the less fat in our diet the better, and get rid of saturated fat altogether.

Consider this: heart disease was virtually unknown one hundred years ago in the US. Most researchers say that heart disease developed as we began to eat more saturated animal fat. But we also began to eat more refined flour, white sugar, and processed vegetable oils (hydrogenated oils and margarine). Most importantly, we stopped eating foods that contain *essential fatty acids.*

Today, the theory that saturated fats cause heart disease has been contested by various doctors, researchers and scientists, whose research has led them to different conclusions.

Uffe Ravnskov, MD, researcher and author of *The Cholesterol Myths*, has published 40 scientific papers on fatty acids and their impact on health. Ravnskov has also reviewed research on cholesterol. He discovered that studies that link saturated fats to heart disease are brought to the public's eye, whereas the equal number of studies that discover the opposite—that saturated fats have no effect, or that people who eat more saturated fats have less heart disease— are ignored so that we never hear about them[9]. Moreover, he found that people who took low fat diets had more depression and suicide. *Fat is important to the healthy functioning of the brain and to emotional stability.*

Mary G. Enig, Ph.D., author of *Know Your Fats* and co-author of *Nourishing Traditions* with Sally Fallon, points out that cholesterol is used by the body to repair damaged tissues—like a Band-Aid on a wound. The goal, they say, should not be to tear off the Band-Aid, but to discover what is damaging the body and deal with that.

Unexpected Facts on Fats:

- In a clinic in Austria, doctors once prescribed fasts of raw milk to heal people of various diseases. The esteemed late physician, Henry G. Bealer, describes the use of raw milk in healing regimes in his book, *Food is your Best Medicine.*
- The Masai tribe and other tribes in Africa whose traditional diet consists mainly of meat, blood and milk, are known for their lack of disease, including heart disease and cancer.

- Naturopaths and allergists find that people with milk allergies often have no symptoms if they take raw milk—probably due to the live enzymes in the milk and to the high content of fat.

Overweight is commonly thought to result from eating fatty foods, though we know that many people who are obese actually avoid eating fat. (These are the people who say they gain weight just by looking at food.) Extreme overweight, while having many causes, is chronified when insulin function (sugar metabolism) gets out of whack. These persons then can't lose weight regardless of how few calories and how little fat they take.

Many factors in our culture contribute to what is called *insulin resistance*, including overeating refined floor, pasta, and sugar, taking too many *processed* fats, poor diet generally, weightgain, lack of exercise, and irregular habits of sleep.

Dietary fat actually keeps blood sugar levels steady, because the body digests them so slowly. Interestingly, any food—including fat—that keeps blood sugar levels steady has the potential to be a fat-reduction food. As if to prove this point, a new weight-loss diet has been shown to be effective that prescribes taking a swig of olive oil at regular intervals throughout the day[10].

Now let's look at nuts—a fatty food that is healthy for us. A study from California looking at 25,000 Seventh-Day Adventists found out that those who ate the most nuts were the least likely to be obese. Nuts help keep blood sugar levels steady—plus their healthy fat content satisfies the normal craving for fat, so that people are less likely to overeat sugary and starchy foods. Another study, this time looking at the effect of carbohydrates, protein or fat on people's ability to concentrate, showed that fat helps people remain the most focused—precisely because it keeps blood sugar levels stable[11]. In other words, fat helps us get what we desire most from food: a focused mind plus emotional satisfaction.

A body of recent studies also shows that natural fats, such as the oils found in avocados, nuts, seeds, and olives, actually improve cholesterol levels and prevent heart disease[12]. Avocado oil is protective of the liver[13]. All this flies in the face of what we've believed to be true for decades.

A Fresh Look at Fats

Healthy fats have crucial functions in the body. They are the building material for cell walls, nerves (including brain tissue), hormones, and hormone-like substances. Fats in a meal serve to slow down the digestion and the absorption of food, keeping blood sugar levels steady, protecting us from mood swings, and staving off feelings of hunger. Finally, the fat-soluble vitamins A and D, found in butter and fish-oil, enable us to absorb minerals from food. Because these vitamins are required for mineral absorption, it can be said that these animal fats promote the uptake of minerals.

It turns out that many early studies on saturated fats are flawed because they lumped together natural, healthy saturated fats and unhealthy hydrogenated fats, such as hydrogenated lard or coconut oil[14]. We now know that hydrogenated fats are unhealthy because hydrogenation changes the chemical structure of fatty acids, rendering them harmful to the body. Saturated fats in themselves are healthy, especially products made from raw milk, like those from Switzerland and France—countries that have bewildered researchers because these populations do not have high rates of heart disease in spite of their diets being high in saturated fat. Indeed, organic milk from grass-fed cows contains high levels of conjugated linoleic acid, a potent anti-cancer agent.

It is interesting to consider that our ancestors did not process their fats. Raw, unpasteurized dairy was fermented into naturally probiotic clabber, cheese, yogurt, and kefir. Coconut oil was cold-pressed. Traditional vegetable oils were cold-pressed. These oils had a long shelf life due to the high levels of monounsaturated acids and vitamin E naturally occurring in the oils.

Studies from Switzerland, Germany and Austria have shown that children raised on farms have significantly less eczema, hay fever and asthma than children growing up in villages do. At first it was thought that this is due to their exposure to animals from an early age. But then it was discovered that village children drinking raw farm milk (not pasteurized) had nearly the same low rate of allergy. Could the immune substances in raw milk provide the healthful effect?[15]

A study from Finland shows that mothers who ingest probiotics (lactobacilli) during pregnancy and while breastfeeding offer their babies more protection against eczema[16]. Well, lactobacilli are naturally present in raw milk products.

And still another Finnish study shows that butter may prevent skin allergies in children: in comparing healthy children and children with skin allergies, the consistent difference is that healthy children took butter, whereas children with skin allergies took margarine, made with processed vegetable oils[17], before the outbreak of their disease.

Studies show that polyunsaturated vegetable oils are not useful in preventing heart disease. Because these oils quickly become rancid in their natural state, they are routinely hydrogenated to give them longer shelf life. This creates trans-fatty acids that raise "bad" cholesterol levels, decrease "good" cholesterol levels, and promote heart disease[18]. Simple saturated fats, however, found for instance in butter, coconut oil, and in dark poultry meat, do not have this negative effect on cholesterol[19]. Monounsaturated fats, found in avocado, olive, and sesame oil, improve cholesterol levels, and raw nuts decrease the risk of heart disease.

Essential Fatty Acids (EFAs)

> *"If we optimize our intake of essential fats ... in the right ratio of omega 3 to omega 6, then we can use saturated fats in moderation without fear. We can then use whipping cream in our coffee, butter on our bread, and sour cream on our potatoes....*
>
> *"This is, in fact, another key point you need to understand. It is more important for health to optimize the consumption of essential fats than it is to avoid the bad fats. The fats that heal protect us from the fats that kill. If you removed all the bad fats from your diet, and did not bring in the good ones, you would still die from degenerative disease, because you cannot live without the good essential fats."*
>
> — Udo Erasmus, Ph.D., from "Fats That Heal Fats That Kill"

Essential fatty acids (EFAs) are essential both because the body cannot make them on its own—we must get them from food or from supplements—and because of their importance to the health of our body and mind. EFAs play crucial roles in the brain and body. Cell membranes are comprised of well-organized rows of different sorts of fatty acids, including cholesterol. While saturated fats give the cell membrane its stability, EFAs furnish permeability, so that nutrients can enter and toxins be filtered out. EFAs also promote oxygenation of the cell, helping to prevent cancer. It's when unhealthy fats, such as trans-fatty acids, take the place of EFAs in the cell membrane that toxic conditions develop.

EFAs have received a lot of attention in recent years from allergists, oncologists, neurologists, and also psychiatrists. It turns out that EFAs are metabolized into a hormone-like substance called *prostaglandins* that inhibit or promote inflammation in cells. If we do not have the right balance of prostaglandins, our cells become prone to inflammation, promoting allergic, or autoimmune diseases.

The nerves in the brain are also comprised of EFAs. According to Patricia Kane, Ph.D., author of *The Neurochemistry and Neurophysics of Autism*, what we eat affects how we think. Unhealthy fats congest nerves in the brain, but even healthy fats in the brain may be injured by toxins (particularly mercury) and be in need of repair through a fresh supply. *To put it simply, injured neural cells cannot transmit key neurotransmitters, and this affects the way the brain works.* This is one reason why supplementing with EFAs is frequently effective in the treatment of depression, bipolar disease, schizophrenia, and dementia, in patients where medication is ineffective. EFAs are also used in treating autism, learning disorders, and hyperactivity syndromes in children.

Summary:

- Fats affect allergic and autoimmune reactions through their impact on prostaglandins.
- Fats may inhibit the development of cancer through their role in the oxygenation of cells.
- Fats affect the way the brain works through their impact on neural cells.

We can get EFAs from foods such as eggs, whole-fat dairy, fat from meat, dark green leafy vegetables, legumes, nuts, seeds, seaweed, and fish (fish is cautioned against for pregnant and breastfeeding women due to their concentrations of mercury and other contaminants). Unfortunately, because most people do not eat many of these foods, most of us are sorely deficient in EFAs.

Most packaged and fast foods contain vegetable oils that *should* be rich in EFAs. The problem is that these oils have been processed and damaged by heat, and the EFAs have been transformed into dangerous trans-fatty acids. Trans-fats prevent EFAs from doing their work by inhibiting the action of key enzymes. They also slip into their slots in cellular walls, decreasing the permeability of cells.

With the central roles that EFAs play in the brain and body, some experts believe that the last few generations of Americans have not been able to develop to their full potential, and that we have become vulnerable to allergy, mental illness, heart disease, and cancer—all because we lack these EFAs! It's even thought by some experts that postpartum depression occurs more prevalently in cultures with low intake of omega 3 EFAs. Fortunately, the body responds quickly to EFA supplementation. After only three weeks, their levels are significantly higher in blood, tissue and breastmilk.

Omega 3 and Omega 6

EFAs are divided into two main structures or types: omega 6 and omega 3. Remember, the body cannot make these fatty acids itself. It needs to ingest them through foods. *Healthy food sources for omega 6 are whole-fat milk, butter, cream, eggs, meat fat, grains, and nuts. Healthy food sources for omega 3 are green leafy vegetables, flaxseed oil, walnut oil, legumes, and organically raised eggs and fish.* Looking at these food sources, it's obvious that people get higher amounts of omega 6 than omega 3 from the foods that most people eat.

Now, experts have long been saying that we should get about four times as much omega 6 as omega 3 in our diet. However, more recent opinion is that we should have equal amounts of each, as this better reflects the diet of stone-age people who relied heavily on fish.

Estimates for the typical American diet however show that most of us have a ratio of 20:1, or 20 times as much omega 6 as omega 3 in our diet. *Still, not everyone has enough omega 6.* People who have so-called *silver fillings* (amalgam fillings) in their teeth have a greater need for omega 6, due to the way that mercury, leaking from these fillings into the body, damages omega 6 fatty acids in their nerves. The babies of mothers who have amalgam fillings may have a higher need for omega 6 as well.

As you see, the situation revolving around EFA deficiency is not that cut and dry, and sometimes experimentation is called for to explore which EFAs are deficient. This is described on page 45. The most obvious symptoms of an EFA deficiency are *dry skin and hair, thin, brittle fingernails, itching, reddish or dry patches of skin, a rash-like appearance of little lumps on the backside of the arms or on the thighs, and dry scaly skin on the knees and elbows.* Less obvious symptoms include autoimmune diseases, such as eczema, and mental problems such as depression or an inability to concentrate.

Increasing Levels of EFAs in Breastmilk

Breastmilk is a baby's source of EFAs. *However, breastmilk can only contain as many EFAs as we have available in our bodies.* Since most of us in the US are deficient in EFAs, there is some cause for alarm. To complicate matters, many of *us lose the ability to metabolize* EFAs into their long-chain derivatives that are important for the brain, nerves, and immune system. If we cannot metabolize EFAs into their derivatives, these derivatives will not be available to be transferred into breastmilk. This makes it even more important that we have a good source for **both basic EFAs and their derivatives** in our diet every day.

Flaxseed Oil

The least expensive way to increase our intake of *basic* EFAs is with flaxseed oil. Flaxseed oil contains both omega 3 and omega 6; indeed, there is no other vegetable source containing such high levels of omega 3. Since flaxseed oil is lactogenic, mothers with high milk supply may wish to take very little flaxseed oil, or take fish oil, legumes and eggs instead, to get the whole range of omega 3s for her baby's best development.

Flaxseed oil does not, however, increase levels of the long-chain omega 3 derivatives, EPA and DHA[*] in breastmilk. It is necessary to take fish oil or algae extract to get these derivatives. While flaxseed oil cannot replace fish oil or algae extract in a mother's diet, taken together, they provide ample amounts of the whole range of omega 3 EFAs.

---

[*] **docosahexaenoic acid (DHA); eicosapentaenoic acid (EPA) These long-chain fatty acids are important for the development of the baby's brain and nerves.**

Look for bottled organic flaxseed oil. Do not confuse this with linseed oil, which is found in hardware stores and is poisonous. Keep the bottle of flaxseed oil in the fridge. EFAs are highly volatile – they rapidly become rancid. If your oil smells 'off,' throw it out[*].

Dosage: 1–2 teaspoons of flaxseed oil a day.

Sunflower, Safflower -- Sesame and Olive Oil

Sunflower, safflower and sesame seed oil are good sources for omega 6. However, sunflower and safflower oils are frequently over-eaten, contributing to an imbalance with omega 3. Rather than using these two oils, in salad dressing, for instance, it is more beneficial to combine equal amounts of sesame and flaxseed oil. This combination provides a one-to-one ratio of omega 3 to omega 6; it can be used in salad dressing, but it should not be heated. Use olive oil instead of sunflower seed oil in cooking.

Store-bought "Balanced Omega Supplements"

Supplements of EFAs that contain a careful balance of omega 3 to omega 6 derivatives are available commercially. Some are advertised as being perfect for pregnant and breastfeeding mothers. If you and your baby have **no** signs of EFA deficiency, taking these is fine[†]. If you do have signs of EFA deficiency (see page 41) it may be wise to initially follow the advice on page 45.

Sources for Omega 3 Derivatives DHA and EPA[‡]

Cod-liver oil, fish oil, and algae extract are excellent sources of omega 3 derivatives *DHA* and *EPA*. These derivatives promote higher IQ and better visual abilities in breastfed babies. DHA may help prevent depression in mothers (see below).

Cod-liver oil contains a lot of vitamin D and A. These vitamins enable a mother to absorb minerals from her food, including calcium. Cod-liver oil is the supplement of choice if mothers don't get enough

---

[*] Some experts suggest emptying vitamin E capsules into bottled flaxseed oil to prevent it from becoming rancid.

[†] For instance, Udo's Choice Oil Blend™, designed by Udo Erasmas.

[‡] docosahexaenoic acid (DHA); eicosapentaenoic acid (EPA)

vitamin D from sunlight, for instance, in winter, or if a mother cannot get outside into the sunlight often, or if she usually wears sun-screen.

Now, as previously mentioned, it turns out that not all adults are able to metabolize these derivatives in their own bodies. Stress, trans-fatty acids, and a lack of key enzymes, vitamins or minerals can impede this sensitive process. This is why some experts suggest that *all* adults supplement with algae extract, cod-liver oil, fish oil, or DHA/EPA supplements, or a commercially available balanced mixture of all the EFAs. However, after about 3-4 weeks of supplementation, it is no longer necessary to take a high daily dosage. A few capsules a week are then sufficient.

In 2000, a study in Texas demonstrated that supplementing with omega 3 derivatives, DHA and EPA, 200 mg per day, doubles the DHA content of nursing mothers' milk[22]. Three sources for DHA were used in this study: 1) supplements of DHA derived from algae, 2) from fish oil, or 3) from eggs. DHA derived from algae produced the quickest results.

Sources for the Omega 6 Derivatives (GLA and ARA)*

Many adults cannot metabolize omega 6 into its long chain derivatives, ARA and GLA. ARA (page 49) is important for the functioning of the brain and nervous system. It can be found in cream, butter, whole milk, egg yolks and animal fat. GLA is important to the immune system. It can be found in certain vegetable oils:

A daily adult dosage is 240-300 mg of GLA, found in:
3,000 mg of evening primrose oil
1,000-1,300 mg of borage oil
1,500 mg of black currant seed oil

Buy only a high-grade product, such as Efamol®. Less expensive products do not contain enough oil for the money.

---

* gamma-linoleic-acid (GLA); arachidonic acid (ARA).

Allergies, Maternal Depression, and EFA Deficiency

Allergies and auto-immune diseases are thought by many experts to have their root cause in a lack of EFAs during pregnancy and early childhood. For instance, a review of studies showed that if breastfed babies have eczema (formula-fed babies have eczema more often), the mother commonly has low levels of EFA derivatives in her blood and breastmilk, indicating that the mother is not able to metabolize these derivatives from the omega 6 and omega 3 in her diet. In one study, giving the mother supplements containing omega 3 derivatives greatly improved the baby's eczema[20]. Today, holistic MDs and allergists commonly prescribe EFA derivatives to breastfeeding mothers of allergic babies, *but they stress that foods containing the basic omega 6s and 3s are also very important* (see page 40).

Unless a mother has a continuously superb diet, she will benefit by supplementing with EFAs, even if allergies are not an issue in her family. During pregnancy, a mother's EFA reserves are directed into her growing baby, and her EFA-reserves may be low after birth, and will be depleted even more by breastfeeding. These reserves become lower and lower in subsequent pregnancies.

Reduced levels of EFAs, especially DHA, promote depression in mothers. In a cross-cultural study, it was seen that women in countries that eat high amounts of DHA have less postpartum depression[21]. The same study showed that risk for depression in the mother can be assessed by measuring the (low) level of DHA in her *milk* (!).

Omegas 3s appear to help mothers who *don't* have depression, too. In an unpublished study by Anton Llorente, Ph.D., of Baylor University, giving 200 mg per day of DHA to mothers in late pregnancy improved their *cognitive capacity*, or their ability to think complex thoughts (or 'think straight') in the weeks after birth. (Most of us would welcome that!)

Should you be taking omega 3s or omega 6s?

If you (or your baby) have symptoms that indicate a lack of EFAs, you will want to find out which omega fatty acid you are deficient in. Most of us are deficient in the omega-3 group; people who have amalgam fillings are at risk to be deficient in the omega-6 group, as well. Our babies probably share our fatty acid balance (or imbalance).

Allergists suggest that, to explore this matter, you begin to supplement one omega group and then gauge the effect. Within 3 to 4 weeks you should see evidence of improvement—or not—and this will indicate if this was the fatty acid you needed.

For instance, if you suspect that you have insufficient omega 3s in your diet, see the food sources on page 40, and begin supplementing with 1) flaxseed oil and 2) fish oil, cod-liver oil, or with DHA extracted from algae. Organic eggs are also of value. The EFAs in these sources are, in a sense, *pre-metabolized* and ready to be used by the body. After three weeks, if you see no improvement, it is possible that you or your baby need omega 6s. See the food sources on page 40, and in addition take foods that contain ARA: cream, milk, and egg-yolk. GLA can be supplemented with oil from the seeds of evening primrose, black currant, and borage. Again, you should see clear improvement in symptoms after 3–4 weeks of supplementation. You can then lower the dosage as your body becomes saturated with the oils it needs.

Even if your baby or you show no signs of EFA deficiency, you may benefit by occasionally supplementing with a premixed DHA-EPA-GLA supplement, or with fish oil or algae extract together with a GLA supplement such as borage seed oil.

Give Your Baby Additional EFAs

It is possible to give EFAs to a baby with massage. For instance, an allergist may suggest massaging a baby with a quarter teaspoon of flaxseed oil, or with a capsule of evening primrose oil, as part of treatment for allergy.

Indeed, mothers in Asia routinely use oils to massage their babies, and they report that their oil-massaged babies have improved growth and health. The fatty acids in these oils are absorbed directly through the skin, and are measurably higher in the baby's blood. This is particularly good news for mothers who formula-feed their babies (formula does not contain comparable EFAs to breastmilk).

Because oils contains different fatty acids and have different benefits, it is wise to alternate them to get the full range of fatty acids. Oils to choose from are sesame seed oil, coconut fat, clarified butter (or simply use organic butter), and virgin olive oil. If my baby were exclusively formula feeding, I would massage her with three drops of fish oil mixed with a half-teaspoon of olive oil twice a week. (Take the rest of the fish oil from the capsule immediately yourself as it will soon become rancid.) Massaging with evening primrose oil is frequently helpful in treating infant eczema. An infant's daily dosage is one capsule (500 mg). It can be opened and rubbed directly onto the skin, or onto the areas of eczema.

- Any time you give your baby something new, whether herb, oil, or food, orally, or on her skin, begin with a tiny amount and increase gradually to test whether your baby has an allergic reaction.

Overcoming Low-Fat Breastmilk and Low Milk Supply:

Diets that are low in fat, EFAs and cholesterol can sometimes cause milk-supply difficulties. Patricia Gima, an IBCLC with long years of experience, has discovered that mothers who are on a low-fat diet, and who have low milk supply, often see a dramatic increase in their milk quantity and in their milk fat if they simply eat more healthy fats.

> *"Lack of fat in mother's milk is shown when the baby has enough wet diapers but infrequent stools and is not gaining weight."* – Patricia Gima

Gima recommends that mothers take:

1) ¼ teaspoon of olive oil (added to food) at each meal,

2) foods high in cholesterol and ARA (butter, eggs)

3) ¼ teaspoon of cold-pressed flaxseed with each meal.

4) fish oil, cod-liver oil, DHA algae extract, or other DHA/EPA supplement.

Gima has repeatedly seen that these babies rapidly gain weight, while mothers notice that their refrigerated pumped milk has an increase in the creamy layer on top.

Gima is not alone in her observations. A study from England in 1991 showed that whereas usually, the fat content of breastmilk drops over several months of breastfeeding, mothers who supplement with EFAs have an *increase* in the fat content of their milk[24].

- Improving the fat content of a mother's milk may solve the "failure-to-thrive" syndrome, especially when babies do not gain weight even when seeming to breastfeed efficiently.

- Increased fat intake may also relieve a baby's colic—his indigestion may be due to getting too little creamy milk.

- Mothers with low-fat breastmilk should not use margarine or processed oil (these are also found in packaged foods). One study (see below) on mice showed that trans-fats lower the fat content of mice-mothers' milk, and an unpublished study by a graduate student showed the same results in humans—the anti-fat effect was equal to the base-line of trans-fatty acids in the mother[25].

Fats as Galactagogues

Around the world, mothers know that the fats they use can improve the quantity and quality of their milk.

- Extra portions of olive oil are given to breastfeeding mothers in Mediterranean cultures to improve the quantity and the quality of their milk.

- In the South Pacific, breastfeeding mothers take fresh coconut-milk, rich in coconut fat, as well as special combinations of herbs cooked in coconut oil, to increase their milk production.

- In India and China, sesame seed and sesame seed oil is used to increase milk supply.

- The Masai—an isolated, African tribe that sustain themselves largely through meat, milk and blood—anoint a new mother's breasts with butter, considered the most sacred of foods.
- Mothers in the US frequently find flaxseed oil, evening primrose oil, or borage seed oil increases their milk supply. These oils have hormonal components as well as containing essential fatty acids.

Margarine, Processed Oils, Trans-Fatty Acids

Margarine, processed cooking oils, and salad oils contain *partially hydrogenized* fat, so-called *trans-fatty acids.* These fat molecules have been forced, either by heat or by hydrogenation, into a molecular form that is not found in nature. Trans-fatty acids clog the membranes of cells all over the body, altering their permeability and preventing enzymes from doing their work. They interfere with the work of EFAs (see above), promoting inflammation and allergic reactions, including asthma[26]. **Trans-fats may cause lactation problems by interfering with the production of fat in mother's milk**[27]. Finally, trans-fats promote non-communicative diseases including heart disease and cancer.

What about all the new studies showing that margarine reduces cholesterol? These studies focused on a new kind of margarine with added *plant*-sterols that reduce cholesterol absorption in the intestine. These margarines still usually contain 20–25% trans-fatty acids.

Many researchers try to justify trans-fatty acids by saying they are not dangerous if one's diet also contains sufficient amounts of essential fatty acids. Recently however, an expert panel at the Institute of Medicine conducted a detailed review of research into trans-fatty acids, and concluded that *there is no level of trans-fatty acids that is safe to consume*[28].

The positive statement we *can* make is that it is not dangerous to include moderate amounts of saturated fats in our diet, *if* we also include essential fatty acids. That's because saturated fats, in contrast to trans-fatty acids, do not interfere in the metabolism of essential fatty acids.

The bad news is that trans-fatty acids pass into our milk. Because in the US we have been eating margarine instead of butter for decades, and have been eating processed foods that are saturated in partially hydrogenized oil, our breastmilk is far higher in trans-fatty acids than breastmilk in other parts of the world.

We can take steps to lower the content of trans-fats in our milk. We can avoid trans-fats in our diet, lowering their levels almost immediately in our milk. We can also avoid sudden weight loss. Trans-fatty acids are stored in fat cells; if a mother loses weight quickly, the level of trans-fatty acids in her milk will sharply increase and her baby will get a mega-dose of trans-fatty acids. Losing about one pound per week is considered to be safe.

Eggs and Cholesterol

Eggs, one of our most nutritionally dense foods, do not increase cholesterol levels significantly, even when eaten every day[29]. In fact, if a healthy person overdoses on dietary cholesterol with butter and eggs, their body will respond by not absorbing the extra cholesterol from the intestine[30]. Eggs contain cholesterol, but also ARA (see below), choline (see page 51), and small amounts of the omega 3 derivatives DHA/EPA.

Saturated Fats

It is not dangerous to include moderate amounts of saturated fats in our diet, such as from cheese or meat, *if* we also include EFAs in our diet, from nuts and grains and oils. It may however be appropriate to limit saturated fats if you have **allergies** or an **auto-immune** disease. You may also reduce them if saturated fats have been a dominant source of fats in your diet. Limiting their use will give your body 'free space,' as it were, in which EFAs can unfold their full effects.

ARA – Arachidonic Fatty Acid

Arachidonic acid (ARA), an omega 6 derivative, is metabolized in the body from the basic omega 6 substance. Not everyone is able to derive ARA, however, so that it may be wise to get ARA already pre-metabolized in animal products. Butter, whole milk, egg yolks and animal fat are sources of ARA.

ARA is important for the brain and nervous system. Patricia Kane, Ph.D., a neurobiologist, refers to ARA as the leading omega 6 for neural function. Kane has studied fatty acids in relation to neural diseases such as Alzheimer's, Parkinson's and autism. She has seen some reversal of these conditions with the chelation of metals from the brain and the balancing and replenishing of EFAs. She recommends that people get plenty of ARA from food since we are all exposed to toxins that affect our nervous system.

ARA is also important in preventing eczema in breastfed babies. However, too much ARA, if not balanced with the full range of EFAs, can lead to inflammatory conditions, as it provides the building blocks for the inflammatory prostaglandin. Experts point out though that it is not the level of ARA in the body, but its relation to levels of other EFAs, that promotes or prevent conditions such as eczema. .

What to do? One study showed that if a breastfeeding mother's diet contains too much ARA (too many animal products), the ARA will compete with the omega 3s and lower their levels in her milk. The mother will have too much ARA. But if she is getting good levels of omega 3s (fish oil, algae extract), *and* is also taking some ARA, the levels of all three become higher in her breastmilk[31]. Remembering to get enough of everything seems to be the trick.

Lauric Acid

Lauric acid has potent antimicrobial properties. It is the building block for the body's own antimicrobial fatty acid, monolaurin, which is made from lauric acid in the intestine. Monolaurin is anti-viral and antibacterial, and it kills the AIDS virus.

Lauric acid is found in coconut oil, in palm oil, and in breastmilk. Normally, lauric acid makes up about 3% of the saturated fats in breastmilk, according to the authority on fats, Mary G. Enig, Ph.D. According to Enig, in countries where mothers eat coconut every day, lauric acid may multiply to 18% of the saturated fat content of breastmilk. Enig encourages breastfeeding mothers who have AIDS or suppressed immune function to take a couple tablespoons of coconut oil every day so that their milk will have high levels of antimicrobial lauric acid and provide more protection to their babies.

The Ayurvedic scholar, Dr. Vinod Verma, suggests alternating the use of coconut, clarified butter, sesame and olive oil in our foods. This way, we get the benefits of each. Dr. Mary Enig says essentially the same thing. She suggests that we prepare stir-fry oil using a combination of coconut, sesame and olive oil in equal parts.

Choline – Brain Food

A nutrient called choline—found in many *mother foods*—may keep the brain running strong. Choline is a precursor to the neurotransmitter acetylcholine, important to memory and learning. Too little acetylcholine is known to be a factor in the development of Alzheimer's disease.

Pregnant and breastfeeding mothers should take note. Studies on rats show that foods rich in choline, taken during pregnancy and lactation, will boost a child's level of acetylcholine as well as increase the development of bigger brain cells in vital areas of the brain. Rats whose mothers took choline remain smart into old age, but a lack of choline in the mother rat's diet leads to mental impairment in the offspring at a young age[32].

Interestingly, studies done in the mid-1980s showed that taking extremely high dosages of choline had the opposite effect, leading to severe disturbances in the neural development of the baby rats. This seems to say that too much of a good thing can sometimes backfire. Feel free to take mother foods rich in choline, or to supplement with the daily requirement of lecithin or choline.

Good sources of choline are:
Animal product: egg yolks
Grains: barley, oats, wheat
Vegetables: onion, garlic, potato, eggplant
Seeds: sesame seed, sunflower seed, flaxseed
Legumes: soybeans, adzuki beans, black beans, black-eyed peas, chick peas, fava beans, field peas, kidney beans, lentils, navy beans, peas.
Herbs: fennel seed, dong quai, fenugreek seed, nettle
Supplement with *lecithin* (16% choline) –follow dosage directions on the package.
Choline supplement—follow dosage directions on the package.
Take foods that are rich in vitamin B-complex, especially pantothenic acid (B5), as this nutrient also contributes to levels of acetylcholine. B5 is found in oatmeal, brown rice, lentils, broccoli, mushrooms, avocado, and peas.

SUMMARY

In this section you can learn how foods, fats, oils and supplements can be used to optimize a mother's intake and balance of essential fatty acids. If you found this chapter too technical to absorb (after birth, mothers tend to find it difficult to concentrate), these rules will tell you everything you need to know.

The Correct Use of Oils and Fats

- **Good fats**. Look for organic butter at your health food store; if you can't find it, normal butter will do. Look for high quality coconut oil such as Spectrum or Omega. Buy cold-pressed sesame oil and cold-pressed virgin olive oil. These good fats do not compete with essential fatty acids in the body and can therefore be used freely. Although these oils are more expensive, you only need a small amount each day to gain their beneficial effects.

- **Unnecessary fats**. Avoid or limit the use of vegetable oils such as thistle seed oil, sunflower seed oil, safflower oil, or canola, as their fatty acids compete with essential fatty acids in the body.

- **Peanut oil** should be limited or avoided because it can trigger severe allergy. (Persons allergic to peanut may also be allergic to sesame seed.)

- **Bad, Trans-fats**. Avoid using margarine or processed or partially hydrogenated oils as they contain trans-fatty acids. This includes so-called *cooking oil* and *salad oil*. Beware of packaged foods such as pastry and potato chips, and store-bought pre-prepared meals, and also fast foods, as these all contain high amounts of bad oils. Overheating oil or butter while frying also leads to the development of trans-fatty acids.

- **Basic Balance of Healthy Fats**, take:
  1) 1/4 teaspoon of virgin olive oil at each meal,
  2) foods high in cholesterol and ARA (cream, butter, eggs)
  3) 1 teaspoon of flaxseed oil per day
  4) a supplement of fish oil, cod-liver oil (see below), DHA algae extract, or DHA/EPA.

- Take **cod-liver** oil in your basic mix (above) for its extra vitamins D and A if you do not get much sunlight. These vitamins are important for the uptake of calcium and other minerals from the food you eat.

- **Choline**: Supplement with lecithin or choline (follow dosage recommendations on package) to ensure that you have a good supply of its brain-strengthening choline, or, regularly eat foods containing choline (see page 51).
- Combine your own **stir-fry oil**, using equal parts of virgin cold-pressed olive oil, cold-pressed sesame oil, and coconut fat.
- Make **salad oil** by combining equal parts of cold-pressed sesame seed oil and flaxseed oil. (Do not heat this oil.)
- If you or your baby has signs of **EFA deficiency** (see page 41), follow the suggestions on page 45 under the guidance of your allergist or doctor to ascertain which EFAs are missing.
- If you have an illness that impairs your immune system, such as AIDS or Lyme disease, you may want to follow Dr. Mary G. Enig's advice and each day add 3-4 tablespoons of the potent anti-microbial **coconut oil** to your fat intake. (Breakfast is a good time to add coconut flakes and coconut milk to cereal; check out the recipe for coconut spread on page 223).
- Butter, cream, animal fat and cod-liver oil contain **vitamins D and A that enable the absorption of minerals**. These fats also enable the absorption of fat-soluble vitamins from food. Adding cream or butter to vegetables and grains insures that you are able to absorb the minerals in these foods.
- If you **sauté or stir-fry** vegetables, use the stir-fry combination of oils and fats mentioned above. The oil should not smoke—do not cook at the highest temperature.
- If you **simmer or steam** your veggies in a small amount of water, add olive oil, flaxseed oil, sesame oil, or butter to taste when the vegetables have finished cooking.
- Coconut oil and coconut milk works well for baking and in soups. Olive oil and sesame oil can be added to salads, or dribbled over vegetables *after* they've been cooked, so that the oil is not damaged. Flaxseed oil can also be mixed into any dish *after* it has been cooked.

Guidelines to Ensure the Uptake of Essential Fatty Acids (EFAs)

- **Avoid** fabricated, packaged and processed foods, fast food, store-bought cookies, pastries, crackers, chips, and pizzas. These contain trans-fatty acids that interfere in the metabolism of healthy fats.

- **Use** mainly virgin olive oil and smaller amounts of cold-pressed sesame oil, butter and coconut fat in meals, as these particular *oils do not compete with EFAs* in the body and are healthful fats.

- If you have allergies or if your health is compromised, it may be wise to **supplement with vitamins and minerals that play a role in the metabolism of EFAs**: vitamin C, B-complex, especially B3 (niacin) and B6 (pyroxidine), zinc and magnesium. *Be careful not to take more than 200 mg of vitamin B6 per day; more may reduce milk supply*[23].

- **Eat whole foods that contain omega 6**, such as eggs, milk, raw nuts, seeds, whole grains, and green leafy vegetables.

- If you take a fatty acid supplement, always stay within the prescribed dosage. Taking higher dosages than recommended can produce a boomerang effect, in which the body stops absorbing EFAs.

- Experts commonly recommend that we **take vitamin E** (100 IU per EFA capsule is a safe dose) **if supplementing with EFAs**, to mop up the increase of free radicals in the body from these volatile oils. Many EFA supplements are already combined with vitamin E.

Breastfeeding--Safe Medication and Birth Control Measures

Most medication is safe to take while breastfeeding, and if there are doubts, there is almost always a breastfeeding-friendly alternative. Unfortunately, some doctors suggest that a mother stop breastfeeding rather than make the effort to find that alternative. A lactation expert, on the other hand, will usually go the extra mile to research the precise medical information that you need to continue breastfeeding.

- **Birth control**: Birth control pills or shots that contain estrogen, including mini-pills and combination progesterone-estrogen pills, can suppress milk supply. Even progesterone-only birth control pills have been noted to suppress supply in some women. Mothers are frequently put under pressure during their first postnatal checkup to go onto birth control pills or to have a hormonal shot to suppress ovulation. If you wish to try one of these hormones or hormone combinations, ask for oral pills to test their effect on your milk supply. Have galactagogues at hand to use in case your supply dips, and go off medication immediately.

- **Aspirin**: The American Academy of Pediatrics recommends that breastfeeding mothers take aspirin with caution, as it has been seen to have negative effects on some nursing babies.

- **Decongestants** and **Antihistamines**: Medications for bronchial congestion are often a combination of decongestants and antihistamines. One decongestant, pseudoephedrine (for instance, used in Sudafed®), is known to decrease milk supply. Be sure that pseudoephedrine is not in the medication you use. Benadryl® and Chlor-Trimeton®, two antihistamines, may decrease supply and make a baby lethargic.

- **Antihistamines and decongestants** may cause babies to become hyper-alert, irritable, or have sleep problems. Mothers should watch for adverse events in their breastfed infants.

- **Ephedra**, an herb used in treating asthma, also contains pseudoephedrine. It is not wise to use this herb while breastfeeding.

Caffeine (coffee, tea, soda, chocolate)

Caffeine is found in coffee, black tea, green tea, mate tea, in some herbal tea mixtures, in some supplements, in most soft drinks, in some carbonated water, and in chocolate. Symptoms of caffeine stimulation in babies include over-alertness, nervousness, not able to sleep, hyperactivity, fussiness at the breast, and colicky behavior.

Lactation experts suggest that up to five cups a day of coffee will not affect most babies. That is five cups of coffee, or ten cups of tea, or fifteen cans of soda. (Do not take soda if you can help it: its sugar and potassium deplete calcium; there are health risks if artificially sweetened; and some mothers with low milk supply report problems building their supply if they take carbonated beverages.)

The reality is that different babies have different levels of sensitivity to caffeine. Some become fussy if the mother drinks one cup of coffee, or takes one bite of chocolate while others appear to be completely resistant to caffeine. Even if a baby shows no obvious reactions to caffeine, there may be a problem in the making. This is because caffeine does not leave a baby's body as quickly as an adult's. It can build up, day by day, and gradually lead to high levels in the baby's bloodstream.

A mother to a baby, who originally showed no reaction to caffeine, might believe that her baby is becoming hyperactive and fussy because he is growing up and getting older, when actually the baby is becoming over-stimulated. In my opinion, over-stimulation from caffeine cannot be good for a baby's developing nervous system.

Two rules of caution regarding caffeine can help:
1) only get as much caffeine as you really need
2) put in a caffeine-free day once a week, to give the baby a chance to decrease his caffeine levels.

A morning cup of coffee is important for many persons with low blood pressure. Some need another cup in the afternoon, and elderly persons often need a cup at night to improve their sleep. In this case, caffeine is medication and should be taken with pleasure. It would be wrong to eliminate caffeine from someone's diet who genuinely needs it. However, if a mother craves caffeine and sweets the whole day long, and if she feels that she is on a roller-coaster ride in terms of energy highs and lows, she may have blood-sugar issues and should look into balancing her blood sugar as a way to decrease her cravings for sugar and caffeine. (See pages 99-100.)

Here is some more you should know about caffeine. Caffeine has been linked to higher excretion of calcium in urine, and to bone loss. If you are at risk for osteoporosis, this is a reason to get your consume of caffeine under control. Maureen Minchin, in *Breastfeeding Matters*, writes about a small subgroup of breastfeeding mothers who develop fibrocystic breasts before their periods. These mothers report that their babies become colicky and may even refuse to breastfeed during this time. When these mothers take caffeine out of their diets their breasts become less fibrocystic, and their babies happily nurse.

Some mothers report that their let-down reflex improves when they eliminate all caffeine, including chocolate, from their diets. I believe that these particular mothers are over-anxious, and that caffeine subtly exacerbates their anxiety, leading to constriction of the tissue in the breasts. (A mother may see similar results if she changes her dietary patterns to reduce swings in her blood sugar levels.)

I prefer to get my morning 'boost' from black tea. Tea contains antioxidants that slow aging processes. Tea improves sensitivity to insulin so that we have fewer blood sugar highs and lows throughout the day. Tea has a positive effect on cholesterol levels. Black tea can be used to make delicious and lactogenic chai tea.

Limit or Stop Smoking

Breastfeeding experts agree that smoking is no reason to stop breastfeeding—though breastfeeding is a good reason to reduce or to stop smoking, if at all possible, and here are some reasons why.

Breastfed babies with colic or allergies frequently improve if the mother stops smoking. Children—even those who are not breastfed—who are exposed to smoke are more likely to develop asthma and other allergy-related symptoms, such as increased mucus production, nasal congestion, ear infections, coughs, sore throats, and respiratory disease. (Breastfeeding may offer these children some protection.) Finally, nicotine is thought to affect proteins in the brain that are involved in sleep. Sudden Infant Death Syndrome (SIDS) is statistically higher among babies whose mothers (or fathers) smoke in the home, or in babies who are regularly exposed to a smoke-filled environment, a restaurant, for instance, or a relative's home where smoking is common.

Avoiding smoke-filled environments is a must for all mothers. If you do smoke, smoke outside of the home so that your baby isn't a passive smoker, and so that you get plenty of fresh air which will help detoxify your body.

Studies show that mothers who smoke, or who previously smoked, have less breastfeeding success. Studies are suggesting that nicotine inhibits the let-down reflex. A study on prematurely born babies found that mothers who smoked cigarettes pumped less milk than those who did not smoke, and that their milk production did not increase as much as with non-smokers[33]. This could discourage mothers from breastfeeding. The let-down may be less affected if mothers smoke after breastfeeding, rather than before, and it may be wise for mothers who smoke to use herbal galactagogues and to eat lactogenic food from the start.

It has also been seen that even mothers who previously smoked do not produce as much cream in their milk as non-smokers. This means that mothers who smoke or who smoked should be get extra amounts of healthy fat in their diets, including lecithin, and eat plenty of dark green vegetables or take herbs such as alfalfa and spirulina, (these reputedly also increase fat levels), and should also avoid trans-fatty acids, as these also lower the fat content of breastmilk.

Medication to Stop Smoking

Nicotine patches are considered safe to use while breastfeeding. They release less nicotine into the bloodstream than a strong cigarette, and since the baby does not passive-smoke his lungs are not directly affected.

Zyban™, a drug used to stop smoking, anecdotally occasionally leads to a decrease in milk supply. If you take Zyban™, keep an eye on your supply and stop if you see that it is dropping. Your production should pick up again soon.

Alcohol – Set Your Limit

Today, experts are reevaluating their recommendations regarding alcohol and breastfeeding. Whereas we know that any amount of alcohol *during pregnancy* is potentially damaging to the baby, the risk while breastfeeding is not entirely understood. Alcohol passes into breastmilk in extremely small quantities and it is not clear what effect this has on the baby. The LLL recommends that one or two drinks on occasion are safe.

Alcohol is also a concern because it is addictive. A mother may begin by drinking one glass a day, and after a while may be inclined to drink two, three, or more per day. Alcohol, like any sedative, can lower a mother's inhibitions. Some mothers may then be more prone to be rough with a crying, fussy baby. Keep this in mind. The postpartum is a vulnerable time for mothers. If you do drink alcohol, know your limit.

Also keep in mind that women do not tolerate alcohol as well as men. In Australia—a country well known for it's appreciation of alcoholic beverages—the National Health and Medical Research Council recommends that women do not drink more than two standard drinks a day. More than this is considered hazardous. It is also recommended that women take a three day pause from alcohol during the week, to allow the liver time to recover[36].

Studies on alcohol and lactation tell a perplexing story. In 2000, a study on beer showed that beta-glucan, a polysaccharide found in barley grain (malt), increases prolactin levels significantly 30 minutes after drinking[34]. As well, beer contains phytoestrogen, which in small quantities may support lactation. However, alcohol impairs the let-down reflex so that babies actually drink less milk even while staying longer at the breast[35]. Therefore, drinking beer or other alcoholic beverage on a regular basis could reduce a mother's supply.

In 2000, a study on beer showed that beta-glucan, a poly-saccharide from barley grain, increases prolactin and is responsible for beer's supposed lactogenic effect[34]. A mother could get the same effect by taking large dosages of real barley malt or food containing barley malt, or by making barley-water. See page 193 for a recipe.

Today's mothers tend to prefer non-alcoholic beer, which also contains helpful phytoestrogen and prolactin-enhancing beta-glucan. In addition, mothers are experimenting with non-alcoholic herbal beers such as ginger beer and root beer, brewed with real spices. Check your healthfood store for these and more varieties of lactogenic beverages.

- Mothers in the US can find chemical-free, organic beer, available from many so-called 'microbreweries.'

CHAPTER FOUR

Supporting Digestion; Preventing Allergies; Lowering the Toxic Load

"Specialists in environmental medicine believe that 80 percent or more of the population have food allergies. Many of these, however, are unrecognized...." — Doris Rapp, MD, "Is This Your Child?"

The research of Dr. Doris Rapp, a leading authority on children's allergies, forms the basis of this chapter. Dr. Rapp was a board-certified medical pediatric allergist for twenty years. She then became a board-certified *environmental medical specialist,* convinced that environmental medicine provides a vastly more effective approach to the prevention and cure of children's allergies. In this capacity, Rapp continued to treat children's allergies for another twenty years before authoring books—that are now classics—on environmental sensitivity and allergies in children. Dr. Rapp promotes an intriguing message: *allergy can be spotted at a very early age, even when a baby is still in the uterus.* Rapp, like many others, believes that recognizing and responding to food allergy and sensitivity in children can prevent or limit developmental delays, learning problems, poor concentration, and hyperactivity in children, as well as emotional instability and antisocial behavior in the adults the children become.

Lactation consultants are on the same track as Dr. Rapp about the connection between what a mother eats and her baby's sensitivities. In 1982, Maureen Minchin, an Australian lactation specialist, pointed out in her book, *Food for Thought,* that there are two main causes for severe and chronic colic. The first is the introduction of cow's milk based formula soon after birth. *The second is the pre-sensitization of the baby within the mother's womb to foods in the mother's diet.* Minchin based her assessment on the observations of lactation specialists. Only in recent years have scientists finally confirmed the presence of food molecules from the mother's diet in her milk.

In this chapter, I will look at the early introduction of foods, at factors involved in pre-sensitization, and at ways that mothers can minimize the development of food sensitivities in their babies before conception, during pregnancy, and while breastfeeding.

No Substitute for Colostrum and Breastmilk

According to *nature's laws*, newborns should only drink their mother's best: colostrum, and then breastmilk. These foods contain essential immune substances that settle in the baby's intestine and provide it with protection. Other kinds of nutrition or fluid introduce microbes and non-human proteins and starches before the baby is ready to handle them. This impedes the optimal development of the baby's intestinal flora, contributing to colic and allergy.

Sometimes, however, it is necessary to give a newborn baby supplementary feedings while the mother builds her supply. In the US, expensive hypoallergenic formula is frequently recommended for the days following birth while building supply. In Europe, lactation experts do not recommend hypoallergenic formula in this instance as it still contains allergenic components. The commercial formula, "Good Start" (now by Nestle, formerly by Carnation), is tolerated well by most newborns.

Digestive Weakness – A Key to Food Sensitivity

As we shall see, improving a mother's digestion helps prevent or reduce allergy in both the mother and the baby. Unfortunately, most of us no longer understand the basics of good digestion. We think, for instance, that it is normal to pass gas frequently, throughout the day, when in fact, a person whose digestion is in perfect order may never pass gas at all. If they do, it will not draw attention because it does not smell. Bad-smelling gas suggests a digestive problem.

Today it seems odd, even offensive, to talk about the "bottom end" of digestion. This was not always the case. Decades ago, people in Europe and the US paid close attention to the color, smell, and consistency of their urine and stool. Through self-observation, they gauged the health of their intestine, liver, gall bladder, and kidneys. Not only has this skill of self-diagnosis been lost, today people actually believe that their stool *should* smell bad. Well, the stool of a person with excellent digestion and a balanced diet does not have a penetrating odor. Moreover, because a slippery sheath envelops healthy stool, a bowel movement should be effortless, quick, and perfectly clean. If it is necessary to push hard, or if the toilet paper is soiled, something is wrong.

Today, almost everyone has some form of digestive problem. Common issues include constipation, inflammation of the intestine, fungal overgrowth in the intestine, a lack of digestive enzymes, an inflamed or underfunctioning pancreas or gall bladder, lack of the immunoglobulin IgA, and insufficient hydrochloric acid in the stomach to initiate the digestion of protein. The following sections look at a selection of these issues.

> Signs of indigestion such as heartburn, bloating, flatulence, constipation, and diarrhea, bad taste in the mouth or sudden tiredness after a meal indicate a digestive weakness *in the mother*.

IgA

The immunoglobulin IgA, found in mucosal tissues such as the walls of the intestine, plays a central role in the prevention of allergy. IgA in the intestine attaches to undigested food molecules and prevents them from passing through the intestinal wall. These are the same undigested food molecules that are involved in triggering an allergic reaction through a mother's milk. Whereas a sub-group of people appears to be born with low levels of IgA, others develop this condition over time and become allergy-prone.

Breastmilk contains IgA, and it is largely the settling of this IgA in the baby's intestine that doctors refer to when they speak of the "maturity" of the baby's digestive system. Without IgA, a baby cannot protect himself from undigested food molecules, including those that may be in his mother's milk. Interestingly, *IgA is measurably lower in the breastmilk of babies that have allergies.* In other words, these mothers are not able to provide their babies with as much protection through their breastmilk as mothers with normal levels of IgA[37].

There may be hope for these mothers and their babies. Astragalus root, an herbal galactagogue and valued food in China, has been shown in studies to improve levels of IgA. If a mother takes astragalus root (along with other steps to improve her digestive health), there will very likely be more IgA in her milk. This would enable a baby to develop intestinal maturity more quickly, so that her baby would have less colic, allergy, and earaches—just like babies in China.

Leaky Gut Syndrome and Fungal Infection

When the intestine no longer seals off undigested food molecules, this is called *increased intestinal permeability*, or *leaky gut syndrome*. A leaky gut promotes food allergy by allowing food molecules to enter the bloodstream, lymph nodes, and other tissue. When the body recognizes these food molecules as "foreign," antibodies and white cells are programmed to attack them. The result is food allergy, and it can lead to inflammation in every tissue and organ of the body, including the brain.

The main defense against leaky gut syndrome is a healthy mix of *good* bacteria in the intestine. Every time we take antibiotics, we kill off good bacteria, giving fungus and *bad* bacteria the chance to get the upper hand. In addition, the sugar that most people eat every day is a feast for fungus. In combination, these factors allow fungus to multiply in force, creating tiny holes in the intestinal wall, and making it permeable.

Substances that pass through a leaky intestine include toxins and undigested food molecules, bacteria, viruses, fungus, and the toxic by-products produced by the fungus and microbes. Together, these factors can overwhelm the liver and lead to a feeling "the blahs", to fatigue, confusion, and memory loss.

In earlier times, people had less gut-leakiness. Before refrigerators and fast food, people *fermented* their food to keep it fresh. The acidity of fermentation prevented the growth of bad bacteria in food. This acidity was, in fact, a by-product of the *lactobacilli* in these foods: the same good bacteria that populate the intestine and prevent it from becoming leaky. Examples of fermented foods include sour dough bread such as sour pumpernickel and rye, fermented raw milk products such as yogurt, kefir, and cheese, fermented vegetables such as sauerkraut and pickled cucumbers, and fermented beverages based on vegetables or grains—many of which were traditionally taken as galactagogues. The *lactobacilli* in these common, everyday foods reinforced intestinal flora—preventing the intestine from becoming leaky.

Today, commercial fermented foods are chemically soured rather than fermented. Even so-called "probiotic" yogurt may be processed so that the lactobacilli are no longer alive. Today, unless we make a special effort, we will not find foods that support intestinal flora and prevent or cure the leaky gut syndrome.

- Mothers routinely receive antibiotics during a caesarian birth and should take lactobacilli supplements to prevent fungal overgrowth.
- Many lactation consultants have observed that thrush—fungal infection of the breast—is more prevalent in mothers who receive antibiotics around the time of birth.
- Frequently drinking alcohol contributes to a leaky intestine.
- Anti-inflammatory drugs (NSAIDS), such as aspirin, ibuprofen, ketoprofen, and naproxen, can increase the permeability of the intestine, as can prescription corticosteroids (e.g. prednisone), and prescription hormones such as the birth control pill.

If you are chronically tired, suffer from depression, have allergies or autoimmune disorders, if you have taken antibiotics off and on, or if you eat a diet that is heavy on starches and sugar, you should look into the possibility of fungal infection of the intestine. A good resource is *The Yeast Connection Handbook* by William G. Crook, M.D. Dr. Crook is convinced that fungal infection can be passed from the mother to her unborn baby, and that it is often responsible for the food allergies that lead to chronic ear infections in young babies and children.

Dr. Leo Galland, in *Superimmunity for Kids*, provides dietary suggestions to prevent and treat yeast infection in babies and children. The best measure is to take lactobacilli during and two weeks after having antibiotic treatment; children and babies can take this as well under the direction of their doctor.

The following probiotics promote intestinal health:

- Lactobacillus acidophilus, L. rhamnosus, L. plantarum, and bifidobacterium bifidum are examples of friendly bacteria that build up healthy intestinal flora. In studies, lactobacilli have improved general health in children and adults, and lowered the risk of allergy in infants, especially if the mother takes them during pregnancy. Special mixtures for infants and adults can be found at healthfood stores. Products that must be refrigerated are the most effective.

- Natural yogurt—made with a live culture of lactobacillus. Your health food store will carry yogurt made with a live culture.

- Kefir—live kefir grains quickly turn milk into a thin, yogurt-like, slightly carbonated beverage, rich in various strains of lactobacilli. Live kefir grains can be found through an internet search[*]. Some people give them away for the cost of postage. This is probably the least expensive way to keep a fresh supply of live lactobacilli in your home.

- Sauerkraut—commercial brands are no longer fermented and do not support healthy intestinal flora, or fight fungal infection. Look for fresh, *real* sauerkraut in the refrigerated section of your health food store, or make your own.

Suggestions in this chapter can help mothers prevent food sensitivity and colic in their babies during pregnancy, and help reduce symptoms of food sensitivity in their baby or themselves, after the baby is born. If a mother has serious concerns about her digestion or her baby's symptoms or behavior, she should consult her healthcare provider.

Enzyme Depletion

Allergists say that a one-sided diet will, eventually, lead to a deficiency in the enzymes needed to digest the particular foods that we prefer to eat, so that undigested food molecules will be available to pass through the intestine. This is another reason why *the food that*

---

[*] http://users.chariot.net.au/~dna/kefirpage.html

we eat the most of becomes the food to which we are most prone to be allergic—and the food to which our babies are allergic.

The best prevention is to take a varied diet (it's also best to eat a wide variety of foods before conception). That way, we do not over-tax those enzymes needed to digest any one particular food. Also, a diet containing fresh, enzyme-rich foods will replenish a mother's supply of enzymes. (During spring, summer, and fall, get as many fresh, raw fruits and vegetables as you can tolerate.) For a breastfeeding mother with a food-sensitive baby, it can be helpful to take digestive plant enzymes, as described below. Taking hydrochloric acid, under your doctor's guidance, can also aid in the complete digestion of food.

Digestive Plant Enzymes

Supplements of digestive plant enzymes are useful in treating food sensitivities and allergies. They help the intestine do its job while a mother improves her intestinal health and her diet.

⇨ *Digestive enzymes are prescribed to breastfeeding mothers of babies who suffer from colic or allergies, in particular pancreatic enzyme, to improve the mother's digestion of protein. Often, this alone is sufficient to improve a baby's symptoms.*

Plant enzymes can be taken before, after, and between meals. Taken before a meal, they improve digestion. Taken after a meal, they mop up undigested food particles in the intestine. Taken between meals, plant enzymes enter the bloodstream and digest food particles in the bloodstream—molecules that might otherwise enter the mother's milk and contribute to allergies or a baby's colic[*].

Supplements should include enzymes that aid in the digestion of proteins, fat, and carbohydrates (for instance, Pan-Enzyme). Digestive plant enzymes are available over-the-counter and as prescription medication. If your family has a history of severe allergy, your allergist may suggest that you alternate between several different products, to prevent you or your baby from becoming sensitized to any one of them.

---

[*] Naturopaths sometimes give powdered digestive enzymes directly to babies who have severe, chronic colic or allergies. Seek a qualified NAET practitioner for more information.

Hydrochloric Acid

With your doctor's permission, you may try taking hydrochloric acid to improve your digestion of proteins. Some person's stomachs no longer produce enough hydrochloric acid. Hydrochloric acid is important for the complete digestion of protein.

Intestinal Inflammation

Inflammatory conditions in the intestine develop into leaky gut syndrome. Besides fungal infection, other causes of inflammation include food sensitivity or allergy, bacteria and viruses, and an autoimmune reaction. The organs that participate in digestion—the pancreas and gall bladder—may also be inflamed.

Signs of inflammation include diarrhea, abdominal cramps and pain, blood in the stool, and smelly gas and stool. In a baby, the red, inflamed circle around the anus may signal allergic inflammation in the intestine. See your doctor if you find blood in your stool, or in your baby's stool, as this may be a sign of serious disease.

⇨ Eliminating problematic foods and improving intestinal health is an appropriate response to inflammation. Your doctor or allergist should oversee treatment and therapy.

⇨ Never allow your baby to receive a vaccine if he has signs of a digestive disorder or intestinal inflammation, or if he is ill in any way, as these factors greatly increase his risk for a negative reaction with neurological damage.

Herbs, Spices, and Condiments that Improve Digestion

Many lactogenic herbs can help reduce intestinal inflammation, increase blood circulation in the intestinal wall, and increase bile flow so that fatty foods become easier to digest. Before using an herb, refer to *A Lactogenic Herbal* in Part Four to learn more about its usage.

• Flatulence: dill seed. This lactogenic herb reduces flatulence in the mother and the colicky baby. The baby gets the medicinally active substances through his mother's milk. For a stronger effect, give him a teaspoon of lightly steeped tea (transparent) before feeding.

• Improved digestion of fat: bitter herbs. Turmeric, marjoram, basil, thyme, dandelion leaf and root, endive, and chamomile activate the production of gall and aid in the digestion of fat. These bitter herbs must be tasted to work. Add spices toward the end of cooking, as prolonged heat damages their medicinal substances.

- To increase digestive activity: carminative herbs, such as cumin, caraway, anise, fennel, dill, and ginger root increase digestive activity and prevent the buildup of gas in the intestine.

- Improved digestibility of beans and legumes: two heaping teaspoonfuls of powdered fennel or cumin seed added to a pot of lentils or other legumes can greatly reduce gas. (Fennel powder disappears into the taste of legumes. Cumin spices it up.)

- Intestinal inflammation: onion and garlic are potent antibacterials, antivirals, and antifungals. They help curb inflammation in the intestine—if the mother can tolerate them. All herbs listed in this section have antimicrobial properties, especially: turmeric, chamomile, thyme, garlic, onion, and ginger.

- Antifungals: all herbs and condiments listed in this section inhibit fungal buildup in the intestines. Antifungals are important. As discussed previously, fungal overgrowth in the intestine may cause the intestine to become permeable, so that partially digested food can more easily pass into the mother's bloodstream and enter her milk, leading to food sensitivities and allergic reactions in herself and her baby.

Signs That a Mother May Have a Food Sensitivity

The following list of symptoms is used by Beverly Morgan, IBCLC, to help mothers identify possible food sensitivities: lumps of phlegm in the throat, runny nose, the need to clear the throat often, clicking in the ears when swallowing (fluid in the ears), restless legs (can't keep legs still while sitting or sleeping), heartburn, headache, joint pain, smelly stools, passing smelly gas, burping up food aftertaste, a bad taste in your mouth (should not have a noticeable taste), grumbling sounds in intestines, wind-burned look to cheeks, reddened/itchy chin or other area of the body, eczema, general fatigue, insomnia, fatigue that hits you about 20 minutes after a meal (you were not noticeably tired before the meal), or a feeling like a hangover after eating a food.

Identify Your Problem Foods

In the US, foods commonly involved in food sensitivity and allergy are sugar, cow's milk protein, egg, wheat, fish, peanuts, nuts, wheat, corn, fish, and sometimes tomato, berries, citrus fruits, and currants. Chicken, beef, pork, and potato are infrequent culprits. Any food frequently eaten is suspect, however, and lactation consultants are seeing beef sensitivity come up more frequently.

Foods from the same animal source may trigger similar reactions. For instance, if there is a sensitivity to milk protein, look for a possible sensitivity to beef as well. If there is sensitivity to eggs, look for a possible sensitivity to chicken. Other common triggers for sensitivity include yeast, artificial coloring, artificial sweeteners, chemical additives, monosodium glutamate, (MSG), preservatives, and nitrates in food.

Eat a Whole-Foods Diet

It is easiest to identify your own and your baby's problem foods if you eat a simple, whole-foods diet. Whereas you can never be completely certain of the ingredients in store-bought foods, you know precisely what you are eating if your meals are prepared at home. In the long term, the time we put into preparing a whole-foods diet is worth the health benefits of discovering and eliminating problem foods.

Another reason to take a whole foods diet is that you or your baby may be sensitive to the additives used to preserve, color, or enhance the taste of food. Many of these chemicals have never been tested for safety.

Keep a Journal

It is wise to keep a food journal, recording the time of day both of what you eat (keep a detailed list), and the symptoms you experience. Keep this journal for a week or two. Keep a journal of your baby's symptoms as well, including sleep patterns, crying spells, and other symptoms. By comparing the two journals, you may be surprised at what you discover. Allergists frequently observe that *mothers and babies share the same food sensitivities.* This is logical, since the same undigested molecules are affecting both the mother and her baby.

Familial Predisposition

Other factors in infant allergy include a mother's, a father's, or their baby's genetic predisposition. If there are allergies in your family, or the family of your husband, or if your children have allergies, consult a pediatric allergist before pregnancy if possible. She may suggest that you avoid foods to which family members are allergic during pregnancy and while breastfeeding. She'll make suggestions as to the best time to introduce these foods as solids. She may also suggest that you take lactobacilli, and other measures, to improve your intestinal health.

⇨ By avoiding foods that trigger symptoms in you or members of your family, your baby will have an easier time with less colic and fewer food sensitivities.

Foods that are Common Allergens

Allergies are highly individual. While anyone can be allergic to anything, high exposure to the food or substance tends to precede allergy. This is why, when you study the list of foods that commonly trigger allergies (see page 69), you should be aware that you or your baby may not be sensitive to any of these foods. Your sensitivity may be to some other food or additive that only you can discover.

Foods eaten the most often tend to be the foods that trigger allergies. In the US and Europe, the two most commonly eaten foods are dairy and wheat; they are also the most common triggers of food allergy. (Read about these on pages 137-142.) Dairy is hidden in most store-bought bread, so that all store-bought products made with bread or breadcrumbs are not allowed if you are restricting dairy. Other foods to avoid are salad dressing, soups, sauces, and all foods containing milk, lactose, or casein. Soy and corn are common ingredients in packaged foods, and they have a high rating for allergy. If soy or corn triggers symptoms, avoid these foods, and avoid all packaged foods containing soy and corn.

Another common sensitivity is to yeast, (signaling, usually, yeast infection in the intestine and body), found in bread, bread crumbs, foods made with bread crumbs, fermented cheese, yogurt (not cottage cheese), malt and products that contain malt, mushrooms, truffles, morel, sauerkraut, grapes, dried fruit and raisins (can have mold growth on them), vinegar (not distilled vinegar), and products that contain vinegar, such as catsup and salad sauce, soy sauce and miso, Marmit® and Vegemite®, wine, beer, cider, and other fermented beverages. Unleavened bread, such as pumpernickel, does not contain yeast.

Some foods, such a peanut, dairy, and wheat, are highly allergenic because their protein is particularly difficult to digest. (Peanut can trigger life-threatening allergic reactions.)

Unfortunately, an in-depth discussion on where allergens can be found in common foods (such as that "non-dairy" often designates a food containing milk protein, that wheat is often found in tofu, and modified corn in yogurt) is beyond the scope of this book. For more information, see *Baby Matters,* by Dr. Linda Folden Palmer. It contains a chapter that explores hidden allergens with a focus for the breastfeeding mother. See also the excellent online resource "Parents of Food Allergic Kids," http://groups.yahood.com/group/POFAK.

An Easy Allergy Test

If you are unsure whether a certain food is triggering symptoms, avoid the suspicious food for four days. *Four days gives the body enough time to recover somewhat from the allergic reaction, but not enough time for the body to become so desensitized to the food that a reaction will be too subtle to notice.*

On the morning of the test-day, if you are otherwise well, take your resting pulse. Then eat a double portion of the food in question on an empty stomach. If the food is indeed problematic, your pulse will become markedly swifter, 12-16 beats faster per minute. Because you may have other reactions as well, wait up to six hours before eating again. Be alert to possible allergic symptoms and note them in your journal. Common reactions include restless legs, bright red earlobes, sudden fatigue, and mental confusion. For a more complete list of symptoms, see page 68. If you are not sure about your reaction, re-test the food on another day, again following a four-day interval in which you absolutely avoid this food.

Overcoming Food Allergies

If a mother avoids problematic foods, takes measures to improve her digestion and improve her diet, and if she eats a variety of whole foods plus healthy fats, she may overcome 95% of her food sensitivities or allergies and be able to eat the questionable foods again after about three months.

Breastfed children—if they are not given the food as a solid, and if the mother avoids the problem foods in her own diet for approximately six months—can usually tolerate the food again without showing previous symptoms. It may be wise, however, to omit the problem food from your and her diet for longer, as allergic symptoms can become masked, and the sensitivity may still be present. Indeed, allergy in children frequently goes "under cover" rather than being truly healed. Old symptoms disappear and new symptoms develop, that, because they are so different from the original reaction, go unrecognized as a response to a problem food. These symptoms commonly include hyperactive behavior and learning difficulties.

⇨ Dr. Doris Rapp's audio-book, "Infant Food Allergies," contains detailed guidelines for breastfeeding and formula-feeding mothers of extremely food-sensitive babies.

Pregnancy: Prevent Food Sensitivity in Your Baby

During pregnancy, keep an eye on your baby's reactions to the food that you eat. According to Dr. Doris Rapp, an unborn baby's typical reaction to a problem food or substance that you recently ate, smelled, or touched will be a *sudden and extreme bout of kicking or hiccups*. If your baby has an excessive bout of kicking or hiccupping, ask yourself what you recently had to eat (usually up to about 4 hours earlier). Recall if you were exposed to a strong chemical smell, such as cleaning detergent, furniture polish, perfume, or insecticide? Or did you touch something allergenic, such as nickel?

If there are allergies in your family, you may wish to keep a journal during pregnancy, recording both the foods you eat and any unusual environmental factors that you encounter. In another journal, note the time that your baby has sudden, excessive kicking or hiccupping (many babies become active at night; this is normal). By comparing the two journals, you may notice a correspondence between your baby's excessive kicking and foods you eat, or certain places you visit. This may indicate possible food sensitivity, or environmental sensitivity to a chemical substance in a building or location.

By being observant, you may be able to discover your baby's sensitivities before she is born. This information will help you and your allergist decide which foods to limit or avoid during pregnancy and breastfeeding, and which foods to introduce last as solids. It may also help you understand your child's behavior, for instance, when he becomes hyperactive, or upset, or aggressive in certain buildings, or upon smelling certain chemical odors, or after eating certain foods.

To reduce environmental sensitivities, move chemical substances such as furniture polish, insecticides, and cleaning detergents out of the home, into the garage. Avoid exposure to chemicals when possible (i.e., don't paint or refurbish your home during pregnancy or when your children are young), and tell the gardener to no longer use insecticide or herbicide on your lawn. (More about this on page 76.)

A baby who is being primed for allergies in the womb may show signs of distress such as excessive kicking and hiccupping. A mother from England wrote about her experience:

> *"My hyperactive son was born 7 years ago. Throughout that pregnancy, I was totally exhausted. I felt movement at a very early stage and he was very active in the womb!*
>
> *"In the late stages I was in hospital having his movements checked due to blood pressure. The nurses fell about laughing. Apparently they had never seen such an active baby! He just didn't stop. He also hiccupped a lot.*
>
> *"I noticed that every time I drank milk he would get more active. I did think it was strange but dismissed it as me being neurotic!*
>
> *"The other strange thing was that throughout the pregnancy I couldn't bear to touch fruit, especially oranges. On the day I went into labor though I suddenly had a huge craving!*
>
> *"We use diet and supplements with him now and oranges are one of the few foods he still can't eat.*
>
> *"Although my husband and I don't have allergies we both come from families with a history of migraines, hay fever, eczema, asthma etc.*

> *"The group that helped me in the UK, Hyperactive Children's Support Group, did some research once on this and found that a lot of babies were active in the uterus. A lot of the babies also had colic. I was breastfeeding and found the colic disappeared as soon as I stopped drinking milk and eating oranges."*[39]

⇨   Dr. Rapp suggests that by paying attention to foods that upset you or your baby during pregnancy, and by avoiding these, you help reduce allergies and sensitivities in your baby *before* he is born.

Signs That a Baby May Have a Food Sensitivity or Allergy

According to Dr. Rapp, sensitivities to foods in a mother's diet may cause symptoms in a baby that include colic, frequent screaming, fussiness at the breast, an inability to accept cuddling or physical closeness, restlessness and agitation, over-alertness, climbing out of the crib and walking at a very young age, sleeping problems, digestive problems, a brilliant-red rash on the bottom.

Other signs include dark, deep eye circles, bags, puffiness, or lines beneath or around the eyes, an occasional brilliant red earlobe or cheek, the baby throwing her head back while screaming, and frequent ear infections (especially if the allergy is to dairy). Constant whining, together with her not being able to stand having her skin touched, may indicate hay fever (pollen allergy).

According to Dr. J. Brostoff, MD, allergist and author, another less obvious sign of food sensitivity may be *baby insomnia*, when the baby seems to be hungry all night long and wakes frequently to feed. This is usually caused by: 1) the baby's stomach is small so she needs to feed more often, 2) the mother has low storage in her breasts, so a baby has to drink more frequently, 3) the baby is undergoing a growth-spurt and is trying to stimulate more milk production with frequent feedings, and 4) the mother has low milk supply.

A fifth reason may be food sensitivity. Some mothers discover that by eliminating common allergens from their diet, such as dairy, beef, fish, or nuts (observe your baby's behavior for clues as to which food you should eliminate), their baby sleeps for several hours at a stretch, and wakes up content.

Prevent Allergy – Reduce the Toxic Load

Throughout Part One, I discuss foods to avoid, reduce, or limit in some way. These foods include allergens, unhealthy fats, margarine, dairy, meat, fish, white sugar, white flour, caffeine, and aspartame. I do not discuss food additives in detail. Food additives are believed to actually cause inflammation in the brain of sensitive children, and to cause or contribute to developmental disorders. This subject is beyond the scope of this book[*]—but the simple solution is to eat as many whole foods as possible and to avoid packaged and processed foods.

Another potent source of toxins is the home and garden. It is widely accepted that we can overwhelm and weaken the immune system by surrounding ourselves with chemical odors and pollutants, in combination with environmental allergens such as dust, dust mites, and mold. When the immune system can no longer deal with the hundreds of chemicals and allergens that assault it every day, it succumbs, leading to allergy, and sometimes to chronic illness.

Ideally, children should grow up in an environment like that of traditional farmer's families—rich both in the protective bacteria of raw milk and fresh food, and in the challenging animal proteins that have helped strengthen the immune systems of human beings for thousands of years. Since this is not possible for most of us, our strategy instead is to *limit* our exposure to difficult chemicals and allergens, while providing the immune system with the nutrients it needs to remain strong. Many herbs and foods have a supportive effect on the immune system. They are listed in Part Four, pages 247-253.

The next section contains a list of measures you can take to reduce toxins and allergens in your environment.

⇨ Reducing the toxic load is preventative of allergies, for yourself, your children, and, if you are pregnant, for your unborn child. Since so many children have allergies today—even in families with no previous history of allergy—it is a good idea for everyone to follow these guidelines.

---

[*] For a brief, well-written overview, see *Allergies: Disease in Disguise* by Carolee Bateson-Koch

How to Reduce Irritants, Pollution and Allergens in Your Environment

- Do not move close to strong electric power lines, next to an antenna site for cellular phones, or into a house that is close to a source of pollution, such as a freeway or waste dump.

- Certain kinds of mold, and hidden pesticides in the home, lead to *devastating health conditions with long-term neurological damage* in unborn babies, children, and adults. Make sure there is no mold in the cellar, bathroom, or other rooms of your home. (A freshly painted bathroom may signal that a previous owner tried to cover up traces of mold.) Before you move, ask about pesticides employed in the construction of the house—insecticides may have been inserted into holes in the foundation, or have been dumped around the foundation of the house. If so, do not move into this house.

- Insecticides and herbicides should not be used, especially not by the mother herself, and not within or close to the home. Instruct your gardener that you no longer wish to have pesticides or herbicides used in your garden. Learn alternative methods to maintain your garden's beauty, and to keep your home pest-free.

- If there are any jobs to do in the home or garden that involve chemicals, take a vacation while someone else does the work for you. Wait until your home has aired out and no trace of the odor remains before returning. A study showed that mice exposed in the uterus to chemicals from insecticide had higher incidence of allergy and autoimmune diseases[40].

- Keep your home well dusted and vacuumed to limit dust mites. Vacuum your mattress when you change the sheets.

- Put the bedding, blankets, and pillows outside on a hot afternoon. Sunlight has a sterilizing effect. Dust mites do not like dry heat. Wash sheets, blankets, and pillowcases at a high temperature. Freezing dolls and stuffed toy animals clears them of dust mites.

- *Pregnancy is no time to renovate your home, due to all the chemical odors involved.* Do not paint rooms, refurbish, or polish furniture, or lay new carpets or floors. If you have to put in new floors or carpets, inquire into the chemical contents. There should be no moth poison or formaldehyde in the new floor.

- Avoid perfumed cosmetics, deodorants, creams, or shampoo: what we smell enters the bloodstream. Cosmetics contain plastifyers, substances that penetrate the skin, enter the bloodstream, and harm the liver and kidney. Do not use fabric softeners during pregnancy, as these are always perfumed.
- Flame-retardants, a fat-soluble chemical, are added to synthetic fabrics and to plastics, including the synthetic fabric of curtains, rugs, and furniture. Bras made of synthetic fabric leak flame-retardants directly into breast tissue. Wear bras made of cotton.
- In allergies, there tends to be a crave-repel dynamic. Either you love it, or you hate it—and both loving and hating can indicate sensitivity to a food or chemical.
- It used to be that allergists advised parents of potentially allergic children not to have pets, so that the children would not become sensitized to the animals. Now, allergists believe that having at least two pets in the home during earliest childhood significantly reduces allergies. (Perhaps keeping pets is the closest we can come to giving our children a farm-like environment.) If your family is at risk for allergies, ask your doctor or allergist for the latest guidelines regarding pets.

Countering Fat-Soluble Toxins from Agriculture and Industry

All of us carry concentrations of toxins in our bodies that we have ingested through food, water, and air—since before we were born. Whereas water-soluble toxins leave the body through urine, breath, and perspiration, toxins that are fat-soluble, (neurotoxins, hormonal disruptors, and carcinogens) cannot be rid of so easily. Dieting and exercise do not burn off these toxins. Rather, when fat cells melt, these toxins temporarily enter the bloodstream where they can do harm in various ways.

In nature, animals that are high up on the food chain have the highest levels of fat-soluble toxins in their bodies. In the ocean, the food chain works like this: little fish eat algae (that thrive on toxic heavy metals) and concentrate these toxins into their tissue. Larger fish eat the little fish and receive an even higher concentration into their tissue. The higher up a predator fish is on the food chain, the more toxins are stored in its fatty tissue. To compound matters, pregnant fish pass toxins into the bodies of their unborn offspring, so that each generation of fish is born with a higher starting level.

Human milk contains a higher level of toxins than cow's milk because we are higher up on the food chain than a cow. Just as cows concentrate toxins into their body fat, including their milk fat, we concentrate toxins into our fat and into our milk fat as well. And, like fish, we pass toxins to our unborn children, so that, theoretically, each generation has a higher starting level.

A very effective way for a woman's body to get rid of these toxins is via the placenta, and breastmilk. In the first case, experts agree that the *influence of toxins on the fetus* is potentially detrimental: here toxins act directly on a vulnerable, developing infant. Experts also agree that the influence of toxins in breastmilk on babies *is negligible*. This conclusion is based on the fact that babies fed on breastmilk are still overall healthier than are formula-fed babies. Still, mothers may wish to reduce the levels of toxins in their breastmilk, as we do not know what the long-term effects of these toxins may be.

> First-born children receive the highest levels of fat-soluble toxins from their mothers[41]. It has been speculated that this may explain why firstborns are more prone to allergies[42].

The breastmilk of vegetarians, especially vegans, contains only a fraction of the toxins found in the breastmilk of omnivorous women[43]. A professor of organic chemistry at the Russian Academy of Science, S. S. Yufit, has published an article on the internet[44] in which he urges pregnant and breastfeeding mothers to become vegetarians, omitting dairy, fish, and meat from their diets. Yufit claims that mothers can reduce fat-soluble toxins in their milk by at least 20%.

The provocative writer of *Baby Matters*, Dr. Linda Folden Palmer, also urges mothers to cut out meat and dairy from their diet, or to take low-fat or non-fat products, as fat-soluble toxins are concentrated in animal fat. If you purchase organic animal products, however, it is not necessary to take low-fat or non-fat products to reduce toxins in your milk. (Indeed, animal fat contains nutrients that we need, such as vitamins D and A.)

During pregnancy, many of the toxins we pass to our infants come from our body fat. Only by not burning fat, that is, by always eating regularly, and getting enough calories to ensure that the body does not resort to burning its fat stores, can we at least partially prevent these fat-soluble toxins from passing to the fetus. Of course, it is best to take organic animal and vegetable products, if available and affordable, especially the first trimester when the baby is developing.

Countering Mercury

Heavy metals, particularly mercury, are toxic to the nerves[45]. Mercury literally destroys a nerve's ability to function—both in the body and in the brain.

Dr. med. Dietrich Klinghardt, an expert on heavy metal toxicity, suggests that pregnant and breastfeeding mothers, even if they still have amalgam fillings in their teeth, take 5 pills or 1.25 grams total of high-quality chlorella[*] per day to mop up mercury and other heavy metals from their intestines. Taking a higher dosage of chlorella is risky, according to Klinghardt. It could lead to a large amount of toxic metals flooding out of body tissues and entering the placenta or breastmilk. Taken at the above dosage, however, chlorella will reduce the content of mercury in the bloodstream and in breastmilk[46].

If the mother reacts badly to chlorella, this could be a sign of two things. Most likely, it means that she cannot digest chlorella well. (This should occur less if a highest quality product is used.) However, the other explanation is that her body contains too much mercury for this gentle treatment. She should stop taking chlorella immediately and seek the guidance of a therapist knowledgeable in this field.

Another slow but non-risk way to reduce mercury, according to Dr. Klinghardt, is to take small portions of *real* sauerkraut throughout each day. Mercury is filtered out of the blood by the liver and is deposited in the intestine via bile. Usually, this mercury is reabsorbed into the body through the intestine. Chemicals in sauerkraut bind with mercury in the intestine and lead it out into the stool (this is also chlorella's working principle). By eating sauerkraut, mercury levels are reduced, very gradually, in the body. More importantly, this measure reduces the mercury available in the bloodstream on a daily basis.

---

[*] Algomed® and Bio Reu-rella®, high quality chlorella, are available in Europe. Dr. Mercola sells high quality chlorella at his website: http://www.mercola.com/forms/chlorella.htm

- Studies on animals show that mercury leaches out of amalgam fillings, and, within days, binds to tissue, organs, and nerves within the brain and body. In spite of these studies, some dentists assure patients that mercury remains bonded within the filling. Worse, they continue to give amalgam fillings to pregnant and breastfeeding mothers.

- Mercury is transformed into highly toxic methyl mercury by the bacteria in our intestines. There is no "harmless" mercury.

- Chewing gum, or taking hot drinks, dramatically increases the rate that amalgam fillings in the mouth release their mercury. This is a good reason to rethink the gum habit, and to begin drinking cooler beverages.

- Contamination from amalgam fillings in one's teeth is much higher than contamination from the environment or from eating fish; nonetheless, it is wise to avoid all sources of mercury, especially during pregnancy, when the baby is most vulnerable.

- There is an ongoing debate as to the influence of mercury on the increasing number of children who are autistic, have neurological issues, or learning/concentration disorders. Many mothers of autistic children say that their children were normal but regressed after being exposed to a vaccination that contained mercury. The reaction may have been to other substances in the vaccination, as well.

- Cautionary measures: Before you have a Rhogam injection during pregnancy (contains mercury in the US), or decide to vaccinate your children (children have over 30 'shots' before the age of five, all of which contain mercury), and before you use an anti-fungal spray in your home or garden that contains mercury, inform yourself as to the pros and cons, as well as the alternatives.

A study from 1994 in Colorado showed that women who have amalgam fillings are at significantly greater risk for anxiety, indecision, uncontrolled anger, and depression than women who have no amalgam fillings. The researchers say that mercury may produce these symptoms by affecting neurotransmitters in the brain[47].

Detoxify Through Diet

Because various health problems are increasing in the US, it is wise to incorporate foods into our everyday diet that support gentle detoxification. The following methods are safe to use while pregnant and breastfeeding.

- Essential fatty acids and healthy fats and oil support the immune system and reduce inflammation throughout the body. (See *Get your Fats Right.*)

- Half a lemon squeezed into a cup of boiled water helps the kidney detoxify the blood, according to Traditional Chinese Medicine. Take once a day.

- In India, boiled water is sipped throughout the day to detoxify the digestive system. Mothers, following this advice, have reported feeling more energy.

- Carrot juice is a blood purifier. Its beta-carotene supports the liver. Fresh-pressed is best, one cup a day, in the late morning. Add 1/4 teaspoon of flaxseed oil, olive oil, or cream to the juice so that the fat-soluble vitamins can be absorbed. Swish the juice around in your mouth and mix with saliva before swallowing to make the juice more digestible. Beet juice is also used to clean the blood, and is helpful in preventing cancer. Carrot and beet juice have a lactogenic effect on some women.

- *Green juices* are recommended to improve vitality and stamina as well as for their detoxifying effects. They also have a lactogenic effect. *Green drinks* come in powder form or as supplements. (For recipes and more information, see pages 194-198.)

- The late, renowned physician, Henry Bieler, suggested taking a green soup comprised of zucchini, green beans, celery, and parsley to support the liver and adrenal glands with specific salts and minerals in these vegetables. This soup is an alternative if a mother cannot digest freshly pressed vegetable juice well.

- Dr. Dietrich Klinghardt, an expert in heavy metal toxicity, recommends sauerkraut, taken throughout the day, to detoxify the intestine of mercury. This is a safe way to reduce the levels of mercury available to pass into breastmilk. Sauerkraut, if truly fermented (available in health-food stores) can also help build up healthy intestinal flora and improve digestion.

- Foods high in fiber. Fiber attaches to toxins and excess estrogen in the intestine and bloodstream, enabling them to be transferred out of the body. Fibrous foods include whole grains (whole grain breads and crackers), legumes, nuts, seeds, and most fruit and vegetables.
- Nettle tea: the soluble fiber enters the bloodstream, where it attaches to toxins and helps transfer them out of the body. Nettle also activates and strengthens the kidneys.
- Condiments such as garlic, onions, and ginger are anti-bacterial, anti-viral, and anti-fungal. Cinnamon and coconut oil are anti-fungal. Ginger expands the blood vessels and capillaries so that our tissues are better nourished and toxins can be flushed out. Use these condiments and spices often in your meals.
- In China, mothers take one bowl of specially prepared chicken soup, once a week, to help support the detoxifying action of their body. Researchers have discovered that chicken soup has potent anti-inflammatory properties. See pages 175-176 for a recipe.

Detox Warning

Try to avoid doing what is called a *major detox* while breastfeeding or pregnant. This includes fasting, taking more than one or two cups of freshly pressed juice or green-drinks per day, losing weight too quickly (one pound per week is considered a safe weightloss for a breastfeeding mother), or using strong, detoxifying herbs, including **cilantro** (see below) or high dosages of **chlorella** (see page 269).

When a mother *detoxes*, toxins flood out into the bloodstream where they can cross over the placenta during pregnancy or enter a breastfeeding mother's milk. In pregnancy, this can impede the baby's development. In breastfeeding, this may result in the baby becoming fussy, or coming down with a stuffy nose. Normal-term babies are usually robust and can deal with a temporary increase in toxins, but there is no reason to put a baby to the test!

Cilantro, a leafy vegetable from India that has become popular in the US, contains substances that open the barrier between the bloodstream and the brain. Indeed, cilantro is employed by doctors of natural medicine to help extract heavy metal from the brain. Taken inappropriately, however, cilantro could enable toxins, bacteria, and viruses to invade brain tissue[*]. Because we do not know if cilantro's property is transferred to the baby, it is wise not to take cilantro during pregnancy or while breastfeeding.

Careful – Herbs for the Liver

Liver-herbs have a healthful effect on the mother and *most* babies. Liver-herbs help a so-called *fatty liver* to heal, (women tend to develop fatty liver during pregnancy). In the process, the liver releases its stored fat—and fat-soluble toxins—into the bloodstream, and milk. While these levels are negligible for most babies, *premature babies, or babies with health issues,* might be affected by these toxins. Should your baby have had a premature birth, or have health issues, you may wish to avoid taking these herbs at full dosage.

Lactogenic liver herbs: blessed thistle, milk thistle, dandelion root.

Baby's Jaundice

Yarrow is a very gentle liver herb. 1 cup a day is recommended to mothers whose baby has jaundice. The herb is said to help the baby's liver pick up its work. Yarrow may reduce milk supply in sensitive mothers.

Detoxing Fat-Soluble Toxins

Experts in natural medicine are experimenting to find ways to draw fat-soluble toxins out of the body. An olive or sesame oil massage before bathing or showering, footbaths using a water and vinegar solution, and gargling with sunflower oil, are some of these.

See articles at www.mother-food.com for a description of these methods.

---

[*] Cellular phones and cordless phones may also weaken the barrier between the bloodstream and the brain. This would allow toxins, bacteria, and viruses to enter the brain. There they can lead to inflammation, degenerative neural diseases, and some experts believe to cancer. To be on the safe side, these phones should not be used in the proximity of infants, **nor should central home stations** be located near rooms where children spend a lot of time.

CHAPTER FIVE

Caring For Colic

Colic is a catch-all word. Babies who are upset or screaming at the breast, who are distraught, incessantly crying, or always fussy, and especially babies who pull their legs to their stomach and kick them away, who are gassy and clearly uncomfortable or suffering, are all said to have colic—though these symptoms can mean many things, and respond to many treatments, as we shall explore in this chapter.

Foremost Prevention: feed only colostrum and breastmilk

There are two main causes for extreme and severe colic, according to Maureen Minchin, a breastfeeding specialist from Australia and author of *Food for Thought*. One is the introduction of cow's milk based formula soon after birth. The other is the pre-sensitization of the baby within the mother's womb to foods in the mother's diet.

Indeed, colostrum and breastmilk are the best preventative for allergy and colic, providing the baby's intestine with protective factors. Other fluids introduce non-human proteins, microbes, and starches before a baby's intestine is ready to handle them. This interferes in the optimal development of her intestinal flora, and may sensitize her for food allergy or sensitivities.

Lactation specialists in the US frequently suggest that mothers bring a package of *extensively hydrolyzed* hypoallergenic formula to the hospital, in case it is necessary to supplement-feed while the mother builds her supply. In Europe, lactation experts do not recommend hypoallergenic formula in this instance as it still contains allergenic components. Practical-thinking lactation consultants in the US have found that "Good Start" (formula made by Nestle, formerly by Carnation), is tolerated well by most newborns.

⇨ The first rule of mothering is always: "feed the baby."

Food Avoidance: Broccoli, Lentils and Onions

Most mothers have heard that any food that causes digestive problems in herself, such as flatulence, or allergy, can cause her baby to have problems as well. This isn't always true, but it's often true, so that it may be on the safe side, at least in the early days and weeks after birth (until you get a feeling for your baby's digestive stability) to avoid foods that are difficult for many adults to digest. Avoiding or limiting these foods during a baby's first month of life may help prevent colic and fussiness, especially if these foods affect the mother negatively.

> Cruciferous veggies: cauliflower, broccoli, cabbage, Brussels sprouts
> Legumes: beans and lentils
> Condiments: onions and garlic

Current wisdom in the lactation community is for mothers to freely eat all foods until a baby's behavior signals that something is amiss. In my opinion, this may allow a cycle of digestive distress to develop in the baby that wouldn't have been necessary. Clearly, "to eat or not to eat" is a question that every mother has to answer for herself.

After experiencing colic and constant screaming with my first baby I avoided all foods or food combinations that I knew caused me problems. My later babies were happy and calm, except when I took my problem foods: then they began to cry inconsolably, as my first baby had done.

Too Much Sugar, Not Enough Cream

When a baby appears to have colic, the problem may be related to an overdose of *foremilk,* the extra-sweet milk that flows at the start of a feed. Foremilk contains natural sugars, vitamins, proteins, minerals, and water, but it does not contain much fat. *Hindmilk*, the milk that flows later in a feed, is rich in fat. Hindmilk satisfies the baby's hunger. Just as eating too many sweets can cause an adult to have a stomachache, babies feel unwell if sugar is their main meal. Not only will a "foremilk-baby" be fussy, but she will soon be hungry again as she is missing the high-calorie content of the fattier hindmilk. These babies are caught in a vicious cycle of hunger and pain, wanting to be fed often even while clearly suffering.

In this situation, a mother may try nursing on only one side until that breast is completely emptied, and only then switching to the other breast. Use breast-gland massage and breast compression to ensure that milk is flowing, and inhale deeply through the nose (see pages 8-9). Only when the breast is emptied and only if the baby is clearly still hungry should the mother change breasts at one feeding.

⇨ Babies may require considerable time to remove the thicker, creamier milk from the breast. Changing breasts *by the clock, before the baby has completely emptied the breast,* can exacerbate foremilk-colic.

Mothers with an **overactive milk-ejection reflex** (OMR) may see colic in their babies for the same "sweet" reason: his stomach may be filled by the thinner, sweeter milk of his mother's powerful let-down. Expressing milk before breastfeeding can bring resolution. Pump or hand-express to stimulate the initial powerful milk-ejection reflex. Allow the milk to flow into a container or towel. Now your baby has a better chance of getting a creamier meal.

*If a mother is eating a **low-fat diet**, her milk may be low-fat as well, and this can also lead to symptoms of colic.* She should increase the healthy fats in her diet by taking flaxseed oil, fish oil, olive oil and butter (see page 47). This will lead to creamier milk, and may resolve her baby's fussiness without further changes to her diet.

⇨ A visit with an IBCLC can help identify whether a baby is suckling well and emptying the breast appropriately.

Sugar and Caffeine: Frequent Culprits

If a baby's fussiness or crying continues after the above measures, the mother may try eliminating sugar from her diet and reducing or avoiding beverages that contain caffeine. Sugar (even in small amounts) and caffeine, are not uncommon culprits behind a baby's fussiness and colic. Because they are relatively easy to eliminate from a mother's diet, they can go first, to test whether these are in fact the triggers. A mother will have to avoid all foods that contain refined or natural sugar such as white sugar, maple syrup, honey, cane sugar, molasses, malt, corn syrup, fruit, and dried fruit. *Sugar* is found in surprising places, such as in catsup, soy sauce, and salad dressing. Unfortunately, it is also found in chocolate. (Do not take artificial sugar substitutes.) *Caffeine* is found in coffee, black and green teas, mate tea, in most soft drinks, and in chocolate.

If sugar or caffeine is the culprit, you will probably see your baby's colic improve very soon after omitting these foods—perhaps immediately. At the latest, your baby will be happier within a few days. You can then try to re-introduce these foods to your diet in small amounts. It is wise to wait a week or two if a very young baby is involved. You may find that taking small amounts of your favorite sugar or caffeine food with a large meal, rather than alone as a snack, is easier for your baby to tolerate.

Caffeine, PMS, Breast-Refusal and Recurrent Mastitis

Maureen Minchin, in *Breastfeeding Matters*, writes that some mothers see a cluster of symptoms before menstruation, including recurrent mastitis, that are exacerbated by caffeine. By eliminating caffeine from their diets, these mothers have fewer PMS symptoms, and fewer fibrocystic breast changes. Their babies no longer appear to dislike their breastmilk and they no longer have colic.

Sugar, Starch and Fat

The combination of sugar, starch, and fat is known to be difficult to digest—and it may cause colic. For more information, see *Indigestion after Breakfast and a Baby's Colic*, on page 207.

Exercise and Lactic Acid

Another potential cause of fussiness is lactic acid—a chemical produced during extremely strenuous exercise. Lactic acid can make breastmilk taste sour or bitter. Occasionally, a baby will become fussy or refuse to take the breast after a mother exercises. A very young infant may be more sensitive than an older baby.

Dr. R. Laurence, author of *Breastfeeding—A Guide for the Medical Profession*, advises mothers to shower or wash their breasts after exercise to remove salty perspiration; to pump or hand express a small amount of breastmilk, and discard it; and, if her baby still does not want the breast, to give him milk that she has previously expressed.

GERD

Some babies who appear to have colic actually have gastroesophageal reflux disease (GERD). In this disease, acidic stomach contents regurgitate, or back up (reflux) into the esophagus, (the tube between the stomach and the mouth) causing inflammation and pain (heartburn). When a baby has GERD, she may spit up or vomit large amounts of milk several times a day and have other signs of distress, such as pulling off the breast frequently and arching backward.

Babies with GERD may projectile vomit, spit up, arch their backs, and seem uncomfortable on the breast. Babies with GERD probably feel more comfortable nursing with their bottom well below the level of their head.

GERD causes some babies to drink less milk, and occasionally to refuse the breast altogether. When babies reduce their milk intake, this causes low milk supply in the mother.

Some babies suffer silently from this condition, with no overt symptoms to alert the mother. These babies typically always want to suckle while seeming to remain hungry. They may be upset away from the breast, but once on the breast, the mother notices that the baby doesn't really drink. Sometimes the mother thinks the baby doesn't like her milk—the baby may make a disgusted expression and push the breast away, but then return to the breast for emotional comfort.

GERD can be triggered by something that the mother is eating. While many mothers see improvement in their baby's GERD when they discover the problem food and take appropriate measures (see Chapter Four), other mothers find that these measures do not help their baby's GERD.

- Medication for GERD is available and mothers should not hesitate to request treatment. Not all doctors will prescribe medication unless a baby is losing weight, unfortunately.

- Lactation consultants have observed that when a mother uses domperidone to increase her supply, a baby's symptoms of GERD frequently become milder. This is interesting because the primary effect of domperidone is to improve the *mother's* digestion—showing how closely connected a mother's digestion and her baby's digestive issues can be.

- The same effect may be seen when a mother follows the measures in the last chapter on pages 61-68, to improve her digestive health.
- An excellent online support group can be found at: http://health.groups.yahoo.com/group/breastfeedingreflux

Identify Your Baby's Problem-Foods

Colic is usually caused by a food sensitivity or allergy. The question is—sensitive to which food? It is possible to answer this question during pregnancy. This is described in Chapter Four under *Pregnancy: Prevent Food Sensitivity in Your Baby*, on pages 72-74.

To discover your baby's problem foods while breastfeeding, try the journal-method described on page 69. Record the time of day, what you eat and drink, and your exposure to chemical substances such as furniture polish, gasoline, industrial chemicals, glue, powerful cleansing substances, perfume, and the chemical odors in clothing or furniture stores. In a second journal record your baby's stools, (the color, consistency, and smell of the stool), and your baby's behavior, such as when he begins to cry or show signs of discomfort, or when he has a red ring on his bottom, a red earlobe, insomnia, or other symptoms described on page 74. By carefully comparing the two journals, you will probably see connections that were not obvious before.

Usually, a breastfed baby will react within four hours after breastfeeding or being exposed to a chemical, but *occasionally it may take a day or longer to see a reaction.*

⇨ Babies are frequently sensitive to the foods their mothers eat a lot of, especially foods that we craved and overate during pregnancy. Indeed, eating a varied diet during pregnancy is the first basic step in preventing food sensitivities and allergies in a baby.

⇨ Remember, if your baby is showing complex behavior and possible allergic symptoms, consult a doctor of environmental medicine or a pediatric allergist.

Dairy and Wheat

If you are not able to keep a journal to detect your baby's unique sensitivities to food, you may try eliminating those foods most commonly linked to colic, foremost dairy, followed by egg, wheat, soy, corn, and peanut. Dairy includes all cow's milk, cream, ice cream, butter, yogurt, cheese, and *casein* or *lactose* as an ingredient in packaged foods. (Infants and children who are sensitive to dairy are sometimes also sensitive to beef and cow-based products such as gelatin.) For more information on dairy, see pages 138-142.

If the mother sees no improvement after eliminating dairy for 3-4 weeks, she should pay attention to her baby's reaction to her diet and eliminate what she believes is the most likely trigger from the above list. If these foods do not seem to be the problem, see page 69 for a list of common foods that trigger sensitivity or allergy, and remember this clue: we can be allergic to any food, and it is usually the foods the mother craved and ate the most of during pregnancy that the baby cannot tolerate.

Wheat contains high levels of gluten, a gluey protein that is difficult to digest. Rarely, it is necessary to eliminate all foods that contain gluten. For more information on gluten, see page 137.

⇨ Major dietary changes should be overseen by your healthcare provider.

Calming a Baby

It has been documented that babies who receive lots of holding and carrying from day one—even when they aren't crying or hungry—are less likely to develop fussiness and colic. This hints at the importance of physical contact, and of good bonding with primary caretakers, for the healthy development of the digestive and the immune systems. That's good news, though it comes too late for many first-time parents of colicky babies.

Fortunately, there are countless ways that mothers and fathers can help ease their baby's discomfort. Ask your LLL-leader or experienced mother or healthcare provider for suggestions, or read up on these techniques in baby-books. These methods include special holding positions, burping tricks, baby massage, music, dance, stories, and songs (try singing both soft and loudly). Breathing deeply, and concentrating on being calm within oneself, can also help your baby relax: he feels that somewhere out there, beyond his pain, is a source of balance and wholeness: it is you.

⇨ Before trying any of the below, look at the dietary approach described in Chapter Four. Treating a baby's colic is a learning process, leading to insights into a mother's digestive health and other health issues.

- A mother can give her colicky baby one teaspoon of a very lightly steeped tea before breastfeeding. Try fennel, anise, or dill seed tea. It should be lukewarm, or just slightly above room temperature.
- Doctors may prescribe lactobacilli for a colicky baby. Commercial products specifically for infants are available. Digestive enzymes should only be given to babies under the direction of a doctor.
- Some mothers swear by "gripe-water", made of oil extractions from digestive herbs. A mother may try taking gripe water herself first; sometimes this helps her baby. If you do give gripe water to an infant, carefully follow the dosage directions on the package.

⇨ Some babies will not be calmed. Then there is nothing to do but hold him, breathe deeply, and wait out the spell of distress. Earplugs may also help. *Don't leave your baby alone!*

Earplugs to Protect Yourself and Your Baby

Babies who suffer from pain have a different scream from those who cry because they are hungry. A baby in pain has a piercing overtone to his scream that jangles and frazzles his parent's nerves— no matter how much they love their baby. This high-pitched scream can bring parents close to shaking the baby (fatally dangerous), or to putting the baby in his crib and closing the door (also dangerous—for his emotional and mental development). Indeed, babies who have colic and who scream a lot are abused more than babies who do not.

If you feel as though your baby is driving you out of your mind with his screaming, you can resort to *earplugs*. If you have no earplugs, crumple up a largish piece of napkin or toilet paper and stuff it into your ears (it should be large enough to extract easily). Next day, buy the best ear-plugs you can afford. You'll be amazed at how much better you feel. Be kind to yourself and protect your nerves while holding and comforting your suffering baby. He won't be offended.

Colic and Possible Developmental Problems

Not all babies who have colic go on to have developmental issues, though children with developmental problems usually have colic as a baby. It is therefore a sign to be taken seriously.

One proactive thing you can do is to become aware of experiences in your home that the baby cannot *assemble* and integrate. For instance: noise. Babies want to connect the sounds they hear to things going on in their environment: a mother's voice indicates that she is near; a meow means a cat, and so on. With noise from television, however, it is impossible for a baby to connect what he hears to people and things in his world. The same pertains to radio[*].

A sensitive baby who is finding it difficult to figure out his world may become worked up, overly alert, nervous, introverted, or colicky if there are too many sounds or other kinds of information around him that he can't figure out. His developing brain may be impressed by confusion and helplessness regarding the process of learning.

Here are a few recommendations to avoid over-stimulating and falsely stimulating a potentially sensitive baby. (I would follow these measures for all babies, but especially boys, as they are more prone to have developmental difficulties.)

- Protect his eyes. Take out strong light bulbs and replace them with moderate bulbs throughout the house.
- Protect his skin. Do not use woolen, scratchy or synthetic materials on your baby's skin. Use ultra-soft pure cotton underclothing, socks and pajamas.
- Protect his nose. Do not use perfumed baby creams and powders, or strongly scented cosmetics, aromatherapy, cleaning detergents, etc., in the home.
- Protect his ears. If you watch TV or listen to radio with your baby on your lap, do so with ear-phones on, and turn his face away so that he doesn't see the TV. Hum melodies at the same time so that he hears you and feels close to you.

---

[*] A study from 2004 on twins, by Stephen Petrill and colleagues at Pennsylvania State University, showed that children whose homes are the most disorganised and noisy have lower IQs and more learning problems. *Intelligence* (DOI: 10.1016/j.intell.2004.06.010

- Provide emotional protection. Be there for your baby; respond quickly to his cues, so that his brain doesn't experience the stress of unanswered signals.
- Provide 'layers.' Your very new baby recently was within your womb, deep within your body. Now he is out in the open. Providing layers promotes a feeling of familiarity and comfort. Wrap your baby loosely in a small cotton blanket while you carry him throughout the house. Let the corner of the blanket form a hood over his head. In most cases, a very young baby finds this tremendously relaxing—even while nursing[*].
- You may also provide some comfort to yourself by nursing in bed under covers, or by wrapping yourself and your baby in a blanket or sheet while nursing.
- For early diagnosis of a baby's developmental issues, contact an occupational therapist with experience with infants and training in sensory integration.

Colic and the Decision to Breastfeed

Mothers whose babies scream for hours on end, or who seem to dislike their breastmilk, may be tempted to stop breastfeeding. However, not all babies do well on formula. Sensitive babies can become sensitive to formula with time, as formula is based on foods that are highly allergenic.

Even babies who apparently do better on formula may be missing a unique opportunity. Breastfeeding mothers are usually able to discover their baby's problem-foods. By avoiding these foods, their breastmilk will provide their baby with perfect, non-allergenic nourishment. Long, exclusive breastfeeding gives the baby's intestine time to heal, and gives him time for his immune system to mature.

When the mother introduces solids to her baby, the baby's problem foods will be the ones she introduces last[†]. By avoiding these foods until her baby is at least a year old, her baby will have a chance to

---

[*] Tight wrapping should only be done under the direction of an occupational therapist. Loosely wrapping a baby in a cotton blanket is sufficient to calm most babies. The sooner comforting measures of this kind are taken after birth, the more preventative it can be of colic and nervousness.

[†] Consult your doctor for the latest recommendations regarding the introduction of sensitive foods.

outgrow his sensitivities. This way, a breastfeeding mother may prevent, avoid, or minimize long-term food sensitivities and allergies that might otherwise develop into health and cognitive issues later in life[*].

- Infant allergies that appear to go away often mask themselves, reappearing as behavioral and learning problems later on. Sticking to breastmilk may ameliorate the allergy at its root.

- An allergy to breastmilk is extremely rare. Doctors who diagnose breastmilk allergy often do so because they are at the end of their wisdom—health professionals learn very little about food allergies and breastfeeding in their basic education.

- Check out the section, *Get your Fats Right* and subsequent sections in Chapter Three, to see how the fats we mothers eat can help our baby's immune system to overcome allergies. Read *Leaky Gut* and subsequent sections in Chapter Four to learn about improving digestive health. Remember: good digestive health can help a mother's body make milk that is easier for her baby to digest.

- For mothers of allergic infants who decide to change to formula, the pediatric allergist and author, Dr. Doris Rapp, suggests rotating formulas every day that are based on different foods, to avoid sensitizing the baby to any one food. (For instance, formula based on: wheat, corn, soy, and modified bovine milk[†].) Talk to your pediatric allergist about your options.

---

[*] I am looking forward to the study that will reveal the true influence of breastmilk on allergies in allergy-prone families—using mothers who eliminate trans-fats from their diets, who enrich their milk with healthy fats, who treat their digestion with digestive herbs, lactobacilli and digestive enzymes, and who use astragalus to enhance their production of the immunoglobulin IgA. In other words—studies done with mothers whose milk resembles the milk of mothers from the pre-industrial world—where allergies and colic are almost unknown.

[†] Order Dr. Doris Rapp's audiotape "Infant Food Allergies" from the following number: (716) 875-5578. This audio-tape contains information for both breastfed and formula-fed allergic babies.

CHAPTER SIX

Keep Your Health the Best It Can Be

This chapter addresses postpartum depression, thyroid problems, and blood sugar issues.

Postpartum Illness and Depression

Katharina Dalton, a British medical doctor, once suffered from a severe case of the premenstrual syndrome. She became the first medical person to explore women's hormonal ailments in the 1950s. Today, decades later, her discoveries and recommendations are still highly regarded and widely implemented.

Dalton invented the phrase *postpartum illness* to denote the range of physical, mental, and emotional unwellness that mothers may experience the year after birth—from the third-day blues, to muddle-mindedness, irritability, anxiety, exhaustion, depression (PPD), and even the rare form of psychosis that about one in five hundred women experience within the first two weeks after birth.

Although much has been written about postpartum depression, it is important to go into it here briefly because medical treatment for postpartum depression can impair milk supply—and dietary habits can help prevent or minimize postpartum exhaustion and depression.

In England, mothers with postpartum depression are treated with natural progesterone at Dr. Dalton's suggestion; in the US, doctors frequently treat with estrogen. Both hormones can impair milk supply in vulnerable women—though estrogen will impair supply in almost every woman.

Several antidepressants are considered to be safe for breastfeeding mothers and their babies. Prozac is controversial because it commonly causes fussiness and insomnia in babies. Zoloft and Paxil have a good reputation and are usually well tolerated. Wellbutrin anecdotally can impair milk supply and therefore should be taken cautiously. The herbal antidepressant, St. John's Wort, has not yet been approved for breastfeeding mothers due to lack of studies, though some well-known herbalists do treat mothers with St. John's Wort.

Postpartum depression can gradually develop out of postpartum exhaustion. A mother may hardly notice that she has slipped from feeling bone-tired to being irritable, anxious, crying all the time, depressed, or even suicidal. *If you ever feel that you might harm yourself or your baby, don't wait—seek medical help immediately.*

If you are suffering from depression, do not hesitate to take antidepressants if necessary. I would like to mention though that I have seen mothers who were ready to take antidepressants, but whose depression turned around when they received concrete help for their breastfeeding problems. Abrupt weaning, on the other hand, can trigger hormonal imbalances, and cause emotional grief. Both of these factors are likely to intensify depression. Sometimes, just having a good talk with a lactation consultant and developing a strategy for breastfeeding is enough to lift a mother's spirits. She again feels in control of her life. Half the battle is won.

PPD and PMS

Katharina Dalton observed that postpartum depression frequently develops out of postpartum exhaustion. She was the first to note that both postpartum exhaustion and depression have *symptoms in common with the premenstrual syndrome* (PMS), i.e., that these illnesses share a common underlying hormonal imbalance. Her next discovery was that women who suffer from extreme exhaustion or depression in the year after birth are at high risk to develop maternal PMS, *in which postpartum symptoms reappear the week or two before menstruation.*

Usually, maternal PMS is self-limiting, meaning that the mother recovers without treatment. PMS can however become chronic, severe, and debilitating. At worst, symptoms become what are called 'pervasive,' meaning that they are no longer restricted to the premenstrual phase.

One of Katharina Dalton's most valuable contributions, in my opinion, was her discovery that dietary measures can greatly ease the symptoms of these illnesses. I have based this section on her premises about diet in the postpartum.

⇨ Take postpartum illness seriously. Learn life-style changes to help prevent it from developing, from becoming worse if you have it, and from becoming a severe form of PMS.

A Support Net – Our First Line of Defense

The emotional vulnerability of the new mother (after each birth, we are always again a new mother) cannot be described in words. Tactless or thoughtless remarks made by people around us, (including doctors and nurses), or unexplained behavior in our baby, can throw us into a morass of self-doubt and anxiety. This is why it is so important to have a network of other mothers who have *been there* and survived, and who can provide unflinching support.

In any group you join, however, there are bound to be mothers who believe that "every woman can nurse" and that breastfeeding failure is always a mother's fault. Do not let these women intimidate you, or deny you the support group you need[1]!

One of the most accessible sources for support is mothers' meetings organized by La Leche League (LLL). You can join these meetings when you are still pregnant. If the mothers there look blissful with their infants at their breasts, you can be sure that many had to travel a hard road to arrive at their bliss. Feel free to ask

---

[1] In my opinion, these groups should also be open for formula-feeding mothers who are working through their grief of not having been able to breastfeed, and who wish to belong to the breastfeeding community and profit from the atmosphere of attachment parenting.

questions, to make friends, and to take telephone numbers so that a familiar voice is near at hand when you need it most. The women who organize these groups, LLL-Leaders, have a wide range of experience and knowledge. They offer support by telephone as well. Have the telephone numbers of a few LLL-Leaders at hand, in case one leader is busy when you need help.

LLL-Leaders can assist mothers most of the time, but it is sometimes necessary to refer a mother to an *International Board Certified Lactation Consultant* (IBCLC), who has the equivalent of a master's degree in the science of breastfeeding support. It is of course possible that the IBCLC in your area may not be available when you need her most. Hopefully, your LLL-Leader will recommend other competent lactation experts, or help you find the information that you need.

LLL-Leaders should also be able to refer you to a local pediatrician who is knowledgeable and supportive of breastfeeding. Many pediatricians understand the benefits of breastfeeding, and they support breastfeeding, but unfortunately are not educated on the maternal side. Pediatricians without much experience in this area can unknowingly give mothers advice that is ultimately harmful to the breastfeeding relationship.

It is likely that your LLL-Leader will also know about local milk banks and pump rentals and about resources for babies who need additional help, such as cranio-sacral therapists, osteopaths, occupational therapists, and chiropractors who have experience treating infants. These therapies often help babies who are lethargic, uncomfortable (in pain), fussy, or who have a weak suck or other suck issue.

Truly, having a community of breastfeeding mothers, the support of an LLL-Leader, a breastfeeding-friendly doctor, and an IBCLC, can mean the difference between a mother maintaining her self-confidence, optimism, and zest for motherhood, or her succumbing to a feeling of it all being too much to bear—especially during the early weeks when so much is new and, for many mothers, very difficult.

Common Health Problems in the Postpartum

Dr. Katharina Dalton writes that four common health problems contribute to postpartum illness: anemia, low levels of potassium, low blood sugar and low thyroid function. These can lead to exhaustion, irritability, and depression. The good news is that these problems can be countered by simple dietary measures.

Anemia

Low iron levels during pregnancy and blood loss during birth contribute to postpartum fatigue, exhaustion, depression, and low milk supply. Because anemia impairs the mother's mood and lowers her energy, it has been observed to impede bonding with her baby.

The importance of increasing a mother's iron levels during pregnancy and after birth cannot be stressed enough. The lactogenic, iron-rich herb stinging nettle is traditionally given to alleviate anemia. Dong quai, a potent blood-tonic is taken in China after birth by mothers who experience blood loss. It is said to build blood, prevent depression, and support milk supply.

Foods that provide iron include prunes, pears, black cherries, blackstrap molasses, dark greens, beet root, beet juice, dried beans, red meat, organ meats, poultry, miso, nuts and seeds. Persistent iron deficiency anemia can be treated with Floridex with iron, available at healthfood stores. Floridex usually brings quick results, without the constipation associated with iron supplements.

Lack of Potassium

The exhaustion mothers feel after birth may be linked to depletion of potassium. Foods rich in potassium that probably won't contribute to a baby's colic include bananas, potatoes and dark green leafy vegetables.

Low Blood Sugar (reactive hypoglycemia)

Low blood sugar may occur after eating a refined carbohydrate such as pasta, potato, juice, white flour or sugar that the body can speedily digest and use as energy. These foods lead to a *sugar high* that feels good emotionally, but is potentially lethal to the body.

In response to the excess sugar, the pancreas releases insulin, a hormone that orders the body to remove sugar from the bloodstream. When, in this situation, a *lot* of sugar is *suddenly* removed from the bloodstream, we speak of having low blood sugar in response to what one eats, also called *reactive hypoglycemia.*

Everyone has phases of low blood sugar, but not everyone *suffers* from it. Women who are premenstrual, and mothers in the postpartum, tend to be ultra-sensitive to low blood sugar. Symptoms include irritability, mood swings, and exhaustion.

Sensitivity to low blood sugar tends to go hand in hand with cravings for sugar and caffeine. When our energy is gone, we lunge at that cup of coffee, or at that piece of chocolate cake. The bad news is that sugar and caffeine exacerbate the problem: now the mother suffers from sugar highs and lows the whole day long, as well as accompanying mood swings.

Reactive hypoglycemia is fairly easy to overcome. The solution is to avoid or greatly limit refined carbohydrates (white flour and sugar) and sometimes also high glycemic foods, (potatoes, pasta, pizza) and also stimulants such as coffee and chocolate. Eat a complex, unrefined carbohydrate, plus a protein, every 2 to 3 hours. Examples include whole grain bread or crackers, oatmeal, an apple, or a handful of nuts. Avoid concentrated sources of sugar. Be sure to add protein to each meal or snack, such as nut-butter, sunflower seeds, tofu, egg, meat, cheese, goat's cheese, or unsweetened, probiotic yogurt.

A few progressive doctors and psychiatrists now treat their patients by teaching them how to avoid low blood sugar. Panic attacks, irritability, emotional over-reacting, and even mental illness may improve when people learn how to keep their blood sugar stable.

- Prevention is the best way to avoid blood sugar swings. Eat by the clock, before you are hungry, and before you feel a drop in your energy.

- For suggestions on balancing *insulin resistance*, a common complication in hypoglycemia, see pages 104-105.

- For suggestions on overcoming sugar and caffeine addictions, see pages 111-117.

More About Sugar: Craving Sweet Food in the Postpartum

Women after birth tend to crave sweet food. Milk production removes sugar from the blood, which we need to replenish. Traditional systems of medicine from India and China say that naturally sweet food is particularly lactogenic and healthful for mothers. These foods include: grains, legumes, coconut, almonds, sesame seeds, apricots, dates, figs, as well as sweet potato, fennel, lettuce, carrots, and beet root.

Because most of us are used to the extreme sugary taste of cookies and candy, we may not be able to savor the more subtle sweetness of these foods. Our taste buds can become more sensitive if we eat fewer foods containing white sugar. With time, anyone can learn to appreciate the subtly sweet taste of natural foods.

For mothers with a sweet tooth: you do not have to stop eating your favorite desserts altogether if you are not ready to give them up. Here is the trick: by eating your sweets along with a meal or snack that contains a good portion of protein, the sugar will have less of a negative effect on your blood sugar level.

- If you crave sugar, be careful that your intake of sweet food does not lure you into a hypoglycemic cycle (see above).
- White sugar robs the body of minerals. You need your minerals, both for your health and for your milk production.
- See "Sweets" and "Snacks" in *Recipes* for naturally sweet foods that satisfy a sweet tooth.
- Remember: sugar, starches, and caffeine do not support your physical and emotional health. Just the opposite: they can lead to a mother feeling irritable, exhausted, and depressed. (The same is true for foods containing artificial sweeteners.)

More About Sugar: Sugar and Colic

As if to complicate matters still more, many babies respond to sugar in the mother's diet—even small amounts, and even to natural sugars—with crying, fussiness, or colic. Fortunately, if sugar is the problem, your baby will show discomfort within a very short time, probably one to four hours after you ingest a sugary food, so that it's relatively easy to tell if sugar was the cause.

Because many babies are sugar sensitive, it may be wise to wait four weeks before using large amounts of natural sweeteners in your drinks or on your cereal, such as honey, molasses, or malt syrup (not to mention your favorite white-sugar desserts). Start with one-quarter teaspoon a day and increase the amount, keeping an eye on your baby to see how she deals with the increase of natural sugar in your diet.

Some babies may do well with one kind of sugar (say, maple syrup), but have a strong reaction to another kind (say, corn syrup, dried fruits, or chocolate). This is something to be mindful of as you experiment with sweet food.

Colic commonly begins sometime during or after a baby's second week of life. If you are careful to avoid colic-causing foods during this sensitive first month, you may save both yourself and your baby a lot of stress later on. (I would be particularly careful if my baby is a boy, as boys tend to have more digestive problems.)

Low Thyroid Function (Hypothyroidism)

It is normal, after giving birth, for a mother's thyroid to require time to pick up its work. It may not function at normal levels for several weeks, leading to dry skin and hair, to hairloss, weightgain, and to fatigue.

Although mild hypothyroidism is common after birth and does *not* affect milk supply, severe hypothyroidism (and also, hy*per*thyroidism) will lead to milk supply problems. One telling sign of hypothyroidism is if you feel cold all the time, even when people in the same room feel warm.

There is a simple test you can perform to see if your thyroid is underfunctioning. Keep a thermometer by your bed. In the morning, before getting up, lie entirely still while taking your temperature for fifteen minutes. Any motion can upset your results. If your temperature remains beneath 97.6 for five consecutive mornings, your thyroid may be underfunctioning. Consult with your doctor. She may wish to test your thyroid levels.

Thyroid related milk supply problems may be resolved when a doctor prescribes thyroid hormone, and the mother builds her supply through pumping, herbs, foods, and by supplementing with a supplemental nursing device if necessary until her milk supply is strong.

The good news is that a mildly underfunctioning thyroid usually kicks in on its own, sometime during the first year after birth. Again: a mildly underfunctioning thyroid will *not* interfere with milk production.

- Iodine is a substance that the body uses to make thyroid hormone. Different geographical areas have different amounts of iodine in the soil, and iodine is commonly added to table salt in areas where it is lacking. The problem is—as in Germany and Switzerland— that too much iodine, found in all foods containing iodized salt and sometimes added to other foods as well, can lead to hyperthyroidism: feeling warm all the time, weightloss, nervousness, insomnia. Be aware of potential problems, and check out your sources of iodine.. (A local naturopath may be able to help you understand the iodine status of the vegetable produce in your area.)

- If you believe you have symptoms of hypo- or hyperthyroidism, you may wish to inform yourself before talking to your doctor, as many patients believe that thyroid tests are not valid as commonly interpreted. A good resource is: Mary Shamon's *Living Well with Hypothyroidism: What Your Doctor Doesn't Tell You... That You Need to Know*.

- Kelp offers an alternative to iodized salt. You can choose not to use table salt, and sprinkle a pinch of kelp onto your meals instead.

- Iodine enters a mother's milk, and becomes concentrated in a baby's body. Therefore, only use minimal amounts of kelp every day.

- According to Dr. and Mrs. Balch's *Prescription for Nutritional Healing*, certain foods affect thyroid function. Those that may suppress thyroid function include: broccoli, Brussels sprouts, cabbage, kale, mustard greens, peaches, pears, radishes, spinach, and turnips. Eat these in moderation if you have symptoms of hypothyroidism. If you have severe symptoms, omit them from your diet.

- Foods that support thyroid function include: apricots, dates, egg yolks, molasses, parsley, potatoes, prunes, raw seeds, and whole grains. Also: chicken, raw milk and cheese.

Dr. Balch and his wife also suggest that people at risk for hypothyroidism filter tap water to extract chlorine, and avoid toothpaste that contains fluoride. Both chemicals are structurally similar to thyroid hormones: they may lock into receptors in the thyroid and prevent thyroid hormones from taking effect.

Insulin Resistance

Many women today suffer from *insulin resistance*, a condition that makes eating normal amounts of carbohydrates tantamount to a weightgain program. Insulin resistance develops when cells resist insulin's signal that it is time to absorb sugar from the bloodstream. When an insulin resistant person eats sugary food, the body has to produce much more insulin than usual to get this signal across. When cells finally do respond, the signal is so strong that they absorb *all* the sugar from the blood, leading to symptoms of low blood sugar, to ravenous hunger, and eventually to weightgain.

Physiological factors, possibly genetic, can play a role in the development of insulin resistance. Hormonal and metabolic imbalances, such as Polycystic Ovarian Syndrome (PCOS) and Metabolic Syndrome X, have insulin resistance as a central component.

Certain lifestyle factors exacerbate insulin resistance, including not getting enough sleep, not getting regular exercise, meal skipping, poor diet, and food allergies or sensitivities even without obvious allergic symptoms.

Overweight persons with insulin resistance frequently resort to high-protein diets, such as the Atkin's diet, that encourage eating large amounts of animal protein and non-starchy vegetables. This kind of diet should not be followed by a pregnant or breastfeeding woman as she will not get enough nutrients. She *will* get an overload of dioxin-like toxins found in high concentrations in meat and dairy. This diet is known to overtax the kidneys and deplete calcium stores, plus a recent study showed that the offspring of pregnant women on this diet tend to have high blood pressure[50].

Insulin resistance plays into low milk supply. Mothers are seeing that taking medication and supplements that improve their insulin resistance leads to an increase in the growth of mammary tissue and to an increase in milk supply.

- Talk to your doctor about medication. Metformin (Glucophage) is showing excellent results in the treatment of insulin resistance. It can be taken while breastfeeding under your doctor's supervision. Metformin frequently leads to an increase of mammary tissue, and to an increase of milk production.

- The herb goat's rue contains chemical substances similar to metformin. Goat's rue also increases mammary tissue and frequently leads to a significant increase in milk production. It can be considered in the treatment of insulin resistance.

- The mineral chromium is important in the metabolism of insulin. Supplementing with chromium can improve insulin resistance and reduce sugar cravings. As of writing this now, one mother is seeing increased milk production while taking chromium.

- Black and green tea appears to positively affect insulin function, and to keep blood sugar levels steady, whereas coffee does not.

- Omega 3 EFAs appear to steady blood sugar levels (flaxseed oil, fish oil).

- Supplementing with zinc, even if there is no zinc deficiency, improves insulin sensitivity.

- Eating raw nuts improves insulin sensitivity and helps prevent type II diabetes.

- Cinnamon has been shown to increase the sensitivity of cells to insulin by up to 20 times in mice. (Cinnamon has other nice effects for lactation as well, such as being anti-fungal.) See pages 269-270 for more information.

- Avocado contains a unique sugar that keeps blood sugar levels steady. (For mothers who have chronic milk supply difficulties avocados are questionable. See page 127 for more information.)

Eat avocado in the morning, rather than the afternoon or evening, so that the fat content does not lead to weightgain.

- Remember to get healthy fats and to supplement with EFAs (see Chapter Three, *Get Your Fats Right*).

- If you emphasize animal protein in your diet, look for organic meat and dairy.

- Green leafy vegetables do not cause an insulin response, so you can indulge in this important, lactogenic food.

- Get into a regular sleep routine—as much as possible. Sleep deprivation contributes to insulin resistance.

- Eat meals and snacks every two to three hours to steady your blood sugar levels and keep your thyroid working optimally.

- Your diet should ideally contain protein at each meal and snack, and also starchy vegetables, whole grains or legumes. Avoid becoming one-sided in your diet.

- If problems persist, see a certified nutritionist.

Diabetes

Women with diabetes will probably see their blood sugar levels helped by breastfeeding. Because breastmilk contains sugar, sugar is constantly being filtered out of the blood into breastmilk. Diabetic mothers frequently go into remission during breastfeeding, and occasionally are healed.

There is a disposition for *breast infection* and *thrush* in diabetic mothers. In fact, chronic breast infection or thrush may be a sign that diabetes is developing.

Two galactagogues, fenugreek seed and goat's rue, are used by herbalists to control blood sugar levels—though fenugreek is thought by some herbalists to be inappropriate for type II diabetes. Women with diabetes should only take these herbs under the guidance of their doctor.

CHAPTER SEVEN

Food Cravings, Food Addictions, and Lactogenic Solutions

Mothers who are trying to improve their diets frequently ask how they can overcome food cravings, especially to soft drinks, sugar, and caffeine. Many also want to know how they can lose weight while learning to eat more healthfully. This chapter offers suggestions.

Focus On the Goal

Hone your attitude. As long as you are giving into a craving, *and feeling bad about it*, you are fighting a losing battle. Focus is all-important. If you think over and over, "I will not eat chocolate, I will not eat chocolate, I will not eat chocolate," you are putting emotional energy into the image of chocolate. This energy can enable the image to grow so strong that at some point, you suddenly feel that you have no choice but to binge on chocolate.

Rather than focusing on what you want to avoid, focus on what you want to achieve: "I want to eat healthy food." Do not tag a negative onto this statement, such as, "I want to eat healthy food, in order to lose weight." Evaluate your motives; reorganize your priorities. You will eventually be able to say, "I want to eat healthy food, for the sake of my health."

We tend to focus on the negative in our culture. We want to lose weight, rather than to gain health. We want to fight a cold, rather than to enhance our immune system. We're always combating the problem of the moment rather than improving the overall situation. In our habitual way, we focus on food that we don't want to eat, and on the weight we want to get rid of, rather than focusing on what we truly need: health, vitality, and the hearty enjoyment of good food.

Cancel the Guilt

As long as you are giving in to cravings, find a way to make it okay. Tell yourself, "I need this right now." Don't whip yourself with guilt. Guilt is the glue that keeps us stuck, so that we can't go forward with what we know is good for us.

"I need this now. I'm still in the grip of cravings and that's okay. In fact, I'll allow myself to really enjoy this, instead of feeling guilty about it."

Become more accepting of your present eating behavior, even as you open up new possibilities to explore what you want for the future. Take zinc supplements if you feel repulsed by the idea of eating fresh food—this is often a sign of zinc insufficiency. Bring home new kinds of food from the market (in this case, food helpful for your milk as well), such as oatmeal, millet flakes, almond butter, extra virgin olive oil, whole-grain crackers and bread, nuts, fruits, and vegetables. Situate them in your kitchen in ways that make them easily accessible and appetizing—a beautiful bowl of fruit, or a basket of nuts, or whatever works for you. You can develop a new approach to eating. This approach does not involve negative body images, guilt, and compulsive behavior. It entails looking at what is good and positive and at what works for you right now.

If you feel entrapped by guilt and negative body image, you may do well to seek the help of a therapist or support group. Medication may also help you emotionally lighten up and let go of negative self-images. Other resources that lend themselves to the postpartum period include Bach Flower Remedies, homeopathic treatment, prayer, yoga, and meditation. To paraphrase Christiane Northrup, author of *Women's Bodies, Women's Wisdom*, it's our self-criticizing voice that puts up a barrier between ourselves and our inner guidance. There's a positive center within each of us that will guide us surely to our goal—but self-criticism and guilt cut us off from that guiding wisdom.

Get Friendly with Fresh Food

It is perfectly natural that depression, stress, force of habit, or an eating disorder can get us to the point where fresh, healthy food seems to come from another planet. While this can be a sign of zinc deficiency, and supplementing with zinc can help, it is a good idea to rethink the role and purpose of fresh food in our lives.

The fact is that for thousands of years, human beings nourished themselves with seeds, nuts, roots, fruits, berries and leaves, plus fish and small animals. *Our bodies and minds are profoundly dependent upon nutrients found only in fresh food.* Nutrients in whole, fresh food feed our nerves, organs, muscles, bones *and* our immune system. They help build blood, keep our mind up to par, and our emotions balanced.

Once you recognize your need for fresh, whole foods, it will be easier to include them, a little more every day, in your menu plans. Concentrate on foods that support milk production, such as oats, rice, millet, almonds, sesame-seed butter, chickpea (hummus), potatoes, peas, green beans, asparagus, carrots, and sweet potato. Remember to include healthy fats in your diet, as well as good sources of protein.

Compromise with Your Cravings

I worked out a deal with myself when I had sugar cravings: I would not eat sweet food in the evening, but would allow myself to have as much as I wanted during morning hours. This enabled me to maintain or lose weight, but most of all it gave me a feeling of being in control.

Although hard at first, I was eventually able to suppress my desire for sweets at night through the promise of something scrumptious in the morning. More and more often, however, I'd wake up in the morning and simply not want the promised treat. Soon I was altogether freed from my sugar addiction.

I first used this trick some twenty-odd years ago, when not yet a mother. I used the same trick to manage my weight after the birth of my first child, when I was twenty-nine. What I am coming to is this: today this trick probably would not work. As we get older, underlying metabolic processes in the body get more out of balance. Today, eating sugary foods in the morning would set me up for a day of mood-swings and irritability. It is no longer an option.

According to Christiane Northrup, a growing number of us become insulin resistant (we gain weight more easily, and are more quickly fatigued) as we grow older. In her audio-book, *Your Diet, Your Health*, she speaks of the blessed 10% who continue to be able to eat whatever they like their whole life long. The rest of us have no choice but to learn how *what* we eat, and *the way that* we eat, can affect our health, weight, mood, and energy levels.

I'd like to recommend this audio-book to mothers with food issues and body-image problems. It explains how the chemistry of the body and the brain are involved in our eating patterns (including chemicals that are involved in milk production: oxytocin and serotonin). According to Northrup, when we eat with relish, and eat in an environment where we feel well, and with people we love, we produce positive-feeling neurochemicals, and we metabolize our food better. This can help us to maintain or lose weight.

The crux of the matter is this: the younger we are, the easier it is to halt an imbalance before it gets worse. Take advantage of pregnancy and the postpartum period as an opportunity to explore how healthy food and satisfying meals can work *for* you, rather than *against* you— for your entire life to come.

Serotonin Foods – Reduce Cravings and Support Milk Supply

Serotonin is the *feel good* neurotransmitter. When serotonin levels in the brain rise, our mood flies. When serotonin goes down, our mood takes a nose dive. When serotonin levels are low, people crave sugar and carbohydrates. Keeping serotonin levels steady is therefore important to overcoming food cravings.

In order to have sufficient serotonin in the brain, we need to eat foods that contain *tryptophan,* the amino acid (protein) that is the precursor for serotonin. Meat, eggs, and dairy contain tryptophan in high amounts. The following vegetables, nuts, seeds, legumes, and grains contain tryptophan as well. These are listed in order from highest to lowest in content of tryptophan.

Foods Containing Tryptophan*

The whole seed of evening primrose (munch on the seeds, or crush them to use in cereal or in baking), sunflower seed, watercress, chickpea, sesame seed, spinach, pumpkin seed, fenugreek seed, chives, asparagus, almond, chicory, cauliflower, lima bean, oats, barley, wheat, black bean, green bean, kidney bean, string bean, fennel, cashew, potato, basil, pepper, buckwheat, celery, onion, Jerusalem artichoke, pea, garlic, lettuce, sugar beet, apricot, corn, root of water lotus†, carrot, rye, sweet potato.

A quick glance at this list reveals that serotonin-foods are lactogenic. Indeed, the supplement for tryptophan, 5-HTP, is sometimes marketed as a galactagogue. This is because *serotonin supports the chemistry of lactation by promoting the production of prolactin.* Don't take tryptophan supplements - eat serotonin-foods. *By eating to support your milk production, you steady your mood and reduce your cravings for sweets.* On page 116 you can learn how to adjust your meals so that you get the full benefit from serotonin in your diet.

About Food Addictions

Sugar, aspartame, caffeine, and dairy can be truly addictive. They directly affect our brain chemistry so that people may suffer symptoms of withdrawal if the foods are abruptly cut out of their diet.

In the case of dairy (milk, cheese, ice cream), it turns out that milk proteins (casein) have a similar shape to the beta-endorphins. These are the brain's own pain-killing and mood-elevating chemicals. There's some evidence that because milk proteins structurally resemble beta-endorphins, they can plug into the same receptors in the brain, boosting our mood.

Problems may arise when the brain lowers its own production of beta-endorphins, believing there are already plenty available from

---

* Taken from Dr. J. Duke's online database.

† Used in India as a galactagogue.

dairy products. When we then don't eat enough dairy, levels of beta-endorphins drop and we grow irritable, jittery, and unhappy. Eating dairy again will relieve the symptoms of discomfort: we're hooked.

Caffeine addiction (coffee, black or green tea, sodas, chocolate) may signal that a person's adrenals are not producing normal levels of stress hormones (levels that we need to be active and happy). While caffeine whips the adrenals into action in the short term, it weakens the adrenals in the long run, leading to constant fatigue.

Aspartame, like caffeine, makes us feel energetic. It stimulates the production of dopamine, a neurochemical of physical and mental activity. Aspartame addicts (to sugarless soda and chewing gum) may also go through withdrawal symptoms.

Refined foods, such as white sugar and flour, exhaust the pancreas. This is the organ that produces insulin in order to remove excess sugar from the bloodstream (where it would be deadly poisonous, even in amounts provided by a few cookies). Overeating sugar and refined starch leads to insulin resistance, weightgain, and fatigue, and it increases risk of heart disease, arthritis and diabetes in the long run.

Sugar also increases the production of beta-endorphins—a feel-happy neurochemical. The result: we come to need a *sugar fix*.

Any food we are allergic to can become addictive as well because the body produces endorphins as a response to the discomfort of the allergic reaction. The good news is that healthy foods also have a *feel-good* effect on the mind and body. Eating well makes it easier to go through withdrawal from food addictions.

Tips for Going through Withdrawal from Food Addiction

- Drink plenty of water throughout the day, and prepare meals that satisfy.

- Drink chamomile tea to help keep you calm.

- In trying to overcome any food addiction, focus on the healthy diet you are trying to achieve, rather than on the foods you are trying to avoid.

- Most important: make time for yourself to go through withdrawal. Begin on a Friday afternoon, so that you have the whole weekend to go through the worst of it, when your husband or friend can be there to offer support.

- Get plenty of vitamin B to help deal with the body's stress—but do not take more than 200 mg of vitamin B6 per day, as B6 may reduce milk supply.

- Take supplements of omega 3 or omega 6 to reduce cravings for fats. Or eat foods that contain these fats, such as almonds, pecans, cashews, sunflower seeds and especially flaxseed.

- If you find that you cannot do without the foods you crave, reduce the quantity rather than eliminating them altogether. Concentrate on the new good food habits you want to create.

- Don't allow yourself to suffer too much—breastfeeding is not the best time to endure stress!

For information about foods that promote the production of the neurochemical serotonin, that may also help you overcome food cravings, see pages 110-111. Read about a kind of diet that helps sugar addicts find balance on page 116.

Balance Your Use of Caffeine

In most cases, breastfeeding mothers do not have to avoid caffeine altogether. Just make sure that you are not using caffeine as part of a sugar-and-caffeine cycle, with your blood sugar taking a roller coaster ride throughout the day. *If you find that, rather than eating properly, you are drinking coffee, decaf, soda, or eating chocolate (also contains caffeine), it is time to limit your use of this stimulating drug.*

How many cups of coffee, tea, or soda are allowed to breastfeeding mothers per day? Both a mother and her baby will react individually to caffeine. While very sensitive babies could react with fussiness or colic to even one cup of coffee or tea in the morning, most babies will be fine, even if the mother takes several cups a day.

A baby's reaction to caffeine may not be immediately apparent, however. Caffeine accumulates in the baby's body, and she may gradually become fussier or hyper-alert from day to day. Omitting or reducing caffeine could lead to a happier baby.

Coffee or Decaf?

Is it better to drink decaf than regular coffee? A study from 2002 found that drinking four or more cups of decaf a day increases the risk of developing the autoimmune disease, rheumatoid arthritis, whereas normal coffee does not increase the risk, and tea has a preventative effect[51]. Clearly, decaf confuses the immune system and is not entirely harmless.

In deciding how much coffee or decaf to take, a mother should look at whether she needs caffeine to boost her blood pressure in the morning, or if she just likes the taste. (Decaf contains some caffeine, and some hyper-sensitive mothers react to the small amount of caffeine in decaf.) She should also look at whether she is using coffee to suppress hunger in order to lose weight, or as part of a coffee-and-sugar cycle. These are not good usages for coffee or decaf.

If a mother takes caffeine to boost her blood pressure, it would be wise to take normal coffee or tea in the morning. If she likes the taste of coffee, she might try taking imitation coffee, especially later in the day. It is full of nutritious, lactogenic ingredients. Blackstrap molasses coffee is another alternative. It is rich in minerals, including calcium.

One breastfeeding mother solved her "coffee or decaf" dilemma by deciding to drink one strong cup of regular coffee in the morning. This freed her from craving cups of decaf throughout the day. Each morning, she looks forward to savoring that one cup.

For myself—I take black tea in the morning to boost my low blood pressure. Black tea enhances insulin sensitivity (evening out blood sugar levels) which helps me beat food cravings throughout the day. Its antioxidant flavonoids protect against diseases of the joints and heart, plus it does not lead to higher cholesterol, as does unfiltered coffee. Green tea has the same or more positive effects, but I prefer the taste of black tea.

My personal advice is to drink coffee or tea in the morning if you have low blood pressure, and to regularly space your meals and snacks throughout the day to balance your energy and reduce the need for caffeine. If you crave the taste of coffee, try one of the healthy *coffee substitutes*, or *Ersatz coffee*, such as Pero®, Caro®, Roma™, or "dandelion root coffee," based on malt, chicory or dandelion root, fig, grains, vegetables and nuts.

If you are using caffeine to help you to lose weight, think again: it is better to eat regularly and concentrate on keeping your blood sugar levels steady. This will reduce stress, keep your thyroid active, your nerves strong—and promote healthful weightloss in the long term. Gently increase your exercise program and reduce your fat intake somewhat (but not altogether while breastfeeding and not your intake of EFAs). This will lead to weightloss without injury to your health or to the quality of your breastmilk.

Getting Off Caffeine:

- Remember that simple carbohydrates (white flour, white sugar) will add fuel to the sugar-caffeine craving cycle, and should be avoided or limited.

- Learn to drink coffee or tea without sugar, so that you are not giving your body two strong drugs at once. Do as the British do, and take it with milk, cream or milk substitute.

- Abruptly going off caffeine can trigger fatigue, headache, depression, or flu-like symptoms. If you go off caffeine altogether, do so over a weekend and make sure you have help at hand. Expect to feel irritable or depressed and to have unpredictable behavior, and let your family know so they can be patient with you.

- The best way to recover from caffeine addiction is to get the rest you truly need. After a few days of *allowing yourself to rest* (yes, really take that nap with your baby in the afternoon), you will have more energy and will need less caffeine—or even none at all.

- Caffeine is found in coffee, black and green tea, mate tea, chocolate, and in most soft drinks.

- Going off of aspartame may cause similar difficulties to caffeine and require similar measures while going through withdrawal.

For more information on going through withdrawal from food addictions, see pages 112-113.

A Resource for Sugar Addicts

Some people have an inherited hypersensitivity to sugar, according to Kathleen DesMaisons, Ph.D., author of *Potatoes not Prozac*. These people lack normal levels of beta-endorphins in their brains. They over respond to sugar with powerful surges of beta-endorphins that lift them up emotionally, only to drop into lethargy and irritability soon afterwards. This pattern sets up an irresistible urge to binge on sugar throughout the day. There is also an increased risk of alcohol abuse, as alcohol is a source of concentrated sugar.

In her book, DesMaisons carefully associates various metabolic imbalances with emotional components. This can help mothers to pinpoint what is going on in their body and mind, and in their reaction to food. For instance, symptoms of low blood sugar, according to DesMaisons, include: tired all the time, restless, can't keep still, confused, trouble with memory and concentration, easily frustrated, more irritable than usual.

DesMaisons advocates taking a daily vitamin, always eating breakfast with protein, and taking protein in all other meals as well. Protein provides a steady supply of tryptophan (for serotonin), plus it keeps the blood sugar level steady. If you're going to eat candy, cookies, or ice cream, DesMaisons says to eat it with a protein-rich meal.

Finally, she suggests eating a potato before going to bed. The potato should not be taken with any topping that contains protein. The potato changes body chemistry during the night in such a way that the brain makes and uses more of its own serotonin. This both lifts depression and reduces sugar cravings. Indeed, the goal of this diet is to balance the body's blood and brain chemistry *before* a sugar-junkie actually tries to withdraw from sugar.

The really good news is that the *Potato not Prozac* program can easily be worked into a lactogenic diet. Nearly all the foods she recommends are lactogenic. Potatoes are lactogenic in themselves, as are all foods rich in tryptophan (see list above in *Serotonin Foods*).

See page 104 - 105 for more information on supplements that help balance sugar levels—and that indirectly act as galactagogues.

Mothers with Eating Disorders or Abuse Issues

Mothers with eating disorders have special breastfeeding issues. Many feel uncomfortable with their increase of appetite due to milk production, or they are uncomfortable with the amount of time required to feed the baby, or by the frequency of his need to be fed. These mothers may also object to his becoming "fat" even though they know that plumpness is a healthy, reassuring sign that a baby is getting all the nutrients he requires to prosper.

If you see yourself here, try to view breastfeeding as a chance to get to the bottom of your issues. You may need the help of a doctor, therapist, or support group to understand and work through these problems[*]. You may also benefit from the guidance of a sensitive lactation specialist who can help you adjust your eating patterns to the requirements of breastfeeding.

Mothers who have been sexually abused may understandably find breastfeeding difficult. Many find it difficult to tolerate having their breasts touched, while at the same time yearning for the affirming experience of breastfeeding. Some may be repulsed by the idea of putting the baby to their breast, but be okay with pumping and bottle-feeding their milk.

Indeed, mothers may have these feelings even if they are unable to remember the origins in childhood that led to their feeling estranged from their breasts. All mothers should recognize that feelings are our friends and guides, and are legitimate. In this case, they signal where we may need to ask for professional help. If you see yourself here, and if you conclude that breastfeeding is too challenging in your situation, know that your decision is okay. You are not alone, you are not a failure, and you are not a bad mother.

The goal—for many mothers on some level, as many of us have issues with food, femininity, and motherhood—is to get to the point where we experience physical closeness and providing nutrition, both to ourselves and to our babies, as an act of love and empowerment, regardless how we feed.

---

[*] Eating disorders are being treated with amino acid supplements that are said to nourish the brain chemistry and pave the path to normal eating patterns. However, amino acid supplements, if not carefully administered, can interfere with the chemistry of lactation.

CHAPTER EIGHT

Foods and Herbs

Lactogenic, Anti-Lactogenic

The following section lists foods, condiments, and spices that mothers can take to support their milk supply. Feel free to photocopy these pages to hang in your kitchen as a reminder, and to take along with you when you shop for food.

The lactogenic foods listed here are discussed in Chapter Nine.

Anti-lactogenic foods are discussed in the next section.

A Shopping List

MEAT AND SEAFOOD

- Chicken
- Turkey
- Wild deer (venison)
- Crab
- Squid (Calamari)

For more information about meat and fish, see pages 143-148.

GRAINS

- Barley (pearled whole barley and barley flakes)
- Oatmeal (flakes and whole grain)
- Corn meal (coarse and fine)
- Buckwheat
- Brown rice and white rice
- Quinoa
- Amaranth

⇨ The following grains are generally well-tolerated by persons on a gluten-free diet:
> buckwheat, corn, rice, millet, tapioca, quinoa, amaranth

LEGUMES

- Chickpeas (canned and dry)
- Lentils (large and small, red, green and dark green— small lentils cook more quickly)
- Mungbeans (whole or halved—halved mungbean cook more quickly)
- Other beans: kidney, black and white beans (canned or dry)
- Lima beans (canned or dry)
- Green bean, peas (fresh or frozen)

UNSALTED NUTS AND SEEDS

- Sesame seeds
- Black seeds (Nigella sativa)
- Almonds
- Optional: cashews, pecans
- Sunflower seeds
- Pumpkin seeds

DRIED FRUIT

- Apricots
- Dates
- Figs

FRESH FRUIT AND BERRIES
- Fruits with pits—but caution with digestion:
- Apricots
- Peaches
- Nectarines
- Plums
- Sweet Cherries
- Figs
- Papaya (green, unripe)
- All berries—but careful if you have low supply

BREAD AND CRACKERS
- Whole-grain bread, crackers (available at healthfood store)
- Pumpernickel, sour-dough
- rye, sour-dough
- Moshi, rice cakes (at Asian markets)

SPREADS
- Tahini (sesame seed paste)
- Gomasio (sesame and salt powder)
- Almond butter

NATURAL, MINERAL-RICH SUGARS
- Malt syrup or powder (malt is especially lactogenic)
- Blackstrap molasses
- Honey (raw, if possible)
- Maple syrup

SPECIAL FOODS
- Coffee Substitute (based on barley, rye, figs, malt, chicory)
- Green-Drink
- Rice-milk
- Almond-milk
- Coconut flakes
- Coconut-milk
- Seaweed, assorted

CONDIMENTS
- Onion
- Garlic
- Ginger root

OILS
- Cold-pressed extra virgin olive oil
- Cold-pressed sesame seed oil
- Coconut oil
- Butter

SPICES
- Sea salt, "celtic salt", "krystal salt"
- Fennel seed powder
- Cumin seed powder
- Fenugreek seed powder
- Fennel seed
- Dill seed
- Caraway seed
- Aniseed
- Turmeric
- Coriander
- Cinnamon
- Ginger powder
- Curry mix (mild)
- Basil (dry or fresh)
- Marjoram (dry or fresh)
- Thyme (dry or fresh)
- Organic seasoned salt
- Black pepper corn

VEGETABLES
- Asparagus
- Artichoke
- String bean or green bean (actually a legume)
- Peas (actually a legume), snow peas, sugar snap peas

- Dark green leafy vegetables, including butter lettuce, romaine, endive, arugula, baby spinach, water cress, dandelion greens, beet greens
- Radicchio
- Fennel
- Carrots
- Beets
- Cauliflower
- Broccoli
- Swiss chard
- Sweet potato or yam
- Potato
- Jerusalem artichoke
- Root of water lotus (Asian stores)
- Kale

QUICK PACKAGED FOODS

- Canned legumes: lentils, kidney beans, chickpea
-
- Frozen vegetables: peas, spinach, green beans, carrot, broccoli and cauliflower

- Quick-cooking rice. Add barley, oats or millet to the rice, plus additional water, for a stronger lactogenic effect.

- Granola (especially if loaded with lactogenic ingredients such as coconut flakes, sesame seed, flaxseed, almond, dried fruit)

- Malted Milk – malt in any form is lactogenic.

- Packaged Cereal: Oat Meal, Malt-O-Meal

THE FOLLOWING HERBS ARE POTENTIALLY ANTI-LACTOGENIC IF TAKEN IN LARGE QUANTITIES:

- Rosemary
- Thyme
- Peppermint, Spearmint (food, candy with mint flavor)
- Sage
- Parsley

POSSIBLE ANTI-LACTOGENIC FOODS FOR LOW SUPPLY

Women with chronic low milk may experiment with avoiding:
- Soft-drinks, carbonated beverages.
- Coffee, black tea, green tea
- Chocolate
- Citric acid in foods and juice
- Vitamin C supplements
- Vitamin B6—do not take more than 200 mg per day.
- Aspartame (avoid this in any case)
- Orange juice; citric fruit juice
- Possibly tomatoes, cucumbers, paprika.
- Possibly apples, bananas and avocado.
- Any food that the baby reacts sensitively to.

Anti-lactogenic Herbs

Certain herbs can decrease milk supply. **Sage** tea is well known to lower milk supply—sage in turkey dressing at Thanksgiving may cause the dip in supply that many mothers experience during that particular holiday. **Parsley** is also noted to dry up the milk. Commonly used herbs that are suspected of drying up milk include **lemon balm, peppermint, spearmint, rosemary,** and **thyme**.

Candy, gum, beverages or foods flavored with extracts of these herbs may also reduce milk supply if taken often. *These herbs can, however, all be enjoyed in small amounts.* A bite of parsley each day will help your supply due to the concentration of minerals and vitamins. In fact, in some herbals, parsley is said to be a galactagogue. Thyme is also lactogenic in moderate amounts, and is also included as a galactagogue in some herbals. I had chronic low milk supply, but still enjoyed a cup of sage tea every now and then with no ill effects.

⇨ Sensitivity to these foods differs from mother to mother. Be aware of their possible impact and observe your own reactions.

⇨ Two galactagogues, **fennel seed** and **verbena (vervain)**, are reputed to dry out the body and lower milk supply when used regularly, according to Traditional Chinese Medicine. It is best not to use these herbs exclusively, but rather as part of a lactogenic program, combining or alternating them with other galactagogues.

Anti-lactogenic Foods: Possible Explanations

Just as there is a list of foods that support lactation, certain foods and supplements have been found to impair milk production in *certain mothers*. Most mothers will see no negative effect from these foods. Exactly why these foods rarely have this effect on some mothers isn't known for certain. I expect it has to do with the following factors.

• Foods that elevate stress hormones, leading to the constriction of the capillaries in the breasts.

Foods that promote an elevation of stress hormones include **soft drinks** that contain caffeine, **coffee, mate, black** and **green tea**. Ironically, caffeine has been seen to increase milk production in research on animals. In humans, however, when women take caffeine in order to deal with stress and exhuastion, it appears to impair the let-down. Even **chocolate,** if used as part of a sugar and caffeine cycle, can increase stress hormones. Caffeine may also influence women hormonally, as is seen through its effect on fibrocystic breasts.

• Foods that are astringent, causing sensitive tissue to constrict, leading to restricted circulation of blood in the breasts.

Astringent foods include **citrus juice, citric acid,** and all fruit juice that contains citric acid; **vitamin C** supplements, very **sour berries** and fruit and **red raspberry leaf tea**. Some mothers eliminate mouth-puckering foods from their diet, such as fresh tomato, paprika, and cucumber, and report that this restriction is helpful in building their supply. Carbonated beverages (see below) have a similar effect.

• Additives and supplements that increase levels of dopamine in the brain; dopamine suppresses the production of prolactin, and reduces milk supply.

Chemicals that increase dopamine are **aspartame** and **vitamin B 6**. Aspartame, (NutraSweet), found in sugarless sodas, candies, and chewing gum, is made of the amino acid phenylalanine, the precursor to dopamine. Aspartame, in any case, is not recommended during pregnancy and while breastfeeding as it promotes seizures in some people.

Vitamin B6 is a co-enzyme in the synthesis of dopamine. A rough estimate is that more than 200 mg of vitamin B6 per day may decrease a mother's milk supply. Women have individual responses, however. Some may see no decrease in milk while taking a high dosage, and others could, theoretically, see a reduction in milk supply with a lower dosage.

• Low-supply mothers also commonly need to avoid **carbonated beverages.** Again, we're not exactly certain why. One German expert has pointed out that carbonation is acidic, and that it may constrict circulation to breast tissue. Soft drinks and even carbonated water commonly also contain caffeine. Mothers frequently use soft drinks to suppress their hunger and reduce their caloric intake. Also, the potassium in soft drinks interferes with calcium metabolism, and this may affect milk supply (see page 153).

Cruciferous Vegetables – a potential danger to supply?

The taste of some foods can make a baby disinclined to drink. The vegetables of the cruciferous family (**cabbage**, **Brussels sprouts**, **cauliflower**) contain sulfur and can make breastmilk less tasty for some babies. It can also make breastmilk more difficult to digest for some babies. Onion and garlic also fit into this category, though many babies actually like their mother's milk better when she eats garlic.

If a baby drinks less milk because it doesn't appeal to him, or because he recognizes a taste that previously led to stomach upset, this may cause his mother's supply to decrease.

Preparing these vegetables with carminative herbs such as dill, cumin, and mustard seeds may improve the milk's flavor and digestibility.

Carrot Juice – a galactagogue?

Carrot juice, taken first thing in the morning, has been reported by the natural doctor and author, Tori Hudson, to help mothers wean. Well, I have often recommended carrot juice to nursing mothers—to be drunk shortly before lunch—without hearing that it negatively impacts milk supply. I recommend carrot juice to help a mother feel less fatigued. It has a remarkable effect on mother's vitality. With interest, I have learned that the clinical herbalist, Karen Vaughan, has used carrot juice on herself as a galactagogue. She believes it works due to its hormonal effects.

- Drink vegetable juice before lunch. As with all supplements, its nutrients will be absorbed better if taken with a meal.
- Carrot juice has a balancing effect on a mother's energy, and can be useful when a mother complains of exhaustion.
- Hypoglycemia: carrot juice is sweet and causes an insulin surge. Combine carrot juice with cream (for slower digestion), or take it in small portions before meals.

⇨ See www.ebay.com for second-hand, inexpensive juicers. (Be sure that you are getting a vegetable juicer, and not a lemon or orange juicer.)

Avocados, Apples, Bananas – Anti-lactogenic?

Avocados, apples and **bananas** are staple foods in many mother's diets. They are nutritious, delicious, and they do not have a reputation for impairing milk supply.

This book tries to provide information that goes beyond what is applicable for "normal" mothers. It is intended to provide insights for mothers who *fall out of all statistics*, as they say in German—for that "1 in 3,000" mother who responds ultra-sensitively to everything she eats. It would be a shame if this woman were to do everything she could to increase her milk supply, and not manage simply because she includes certain foods in her diet every day. I am such a woman[*], and whenever I ate avocados, apples, or bananas on a regular basis, I noted a decrease in my milk-supply[†].

It is most likely that these foods do not suppress milk supply, but rather, that extremely sensitive women have to make sure that all the foods that they do eat are definitely supportive of milk supply. Again—I mention these foods only for those mothers who have a case of chronic low supply that is acutely sensitive to food. To find out if these fruits are somewhat anti-lactogenic for you, avoid them while following the other suggestions in this book. Let me know if avoiding these foods helps to increase your supply.

---

[*] One reason for my extreme sensitivity to lactogenic foods may be that I was suffering from a disease that suppresses the immune system, though I didn't know it at the time. I have Lyme disease, the tick-borne infection that mimics many other diseases and that is difficult to diagnose and treat. Lyme disease causes hormonal imbalances such as insulin resistance and low thyroid, and it also affects the pituitary and thalamus. Women with active Lyme disease almost always develop PMS, with symptoms such as changes in hearing and seeing, extreme mood swings, rage, fatigue, and depression. These can last one or two weeks before menstruation, and sometimes occur during menstruation as well. Lyme disease is more prevalent than many people know, and may be behind unexplained low milk supply in some mothers.

[†] It has no connection to avocado the fruit, but avocado leaf is known to damage mammary tissue in goats[52].

CHAPTER NINE

The Lactogenic Foods

Vegetables

This chapter discusses many matters relating to the preparation and combination of lactogenic foods. It also discusses the ways that these foods work in the body to support lactation. In addition, there are sections on dairy, wheat, meat, protein, iron, vitamin B12, and mercury found in fish and amalgam fillings.

Lactogenic Vegetables

Most vegetables, besides being good for you, are lactogenic. They provide the vitamins, minerals, enzymes, folic acid, and beta-carotene that breastfeeding mothers need.

Watercress, spinach, chives, lettuce, beet greens, dandelion leaves, kale, dark green salads, onion, garlic, asparagus, pea, green beans, beet root, fennel, carrot, potato, Jerusalem artichoke, sweet potato, cauliflower, corn, root of water lotus[*], mushroom, seaweed.

Vegetables can be lactogenic for the following reasons:
- **Sedative**—foods and herbs that contain substances that act as a sedative are often galactagogues. Two sedating actions—that of natural opiates, and of natural dopamine suppressants—increase the production of prolactin. Sedating substances in vegetables and herbs may work through these principles and gently increase prolactin production. Sedating vegetables include lettuce, fennel, onion and potato.

---

[*] Used in India as a galactagogue.

- **Calcium**—almost all lactogenic vegetables are remarkably rich in minerals, especially calcium. Read pages 152-153 to learn how calcium supports milk supply.
- **Serotonin**—foods that contain good levels of the amino acid tryptophan, *the precursor of serotonin*, are lactogenic. This is because good levels of serotonin suppress the anti-lactogenic neurotransmitter dopamine. Tryptophan is contained in dairy and meat, though animal products also contain very high concentrations of tryptophan's competition, the amino acid phenylalanine (aspartame!). Tryptophan is found in a better, more lactogenic balance in grains, legumes, and in some *vegetables*. See *Serotonin Foods* on page 111.
- **Hormones and Saponines**: plant-estrogens (phytoestrogen) and saponins imitate hormones in the body. Lactogenic vegetables include our most 'hormonal' veggies: peas, green-beans (these are actually legumes), carrots, asparagus, and potatoes.
- **Support the liver and kidneys**: the following vegetables support the detoxifying action of the liver and kidneys with beta-carotene, antioxidants, and diuretic properties: dandelion leaves, green leafy veggies, asparagus, carrot, sweet potato, and beet.
- **Sea vegetables** (wakame, Irish moss, kelp, and agar) are potent sources of **calcium** and **omega 3 EFAs**. In Asia, mothers take seaweed soup to ward off depression and support their milk supply. For a recipe, see pages 176-177.

Fruit

Delicious and refreshing, fruit are a rich source of vitamins, minerals and sugar. However, some kinds of fruit may pose problems for a small number of very sensitive low-supply mothers. Among these mothers, citrus fruits are reputed to be anti-lactogenic. Some mothers can only increase their milk supply if they avoid all sources of citric acid. We have even heard of vitamin C supplements being problematic. Very sour berries are also potentially anti-lactogenic for sensitive mothers.

Apples and bananas are most people's favorites, and normal-supply mothers find bananas or apple juice helpful and healthful.

I personally felt that they hindered rather than helped me sustain my milk supply during vulnerable times. This was just my experience, however. Everyone is different, and each mother has to find out for herself what affects her positively or negatively.

Avocado is another fruit that may possibly be anti-lactogenic—of course, only for extremely sensitive mothers. Like all anti-lactogenic foods, nearly all "normal-supply" mothers can enjoy them without reservation.

Some people have problems digesting raw fruit. Steamed fruit are easier to digest and are often recommended after birth to prevent digestive problems from affecting a mother's milk and causing colic or upset in her baby. Try cooking fruit with a slice of fresh ginger root, aniseed, or cinnamon for extra flavor and to improve their digestibility and lactogenicity. But first, see cautions for ginger on page 282-283.

Lactogenic Fruit

Our most lactogenic fruits are figs, dates, and apricots. These are good sources of calcium and other minerals. Figs contain high levels of digestive enzymes.

Green papaya, another potent source of digestive enzymes, is taken throughout Asia as a galactagogue. Green papaya should be steamed. For a recipe, see page 177.

Moderate amounts of sweet cherries and peaches are used in Traditional Chinese Medicine to promote the let-down.

Nuts and Seeds

Nuts have proven to be one of those nutritious, fatty foods that improve cholesterol levels and prevent heart disease—showing again the importance of the right kinds of fats.

Nuts are lactogenic due to their high content of minerals and the amino acid, tryptophan, the precursor of serotonin, a pro-lactation neurotransmitter.

Almonds

Our most lactogenic nut, the sweet almond (the nut highest in calcium) is taken by mothers in the postpartum in the Mideast and India. Snacking on almonds is said to enrich breastmilk and make it sweeter and creamier.

In a study in California, almonds did *not* lead to weightgain when taken in modest amounts every day. This is because the fat and protein in nuts satisfy hunger. They also keep blood sugar levels steady, reducing cravings for sweet and starchy foods[53]. Many mothers find that almond milk increases their milk supply. For a recipe, see page 198.

Sesame Seeds

Sesame seeds are our most lactogenic seed. Just as almonds contain the most calcium of any nut, sesame seeds contain the most calcium of any seed. One cup of sesame seeds more than meets the minimum daily requirement for calcium in the US.

Raw sesame seeds slip through the intestine undigested if they are not crushed open. Sesame seeds are crushed, boiled, or roasted in traditional preparations to improve the availability of its minerals. Sesame seed preparations, *tahini* and *gomasio*, can be purchased at a healthfood store or homemade. *Be sure to buy sesame seed products made of hulled sesame seeds, as substances in the hull interfere with their digestion.*

Flaxseed

Flaxseed is lactogenic.

Flaxseed can be crushed (in a mini coffee grinder used exclusively for flax and cleaned regularly to remove old seed and oil) and added to breakfast cereals.

A tablespoonful of flaxseed, soaked overnight, exudes a slippery slime that relieves constipation. Swallow it straight down, or add it to breakfast cereal.

Lactogenic Nuts and Seeds

Nuts: almonds, cashews, pecans
Seeds: sesame, flax

Oils

As a general rule, cold-pressed oils should be kept in your refrigerator, though coconut oil, sesame seed oil, and virgin olive oil will keep for a long time and not become rancid at room temperature.

- **Extra virgin olive oil,** cold-pressed, is renowned for improving cholesterol levels, improving metabolic syndrome, and preventing heart disease. Olive oil contains mainly monounsaturated fatty acids. These do not compete with essential fatty acids (EFAs) found in nuts, seeds, green leafy vegetables, grains, legumes or supplements, making olive oil ideal for every day cooking.

- **Butter** is an excellent source of the fat-soluble vitamins A, D and E. Taken with vegetables, grains and legumes, these vitamins help the body absorb the minerals in these foods. Butter does not compete with essential fatty acids. (Look for organic butter at your healthfood store.)

- **Sesame seed** oil, cold-pressed, has a high antioxidant and vitamin E content that protects it from becoming rancid quickly. Along with high levels of monounsaturated fatty acids, sesame oil contains about 40% omega 6 EFAs, so that over-using sesame oil could lead to an imbalance of EFAs. A healthy mixture of omega 6 and omega 3 fatty acids can be achieved by combining sesame oil equally with flaxseed oil. This combination should not be heated. Rather, use it for salad dressing.

- **Coconut oil** contains over 90% saturated fatty acids; it is soft in hot, tropical countries, but a thick paste in cooler climes. If you live in the US, try to find 'virgin' coconut oil, especially if you are using it for medical reasons. Coconut oil contains high amounts of lauric acid, a fatty acid with significant antibacterial, antiviral, and antifungal properties. In tropical countries, lauric acid protects food from spoilage—along with the profuse use of herbs. Lauric acid is present in mother's milk. Its levels increase if we take coconut oil in our diets. Lauric acid supports the immune system, and mothers with a suppressed immune system or AIDS should take coconut oil regularly.

- **Sunflower, safflower,** and other vegetable oils. While these oils contain valuable nutrients, their high levels of omega 6s can promote an imbalance in our EFA metabolism if they are overused. Use only cold-pressed oils, and do not heat.

- **Walnut** oil, like flaxseed oil, is high in omega 3. Walnut oil is expensive, but just a dash can add an interesting taste to salad dressing and mayonnaise.

- **Flaxseed oil**—flaxseed oil provides good amounts of omega 3 plus some omega 6 EFAs. Flaxseed oil is a potent galactagogue, perhaps thanks to hormonal components in flaxseed.

- **EFA supplements** that have a lactogenic effect are **flaxseed oil**, **borage seed** oil, **black currant seed** oil and **evening primrose seed** oil, all sold as capsules. The latter three supply the important omega 6 derivative, GLA, or gamma linoleic acid. **Fish oil** and **cod-liver oil** prevent or ease depression and improve "fuzzy-mindedness." For more information, see *Get Your Fats Right* in Chapter Three.

Grains and Legumes

Breastfeeding women in many cultures use grains and legumes to support their milk supply, as is explained in the next section. They also use a combination of grains, legumes, nuts, and seeds for protein, as explained below.

Grains and Legumes as Protein

As vegetarians know, the combination of a grain and a legume, nut or seed provides a wide spread of amino acids, called a *complete protein*. Vegetarians commonly take rice and lentils, or whole grain bread with nut butter, to get a complete protein. Indeed, traditional dishes from many cultures are based on this combination. In Spanish-speaking countries, rice and beans are eaten together. In Africa, sorghum is mixed with black-eyed peas. Native Americans combine corn and lima beans into succotash. In the Mideast, hummus is made of sesame seeds and chickpea (garbanzo), and eaten with wheat (pita bread). In India, mungbean combined with rice is the king of foods, taken once a day for optimum health. In China, soy sauce is fermented from soy and wheat. In Japan, miso—taken for breakfast with rice and vegetables—is made by fermenting soybeans with rice or barley.

Quinoa (pronounced "KEEN-wa"), a seed (not a grain or legume) from the highlands of Peru, contains more amino acids than any other vegetable source, including the amino acid lysine that is not commonly found in plants. It requires fifteen minutes to quick-cook and it combines well with rice, grains, or legumes. Although pricey, quinoa greatly expands in size and is well worth its cost in nutrients. Amaranth is another seed from the Andes that, combined with a grain, provides a complete protein.

To learn more about plant protein, read *Diet for a Small Planet* by Frances Moore Lappe, or her new book, *Hope's Edge*, and *Recipes for a Small Planet* by Ellen Buchman Ewald.

The Lactogenic Properties of Grains and Legumes

Grains and legumes share a worldwide reputation for supporting lactation. In the US, the most commonly used grain-galactagogue is oatmeal, though oatmeal is only one of many lactogenic grains and legumes. Others include millet, barley, rice, chickpea, peas, green beans, lentils, lima beans, quinoa, and amaranth.

Women around the world use grains and legumes to prepare beverages that are famous for building and supporting milk supply (see *grain-drinks* on pages 191-193).

Saponins

Saponins, a sweet, soap-like substance, have immune-stimulating and antibiotic effects. The body can use saponins as precursors to make hormones. Saponins may influence the production of pituitary hormones, which include the hormones of lactation. *Oats* contain a wealth of saponins, and this may partly explain the remarkable effect of oats on milk production. Saponins are also found in *chickpeas*, *asparagus*, and *potatoes* (eaten with the skin)—all of them, lactogenic foods.

Phytoestrogen

Grains and legumes are rich in *phytoestrogen*, or plant-estrogen. Phytoestrogen has a mild estrogenic effect. It is thought to balance a woman's estrogen levels, lowering or increasing estrogen as necessary. Phytoestrogen is not carcinogenic because it does not occupy estrogen receptor sites long enough to stimulate tissue growth—in contrast to chemical substances that mimic estrogen.

In supporting lactation, phytoestrogen may do several things. It may lower the body's own level of estrogen by stealing receptor sites away from the body's much stronger estrogen. This would suppress the chemistry of fertility and support the chemistry of lactation. It may also target receptor sites directly that support lactation. For example, in the pituitary, phytoestrogen may help increase the number of cells that produce prolactin, especially in combination with sedating substances in the same herb or food. In the breast, phytoestrogen may stimulate the growth of milk-glands. Researchers have only just begun to study phytoestrogen and lactation, so we can only speculate at this point.

Polysaccharides

Grains contain natural forms of long-chain sugar, called polysaccharides. These sugars have healing or immune stimulating effects on the body.

One polysaccharide, beta glucan, is in barley, oats, and yeast (three galactagogues). In studies on lactation in rats and cattle, beta glucan was found to measurably raise prolactin in the blood and to increase milk production. This may help explain why *barley-water*—a medicinal in which barley's sugars are released into water—has an ancient reputation as a galactagogue. For mothers with chronic low supply, it should be taken intensively, at least four cups a day, and at least for a week.

Malt—made from spouted, dried, and fermented barley—is also traditionally used to stimulate milk production. In Switzerland, malt extract made from organically grown barley is a traditional gift to mothers after birth.

Before I knew much about galactagogues, I relied on malt. I found that it took at least twelve large soupspoons of malt per day, over four day's time, to see a marked increase in my supply. High-quality malt is expensive (low quality is stretched with corn syrup). I was spending twenty dollars a week on malt! But at least I could breastfeed my baby.

Now I would only use malt as an emergency measure, when a high-quality product is worth the money. Many mothers find that malt-based commercial cereals and beverages boost their milk supply.

Phytic Acid and Enzyme Inhibitors

Grains, legumes, nuts, and seeds contain two substances that make their digestion difficult. The first is phytic acid. Phytic acid attaches to minerals such as calcium, magnesium, copper, iron, and zinc in the intestine, preventing their absorption through the intestinal wall, into the bloodstream. The second factor is enzyme inhibitors that block digestive processes. Enzyme inhibitors present an important survival technique for grains, legumes, nuts, and seeds. They prevent these from deteriorating in the soil before the time is ripe for them to sprout. The same inhibitors prevent enzymes in the intestine from doing their work.

In traditional cultures, grains and legumes were soaked or fermented before being prepared as food. Both soaking and fermentation deactivate enzyme inhibitors and break down phytic acids, so that the food becomes optimally digestible.

Of course, mothers after birth, many of whom scarcely find time to eat, may not feel up to soaking grains and legumes. When you come down to it though it doesn't take much time to pour a half cup of a grain or legume into a bowl and cover it with water. If your baby is suffering from colic, or if you have low supply, you may be motivated to soak your main lactogenic grains such as oats and barley.

In my kitchen, there is a note on the cupboard:

Soak for Tomorrow!!!

Gluten Sensitivity

Some mothers and babies are sensitive to gluten found in wheat, rye, barley, and oats. Gluten is a gluey protein that makes dough stick together as bread. Gluten is extremely difficult to digest; as an allergen, it can cause severe inflammation in the intestine and serious disease, called *celiac disease.*

Wheat contains the largest amount of gluten of any grain. Often, eliminating wheat from the diet is sufficient for improvement, and it is not necessary to omit oats, barley, or rye. However, sometimes it is necessary to omit all gluten-containing grains from the diet.

It is not difficult to eliminate wheat on a home-cooked, whole-foods diet. Packaged and processed foods on the other hand often contain small amounts of wheat. *Wheat is often hidden in sauces and soups.*

Grains that do not contain gluten are millet, corn, and rice—though allergic persons can be sensitive to these as well. Quinoa and amaranth, both protein-rich seeds that are eaten as grains (and that are lactogenic), are usually well tolerated by gluten-sensitive people. Unfortunately, oats and barley, two lactogenic grains, do also contain gluten.

- Signs of gluten sensitivity in the mother may be bloating, gas, bowel trouble (not being 'regular,' constipation, diarrhea or both), *and drowsiness after a meal, feeling too full after eating, and weightgain from water.* Gluten insensitivity will eventually lead to undernourishment and loss of weight.

- Signs of dairy sensitivity in the mother (see below) may be stomachaches, cramping, gas, bloating, belching, diarrhea or constipation, but also *respiratory problems, such as runny noses, asthma, wheezing, chronic earaches and ear infections.*

Gluten is found in wheat, rye, oats, and barley.

Dairy

Dairy is widely considered a good source of protein and calcium, and is promoted as one of our best foods. However, dairy is problematic, and may in fact not be a good food to recommend in large quantities to mothers. I will explain as I go along.

People may become addicted to dairy and consume large amounts, every day. Any one-sided diet can cause to deficiencies in vitamins, minerals and digestive enzymes, and may lead eventually to digestive and other problems.

Many adults lack the intestinal enzyme *lactase*, needed to digest milk sugar, *lactose*. In children, this enzyme is usually present, but the milk protein, *casein*, remains a common trigger for allergy in children and adults. Casein is one of the most difficult proteins to digest, and if not completely digested by the mother will enter a mother's milk. Once reaching the baby, it passes through his stomach and into his intestine, where it may cause or contribute to inflammatory processes in the digestive tract—or other parts of his body. A common symptom is colic. (Some researchers believe it may also increase the risk of childhood diabetes[*].)

Should Mothers Avoid Dairy?

Experts are divided on the question of whether mothers should categorically avoid dairy. Some argue that it is normal for a baby to receive bovine milk protein (casein) in a mother's milk: this could be nature's way of provoking babies to build an appropriate immune response to dairy. According to this point of view, it is not the presence of casein in breastmilk, but the *lack* of certain protective immune substances in certain mother's milk that is the problem.

Others say that no babies, including human babies, were designed to deal with difficult proteins from another mammal's milk. There will always be a considerable number of people who lack sufficient immune substances to casein, and there will always be babies who suffer from reactions to dairy in their mother's diet, or to dairy in formula if they are formula-fed.

---

[*]For more information, see the book, *Baby Matters*, by Dr. Linda Folden Palmer.

Consider this: people with an African, Chinese, or Native American background have more milk allergies[*] because in these cultures, cow milk was unknown until recently. People with a Northern European or Caucasian background are more likely to be dairy tolerant because these peoples were dependent on dairy for two thousand years. During that time, their population became selected for those who could tolerate dairy (i.e., those who could not tolerate dairy died young, before they could reproduce). In a similar way, people from Asia and Africa have fewer allergies to peanut (peanut was unknown in Europe), and people from Asia are more tolerant to grain.

⇨ It would be wise for people with an African, Asian, or Native American background to restrict their use of dairy.

Today, however, because so many women *greatly overeat* dairy, babies of all racial backgrounds may be born with a strong sensitivity to dairy. When the breastfeeding mother eats dairy, the baby develops digestive disorders or other symptoms.

⇨ The majority of breastfed babies with colic improve when the mother omits dairy from her diet.

Consider this: traditionally, people in milk-drinking cultures did not drink much fresh milk. Because they did not have refrigerators, they allowed milk to ferment into naturally probiotic sour milk, sour cream, kefir, yogurt, and cheese. Fermented milk products are easier to digest. Fermentation partially breaks down lactose and it pre-digests casein. Cheese contains less casein, as it separates with the whey. A mother who eats fermented dairy products (before and during pregnancy, and while breastfeeding), may hope to see less milk sensitivity in herself and her infant[†]. In fact, the milk-culture bacteria,

---

[*] This is why there is now a movement to serve soy milk in schools with many children from these backgrounds.

[†] Live kefir grains to ferment milk can be ordered online from private persons, often for the cost of postage. Kefir is easier to make than yogurt (just set it up in a jug and the next day it is finished), and is the cheapest way to keep a supply of live lactobacilli in one's diet.

lactobacilli, helps prevent inflammation and allergies by improving the integrity of the intestine. In other words, traditional fermented products, rich in enzymes and lactobacilli, offset the negative effects of dairy.

⇨ Butter does not contain much of the problematic milk protein, and clarified butter, *ghee,* eaten across Asia, contains none at all.

⇨ There is a movement in the US to rediscover and cultivate traditional ways of food-preparation. An invaluable resource is the book by Sally Fallon and Mary G. Enig, Ph.D., *Nourishing Traditions*.

Some medical experts believe that dairy sensitivity in children is compounded by fungal infection in the intestine. The theory is that if the baby has an on-going cold, if he wheezes, or tends to have one ear infection after the other, he is most likely sensitive to dairy in the mother's diet. If he is then given antibiotics for ear infections, he may develop fungal overgrowth in his intestine. This in turn can increase the permeability of his intestine, leading to more allergies and illness.

Many doctors however do not adhere to the fungal overgrowth theory. For more information, see *The Yeast Connection Handbook* by William G. Crook, MD. Talk with your doctor if you are concerned that fungal overgrowth could be an issue for you or your baby.

How to Use Dairy

Many experts would say do not use dairy at all[*], *especially* if you live in the US where cows only survive—considering rampant infections of their over-demanded udders—through routine injections of antibiotics. Dairy cows in the US are also given injections of growth hormones to increase milk production, and these hormones may not be completely harmless to humans.

---

[*] Such as Dr. Jay Gordon at http://www.drjaygordon.com/nutrition/index.htm#Defining

As for milk providing calcium and preventing osteoporosis, many experts argue that this is not the case. They refer to a study showing that the Mediterranean diet contains low levels of dairy but that people there show no symptoms of low calcium intake. Some studies even show a positive correlation between the intake of dairy and the occurrence of osteoporosis[54]. Indeed, all indigenous peoples eating their native, whole-foods diet have no problems with a lack of calcium, whether dairy is included in their diet or not, according to the detailed documentation of the world-traveler, Weston A. Price, from the early 20th century.

While low-fat milk is said to be good for us, it is precisely our high-protein diet that leads to our deficit on calcium. To compound matters, milk's high levels of calcium and low levels of other minerals can throw our mineral metabolism out of balance.

Importantly, nutritionists agree that mothers who avoid dairy should include other foods that contain calcium in their diets. For more information on calcium, see pages 149-154.

With all this against it, milk is still a treasured food to those who can tolerate it. I applaud organic farmers who grass feed their cattle and who treat their animals humanely. By the way, today in Switzerland, where I live, as in most of the world, it is illegal to routinely give antibiotics or hormones to dairy cows.

- Signs of diary sensitivity in the mother may be stomachaches, cramping, gas, bloating, belching, diarrhea or constipation, but also *respiratory problems, such as a runny nose, sinusitis, asthma, wheezing, fluid behind the ears, chronic earaches and ear infections.*

- If you suspect that you do not digest milk well, or if there are allergies or autoimmune diseases in your family, it would be very wise to restrict your use of dairy, especially while pregnant and breastfeeding.

- The main reason to continue taking dairy is the taste. If you don't like the taste, feel free to omit it from your diet.
- Mothers of allergic children say that the baby with whom they consumed the most milk products while pregnant had the most colic and milk allergies.

- Take butter—preferably organic butter from your healthfood store—rather than margarine. Butter is an excellent source of the fat soluble vitamins A, E, D and B vitamins including vitamin B12, as well as the essential fatty acid, arachidonic acid.

- **Fermented dairy products are easier to digest.** Fermentation partially breaks down lactose and it pre-digests casein. A mother who eats fermented dairy products may hope to see less milk sensitivity in herself and her infant[*].

- Imported cheese made from *raw* milk contains enzymes that make it easier to digest. Cheese is also easier to digest if it has not been cooked.

- Processed cheeses contain additives, including hydrogenized oil (trans-fats), and should be avoided.

- The moderate use of fermented dairy—such as kefir or probiotic yogurt—will help prevent milk intolerance and allergies in babies. But remember—low-supply mothers who eat a lot of yogurt *cold* from the fridge could possibly see a reduction in their supply (see pages 29-30).

In my research I came across references to traditional farmers giving galactagogues to cows. In Switzerland, farmers gave their dairy cows fennel and anise to increase their milk production. In Sweden, stinging nettle increased milk quantity and quality, producing rich, yellow butter. Why not give cows galactagogues that increase their milk supply *and* help boost their resistance to infection—such as nettle, dandelion, and sow's thistle?

---

[*] Live kefir grains can be found online, often for the cost of postage. Kefir is easier to make than yogurt (just set it up in a jug and the next day it is finished). It returns many healthy bacteria and enzymes to pasteurized milk, and it can be taken every day as a mildly detoxifying beverage.

Meat

I was a vegetarian for many years. Today I still do not eat much meat. I abhor the meat industry's exploitation of animals. I do eat some meat, however, (as much as possible from organic farmers) and I make sure that my children get a small but stable supply as well. Although I do not want to alienate vegetarian readers by appearing to be pro-meat, I do feel it is important to look at the positive aspects of animal protein in moderate amounts.

Many health experts today, such as Christine Northrup—who has been on the scene of natural medicine since its inception in the 1960s—have observed that vegetarians frequently, over time, develop problems such as food cravings, overweight, loss of hair, fatigue, and depression. The emphasis on grains, legumes (carbohydrates) and dairy in the vegetarian diet, and a potential deficiency in vitamin B12 and possibly in omega 3 derivatives in pure vegans, may slowly push one's metabolism off balance. This doesn't have to happen, but a vegetarian must be aware of these issues in order to prevent them. If you are following a vegetarian or vegan diet, be sure that you are properly informed and that you truly have the time and energy to invest in the preparation of meals.

The Mediterranean diet is held to be one of the healthiest in the world. In this diet people eat plenty of fruits, vegetables, olive oil, grains and legumes. They have a moderate intake of goat's milk products (much easier to digest than cow's milk). A few times a week they add a small portion of meat or fish to their meals. The Chinese diet, also one of the world's most healthy, follows the same scheme though without milk.

There is no getting around this simple fact: meat and eggs are a source of easily absorbable protein and include all of the amino acids, including all essential amino acids, in one package. While it is not necessary or healthful to eat a lot of animal protein, it can be an advantage to compliment one's diet with small amounts.

⇨ Animal fat contains concentrations of chemicals from agriculture. If you possibly can, find a source for organic, grass fed beef and lamb. Other good meat choices include bison, deer, antelope, duck, geese, pheasant, and wild turkey. Look for eggs from pastured poultry. They are available at many health food stores. In some neighborhoods in the US it has become fashionable to put up a chicken coop in the garden or even on a terrace. Perhaps your neighbor will share her eggs with you.

⇨ Avoid processed meats. Sausage, luncheon meats, and bacon are preserved with nitrates, nitrites, and other meat preservatives that are carcinogens.

Is Protein Lactogenic?

Mothers are frequently told to increase their intake of protein if they are having milk supply difficulties. Is protein lactogenic? One amino acid, tryptophan, is definitely lactogenic, and having sufficient protein may be helpful in itself. Animal protein that favors tryptophan (poultry, especially turkey) may be lactogenic.

There has been an ongoing debate the last forty years as to whether we need to take all the amino acids at one meal, or whether the body holds them in deposit like a bank account that we periodically refill even as we use it to pay our bills. There now seems to be agreement that although we do *not* need to ingest all the amino acids at one meal, we do need to get them all within one day in order for the body to properly utilize proteins.

- Amino acids are important for the upkeep of the body. They help keep the mood stable. They are also important for milk production. Some low-supply mothers see an increase in supply if they increase their intake of protein.

- Even a tired mother can find time to crack open a hard-boiled egg, spread cheese on crackers, or drape a slice of turkey on a piece of toast a couple times a day to cover her need for protein.

- If you are a vegetarian or vegan, be sure that you are knowledgeable about mixing and matching vegetables, legumes, grains, nuts and seeds throughout the day to ensure that you are getting a full compliment of protein.

- See above, *Grains and Legumes, As Protein.*

How Much Protein Do We Need?

If you eat in a way that keeps blood sugar stable, that is, three meals and three snacks at regular intervals each day, each consisting of a complex carbohydrate plus protein (meat or vegetable protein), *you will gradually get a sense for the kinds and amounts of protein and carbohydrates that work best* to keep your energy steady. This ratio may change again when you wean—you are eating now to meet the requirements of milk production.

Iron

Iron is essential in a mother's diet. Iron boosts a mother's energy and her mood, enhancing her ability to interact and bond with her baby. The iron from red meat is thought to be easily absorbed. The iron from vegetables is also well-absorbed (with the exception of iron from spinach), but you have to eat a lot of them to get enough iron. For devoted vegans and vegetarians, this is not a problem. And because vegetables contain a range of minerals, this is a good dietary measure in any case. See page 99 for sources of iron.

Vitamin B12

Vitamin B 12 is also an issue for vegetarians and *especially vegans*. B 12 can be obtained through daily portions of B 12 enriched nutritional yeast, but probably not reliably from spirulina or fermented soy products.

Sometimes the body looses the ability to metabolize B12 from food, in which case sub-lingual B 12, or injections, will direct the vitamin into the bloodstream.

Some signs of vitamin B 12 deficiency are:

- **In the mother**: reduced sensation or tingling in the limbs, memory problems, loss of balance.

- **In the baby**: weakness, drowsiness, lack of tendon reflexes, vomiting, difficulty swallowing, chronic constipation, and tremor.

⇨ Untreated, vitamin B 12 deficiency can cause irreversible nerve damage. Fortunately, symptoms can be reversed in the early stages by receiving proper administrations of B 12. See your doctor *promptly* for treatment.

Fish: Mercury, Amalgam Fillings

Researchers in heavy metal toxicity warn that fish of all kinds are becoming increasingly contaminated with mercury, a potent neuro-toxin, as well as with industrial toxins such as polychlorinated biphenyls (PCBs).

In this section, we'll focus on mercury. Fish themselves can generally tolerate high concentrations of mercury in their tissues and fat. Not so humans. Recent observations from Japan surprised scientists and lay-persons alike: mercury concentration in whale meat is now so high that a single serving taken by a pregnant woman could cause birth defects[55].

Fish are frequently consumed by mothers for protein. In fact, some mothers rely so heavily on fish that they are at a loss as to what else they can take for protein. It seems to me that in the light of the contamination of dairy, meat, and fish today, all people should learn about alternative sources for protein, i.e., combinations of grains, legumes, nuts and seeds (see above.)

Mercury poisoning is an issue in most people's lives. Most of us have had dental fillings of amalgam (50% mercury), or our mothers or grandmothers had amalgam fillings. Mercury is changed into the highly toxic methyl mercury by bacteria in our intestines. From there, it is absorbed into the bloodstream and is stored in fat tissue and nerve cells. Mercury is passed from mother to child through the placenta. Mercury may also affect the DNA in sperm. Dietrich Klinghardt, M.D., an expert in heavy metal toxicity, estimates that it requires two generations of mercury-free mothers and fathers for the effect of mercury to wear off.

There is an ongoing debate today as to the effect of mercury in vaccines on autism in children. Although the jury is still out, a significant number of parents have seen improvement in their children's hyperactivity, concentration deficits, developmental issues and autistic syndromes after chelating mercury and other metals from their bodies (and brains). It is said in medicine that the cure can point to the disease. If chelating (removing) heavy metals improves neural integrity in children, then heavy metals clearly are a contributing factor in these syndromes.

Mercury poisoning is thought to be a contributing factor in food allergies. Also, *candidiasis*, or fungal overgrowth of the intestine and body, flourishes on heavy metal toxicity. Interestingly, food allergies and fungal overgrowth are frequently associated with children who are hyperactive, who have learning problems, delayed development and also autistic syndromes. Surely no coincidence!

About Fish

The Food and Drug Administration (FDA) recently put out a warning for pregnant and breastfeeding mothers. They should avoid swordfish, king mackerel, shark, and tilefish, as these have the highest concentration of methyl mercury in their tissue.

Other agencies objected to this guideline. The National Academy of Science said that it would set the limit four times higher and that the list should be longer, to prevent possible neurological deficiencies in children.

The Environmental Working Group and the United States Public Interest Research Group Education Fund reported that the FDA is encouraging consumption of seafood with dangerous levels of mercury: tuna (in the form of steaks), sea bass, oysters from the Gulf of Mexico, marlin, halibut, pike, walleye, white croaker, and largemouth bass. They recommend that pregnant and breastfeeding women not eat more than one meal a month of canned tuna, mahi-mahi, blue mussels, Eastern oysters, cod, pollock, Great Lakes salmon, blue crab from the Gulf of Mexico, wild channel catfish, or lake whitefish.

The Environmental Working Group also named fish that are low in methyl mercury and therefore *supposedly* safe to eat, including trout, farmed catfish, fish sticks (which are usually made from fish with low mercury), summer flounder, wild Pacific salmon, croaker, mid-Atlantic blue crab, and haddock. Shrimp is on the list, too, though the report says that there are serious environmental concerns related to shrimp farming practices[56]. Also, be wary of farmed fish if there is any question of contamination from local industry.

These agencies are all ignoring a crucial fact, however. Since metallic mercury is changed into toxic methyl mercury in the human intestine, these suggestions really do not help mothers make the decisions they need to make.

The decision to eat fish depends entirely on a mother's certainty that the fish comes from waters that are free of contamination. Since most of us cannot be sure of this, fish is not recommended for most of us.

Now, even though mercury from fish presents a clear danger, most of the mercury that enters our body, and our milk, is leeched from amalgam fillings in our teeth. Higher levels of mercury are leeched out of amalgam fillings when we chew gum or drink very hot beverages. It's therefore a good idea to take beverages at a cooler temperature, and to find ways to get over a gum habit.

As you see from the above, at the present time there are no clear, reliable guidelines on fish for pregnant and breastfeeding mothers. Experts in heavy metal toxicity, such as Dr. Klinghardt, advise pregnant and breastfeeding mothers to avoid fish altogether. A few outspoken medical doctors, such as Dr. Jay Gordon, a breastfeeding advocate, also say that fish are too great a risk for the benefit, and should not be eaten[57]. Nutritionists generally advise taking only young, cold-water deep-sea fish that come from unpolluted waters.

With all this uncertainty, thank goodness for inexpensive, molecular-filtered cod-liver oil or fish oil that provides the brain-building essential fatty acids we need from fish. Vegans may take supplements of DHA and EPA derived from algae.

CHAPTER TEN

About Supplements

This chapter provides general information about the use of vitamin and mineral supplements in the postpartum with a focus on calcium, since calcium has been seen to affect milk supply.

Calcium and Magnesium

Calcium and magnesium work together to maintain healthy nerves, strong muscles, and a rhythmic heartbeat. In the brain, they promote neural activity and act as a natural antidepressant. A lack of calcium and magnesium can lead to insomnia, irritability, exhaustion, mental confusion, heart rhythm problems, and depression, among other difficulties, in adults. In children, a lack of these minerals has been implicated in allergic and behavioral disorders, according to Leo Galland, MD, who provides guidelines for treatment in *Superimmunity for Kids*.

Calcium and magnesium may also be crucial to maintaining a good supply of milk in some women. More on this below.

It is recommended that we supplement these minerals together, in a ratio of two or three times as much calcium as magnesium, or 2-3:1. Some experts, however, suggest we supplement on a ratio of 1:1, as so many people are sorely deficient in magnesium.

1000 mg of calcium is the daily requirement—1200 mg for breastfeeding women—in the US. However, in spite of a diet rich in calcium-fortified foods, many adult women are deficient in calcium.

Remarkably, people around the world get far less calcium than we do. 400 – 600 mg of calcium per day is the norm. Even so, there are seldom signs of calcium deficiency in cultures that have maintained their traditional whole-foods diet. Look at pictures of native peoples before industrialization hit their cultures: their jaws are wide enough for their broad, white teeth, and they rarely had cavities[*].

The reason Americans lack calcium is not because we take too little milk, but because our diet causes calcium to be leeched from our bones and teeth. (More on this below.) We can easily make better use of our daily, non-dairy calcium intake by improving our dietary habits.

Foods that Deplete Calcium:

- **Fibrous bulk** is sometimes taken to reduce appetite and to promote regular bowel movements. Minerals bind to this fiber in the intestine, so that they pass through the intestine rather than into the bloodstream.

- **Protein**. We often eat meals that are too heavy on protein (meat, eggs, milk). Excess protein is acid-forming. In order to protect tissues in the body from acidity, the body uses calcium to neutralize the acid. This is another reason that a high-protein diet can lead to a depletion of calcium.

- **Diuretics**. Foods and medication that stimulate the kidney will cause minerals, including calcium, to be excreted into the urine. Herbal diuretics, such as nettle and dandelion, restore the minerals that they cause to be lost. Excessive *protein* will

---

[*]See Weston A. Price's *Nutrition and Physical Degeneration* for photographic documentation of the teeth of indigenous peoples, before and after they began eating a diet of refined foods.

also cause the kidneys to go into overdrive and will lead to a loss of calcium.

- **Caffeine** causes calcium to be excreted with urine. Caffeine is found in *coffee, tea, chocolate,* and most *carbonated beverages.*
- Excessive **salt** also causes calcium to be excreted with urine.
- **Phosphorus** has to be in *the right balance* for calcium metabolism to work. *Too little* phosphorus prevents the body from using calcium. *Too much* and the excess phosphorus binds to calcium, pulling it right out of the bones.
- Foods that are high in phosphorus are: *dairy, meat, white flour,* and carbonated *soft drinks.* These foods cause calcium to be pulled out of the bones—which is why people who eat meat regularly need to supplement with higher dosages of calcium.
- **Sugar** decreases phosphorus in the blood. After eating *sugar,* phosphorus is so low that the body is unable to utilize calcium.

Keep Calcium in Your Bones

- Reduce caffeine, white sugar, and table salt. Most people overdose on sugar and salt in processed foods, snacks, candy, and junk foods. Use natural sugar sources that are rich in minerals, such as blackstrap molasses, malt syrup, maple syrup or honey, and where possible, take sea salt.
- Limit animal protein—roughly three small to moderate servings a day—balanced with vegetables, grains, legumes, and fruit.
- Sunlight. Twenty minutes of sunlight a day provide the vitamin D necessary to utilize calcium. This is important to mothers who may stay mostly indoors with their newborn babies. Sit close to a sunlit window with a lot of skin exposed, and get out into the sun as often as possible.

- A supplement of 400 IU of vitamin D daily may be valuable if you live in an area with little sunlight. Better yet—get your vitamin D from cod-liver oil or egg yolks.

The following non-dairy lactogenic foods are high in calcium, listed from highest to lowest.

Nuts and Seeds:
Sesame seeds, almonds, sunflower seeds, pecans, cashews.

Vegetables:
Lamb's quarters, collard greens, turnip greens, mustard greens, Swiss chard, okra, kale, dandelion greens, green beans, asparagus, peas, broccoli, watercress, cabbage, spinach, artichoke, avocado, carrot.

Rice, Grains, and Legumes:
Navy beans, pinto beans, garbanzo beans (chick pea), kidney beans, wild rice, whole brown rice.

Seaweed:
Wakame, Irish moss, kelp, agar.

Other sources:
Blackstrap molasses, orange juice (calcium fortified).

To ensure that your calcium intake is sufficient, compliment your diet with blackstrap molasses, use tahini as a spread (crushed sesame seeds in sesame oil), and sprinkle gomasio (roasted, crushed sesame seeds with salt) on your veggies and salad.

Calcium as a Galactagogue

Preventing the Premenstrual Dip in Supply

Lactogenic foods tend to be high in calcium. It would seem that calcium has a positive effect on breastfeeding. Even the Greek doctor, Dioscorides, was aware of the calcium-connection. He tells the following story in his herbal compendium from 70 AD.

On a certain Island near Greece, local shepherds discovered that if they ground a calcium-rich stone into powder, stirred this into water, and gave it to their sheep to drink, their sheep produced more milk. (They probably saw their sheep licking the stone, and thought they would help the sheep get a larger dosage.) Well, when their wives saw how much more milk the sheep produced, they decided to try the beverage, too, with the result, so Dioscorides, that they also made more milk.

We know that calcium supplementation does not increase calcium levels in breastmilk, nor does it increase a mother's bone density while breastfeeding (that will increase later on and become more dense than in bones of women who do not breastfeed). Is it possible that calcium helps women make more milk?

We do know that calcium ties into women's hormone production, though we are not sure exactly how this works. Significantly, calcium supplements can relieve symptoms of PMS if taken over a span of several months—and it turns out that women with PMS truly do have difficulties metabolizing calcium during the latter half of their cycles.

Well, an observant lactation consultant, Patricia Gima, IBCLC, made a remarkable discovery in this connection. It's fairly common for breastfeeding mothers who have begun to menstruate to see a drop in their milk supply during the two weeks before their period. Thinking that this might be related to their impaired calcium metabolism (see above), Gima suggested that these mothers take supplements of calcium and magnesium during that time. It worked: the mothers' milk supply became stable.

Patricia Gima suggests:

200 mg calcium, 3 times per day, before meals.

100 mg magnesium, 3 times per day, after meals.

Mothers who consume a lot of meat and dairy may need to take up to double this amount, or 200 mg calcium and 100 mg of magnesium, 5 or 6 times a day.

Calcium and Lactogenic Foods and Herbs

As previously mentioned, calcium is found in almost all lactogenic foods and herbs. Green leafy vegetables, peas, green beans, legumes, chicken soup, almonds, and especially sesame seeds, are all excellent sources for calcium. Nettle is the herb highest in calcium, and as a medicinal herb it can be taken every day without danger.

One cup of sesame seeds contains 1400 mg of calcium—that's more than the US daily requirement. Indeed, sesame seeds are renowned as a galactagogue. The seeds should be roasted and crushed (gomasio), boiled, or taken in the form of sesame butter (tahini). Taken whole, the seeds slip through the intestines and their nutrients are not absorbed—even if their hulls have been removed.

In Mediterranean countries, mothers use tahini, or sesame butter, to support their milk production. They add tahini to hummus (garbanzo bean spread). In Asia, roasted or boiled sesame seeds are taken.

⇨ **Allergy warning**. Nuts and seeds are common allergens, especially peanut and sesame. Mothers who have allergies or food sensitivities, or whose families have allergies or food sensitivities, should avoid eating nuts and seeds on a regular basis during pregnancy and lactation, so that the baby does not become sensitized to them.

Nutritional Supplements

Many American women are somewhat deficient in vitamins, minerals, and trace elements. For this reason, most experts suggest that mothers take supplements while pregnant and breastfeeding, when our nutritional needs increase. Supplementing is not a substitute for a good diet, however, and supplements are best absorbed in combination with good food.

Supplementing can be tricky. Because vitamins and minerals compete with each other for absorption, taking large amounts of one vitamin or mineral can lead to a depletion of others. Not only that, but high dosages of one nutrient can actually lead to *less* absorption of that particular nutrient as the body says, "Enough is enough!"

Many mothers are wise when it comes to supplements, and have researched and found products that work for them. When health issues are involved, however, it is best to seek the guidance of a healthcare provider who is skilled in nutritional medicine.

Prenatals and Zinc Deficiency

Breastfeeding experts say that mothers may continue to take their prenatal vitamins after birth. Prenatals contain a well-balanced ratio of nutrients, with additional levels for the special needs of pregnancy. Although these levels are different during lactation, the difference isn't significant enough to make the supplement inappropriate.

It is widely thought however that the high iron contained in some prenatal supplements could be harmful. This is because iron competes with zinc in the intestine for absorption. Zinc is important for a fully functioning immune system and for the development of a baby's brain. If iron prevents the absorption of zinc, the body's stores of zinc may become depleted over time, leading to immunity deficiencies and perhaps also to developmental and behavioral problems in the baby.

⇨ If your prenatal contains iron, or if you are supplementing with iron, take an additional supplement of zinc at a different time during the day, to counterbalance the zinc-depleting effect of iron.

⇨ Recent studies indicate that taking additional iron in early pregnancy may benefit the baby, even in mothers who are not anemic. In this case, be sure to take zinc as described above.

In *Superimmunity for Kids* (1989), Dr. Leo Galland states that zinc deficiency is a common problem resulting from prenatal supplements. In this book he provides a well-balanced plan for nutritional supplements during pregnancy and lactation. This is a book that every mother should have, regardless of whether she breastfeeds or formula-feeds, and women looking for a closely defined supplemental plan will find it here.

Food sources for zinc include red meat, legumes, nuts, and seeds (especially sunflower seeds).

Supplementing with Iron

Iron supplements are famous for causing constipation during pregnancy. It would be wise to try to boost one's iron by using natural sources, such as herbs and foods, before resorting to a supplement.

Food sources for iron include red meat and dairy, green leafy vegetables (iron is not easily absorbed from spinach), dried beans and peas, and nuts and seeds. A great source of iron is freshly pressed red beet juice or red beet in any form.

Tips to Taking Supplements

- **Absorption.** Supplements are best absorbed in small dosages, taken before a meal or snack. Taking supplements between meals may cause them to pass through the intestines unabsorbed.
- **Prenatal supplements.** If you continue to take your prenatal supplement, break it into smaller dosages and take it throughout the day before meals. Take an extra dosage of zinc with a snack if your prenatal supplement contains iron.
- **Essential fatty acids** are taken before meals. Experts suggest you also take vitamin E, (100 IU per capsule of EFA) to clean up the free radicals released from the EFAs. Vitamin E is taken after a meal.
- **Timing.** If you take vitamins separately, water-soluble vitamins are taken before meals (C, B-complex), and fat-soluble vitamins are taken after a meal (A, E, D).

Iron absorption is improved when a person's diet includes vegetables and fruit that provide vitamin C.

Large dosage supplements of vitamin C however can damage the iron in the bloodstream, leading to 'rust.'

Calcium and magnesium can be taken together, but for best absorption they should be taken at different times of the day. They can be taken before a meal or between meals. Calcium, taken right before bedtime, is relaxing and helps people fall asleep more quickly.

- **Dosage**. Daily requirements of vitamins are set at a level that prevents illness from occurring. Doctors specializing in nutritional healing maintain that this dose is too low. We not only want to prevent disease, they say, we want to build nutritional reserves that will help buffer us from stress, and from the daily assault of pollution on the body.

These nutritional doctors maintain that we can double or even triple the daily requirement, without danger. *Nutritional Healing*, or *orthomolecular medicine*, as large-dose supplementation is called, may correct chronic health problems or prevent degenerative health problems from occurring.

It is important to consult a doctor of nutritional medicine if you are considering taking supplements to treat health issues. Designing your own supplemental program can be dangerous and lead to more deficiencies.

⇨ Do not take supplements of amino acids, as these directly influence brain chemistry (as does aspartame which is comprised of one amino acid). The chemistry of lactation is sensitive to interference.

⇨ Do not overdose on **vitamin B 6** as it may reduce milk supply! Up to 200 mg per day is a dosage that most mothers can tolerate.

⇨ Be sure to get folic acid, before conception and throughout pregnancy and lactation. (Take daily portions of salad, green herbs, or supplement.)

⇨ As explained in *Get Your Fats Right*, supplementing with healthy fats and essential fatty acids may be one of the best ways to support your milk supply and improve the quality of your milk.

Part Two

Milk Supply Difficulties, Then and Now

CHAPTER ELEVEN

Ancient Remedies

Around the world, women wisely use lactogenic foods and herbs to support their milk production. Only in the West was this wisdom temporarily lost. Today, mothers again work together with their lactation specialists and doctors to understand how herbs and foods can enhance their experience of breastfeeding and motherhood. We are creating new traditions, and mothers again have the option of encountering breastfeeding issues, and their baby's food sensitivities, with herbs and dietary changes.

The loss of this knowledge is centuries old. It ties in to the plight of European midwives who were knowledgeable in the use of herbal medicine, including herbs to prevent pregnancy, herbs for abortion, herbs for birth, for convalescence, and for breastfeeding. In an attempt to disempower women from birth control strategies, midwives were forbidden under punishment of death to prescribe any herb at all. The intention to limit the scope of midwives has extended into our times. About eighty years ago, schools of midwifery in central Europe again required midwifes to promise that they would not prescribe herbal medicine. Herbs for milk production were forbidden as well.

Luckily, lactogenic traditions are persistent. Today across Europe, mothers still use herbs and food to support their milk supply, such as oatmeal, fennel tea, Rivella, malt, and beer (mostly non-alcoholic beer). Commercial lactation teas, homeopathic remedies, and herbal massage oil for the mother's breasts are sold in most pharmacies.

Today in the US, lactation teas, tinctures, and homeopathic remedies are available in various stores as well as online. Lactation specialists may suggest that—only if necessary—a mother support her milk supply by taking herbs such as fenugreek, goat's rue, alfalfa leaf and blessed thistle, plus oatmeal, nutritional yeast, protein, green-juices and green-drinks, supplemental oils, and calcium/magnesium supplements.

In the following sections, I explore the ways that breastfeeding difficulties are perceived and treated within three ancient traditions of medicine. Perhaps we can learn from these cultures, and borrow or adapt some of their remedies and recipes for our use. Unfortunately, the medical traditions of Native America, Africa, and the South Pacific are beyond the scope of this book. Maybe next time!

OUR GREEK ROOTS

The ancient Greeks thought of both breastmilk and semen as a *sublimation*, or higher quality, of blood – an apt description since both fluids are indeed nourished and derived from blood. The health of the organs that clean and nourish the blood were therefore thought to be instrumental to the digestibility of breastmilk, as will become clearer in the discussion of Ayurvedic medicine.

Surprisingly, many of the lactogenic foods and herbs that are used today across the US and Europe today were recorded in a book titled "The Material of Medicine," written 2,000 years ago by a Greek doctor named Dioscorides. Dioscorides traveled with the Roman Legions as a military doctor. He was in a unique position to study and compile information about medical methods from all over the Ancient World. His six books contain over 1,000 different plants, oils, resins, minerals, wines, and animal parts.

Dioscorides made detailed records of women's medicine, including remedies for abortion, menstruation, cancer of the breast and womb, and for breastfeeding problems. Although his books were copied countless times through the centuries, herbals written centuries later tended to omit medicinals for women—including the foods and herbs used to support breastfeeding[*].

There are thirty medicinals for lactation in Dioscorides' great work. Six are for increasing milk, thirteen are to "bring down" the milk, one is to keep the milk "fresh", three are for mastitis, six for engorgement, one to "extinguish" milk-production, and one to re-lactate after milk has been extinguished.

Increasing Milk Supply

To increase milk supply, Dioscorides suggests five medicinals: barley-water; chickpea; astragalus; fig-wine; and chalk-stone.

Barley-water is made by simmering a small amount of barley in plenty of water, and then straining off and drinking the water. It can also be made by cooking a small amount of barley flour in water. In England, barley-water is still used today for conditions of the liver, intestines and stomach, to soothe the nerves, for congestion of the lungs, and for fever. It is said that when a mother drinks barley water, her milk will soothe a baby's digestion.

Dioscorides says: "Barley is best which is white and clean..., yet Ptissana (barley-water) is more nourishing than barley flour by reason of the cream that comes off it in the seething.... It does also cause abundance of milk, being sod together with fennel seed and so supt up."

You'll find a recipe for barley-water in the beverages section.

Chickpea, of all the legumes, contains the very highest levels of a nutrient called inositol. Inositol functions in nerve transmission, in the regulation of enzyme activity and in the transportation of fats within the body. It is also important to the metabolism of calcium, acts as an anti-depressant, and can improve the transmission of neural signals in individuals afflicted with diabetic nerve damage and numbness.

---

[*] An exception is the British physician Culpeper, whose herbal from the early 17th century includes most of Dioscorides' galactagogues.

Low-supply mothers have seen true support with chickpeas. It is most commonly prepared as hummus, a delicious paste used in Mideastern cooking.

Dioscorides says that sprouted chickpea will help "breed milk." Chickpea is also prescribed in an ancient herbal from Egypt: "For the breasts so that they give milk: Take 'falcon's eye' and cook it. The patients are to drink the liquid first, then eat the rest."

Astragalus (sp.): "The tea from leaves, being drunk, is thought to cause more milk." (The root is used as a galactagogue in China and India.)

Fig-wine is made by allowing dried, black figs to ferment in a flask for ten days, covered by "an infusion of the husks and stones of grapes new-pressed." Sometimes fennel and thyme are added to the brew. On the eleventh day, the 'wine' is poured off.

Dioscorides says: "The wine ... draws down the menses, and makes milk abundant...."

Calcium: Melitites Lithos. Honey-stone. Sweet Chalk.

Dioscorides recommends **powdered chalk,** dissolved in vinegar and water, to increase milk in both animals and women. He writes: "The milk of goats and of sheep being extinguished, if any beat the chalk stone small, mixing it with brine (salt water used in pickling), it helps the little flock. They say that it can do the same to women for the breeding of milk, being beaten and drank...."

There is evidence today that calcium supplementation will stabilize milk production (see page 153). Not surprisingly, most lactogenic herbs and foods contain high levels of calcium.

Triggering Milk Flow (the Milk-Ejection Reflex)

Dioscorides provides us with thirteen medicinals for the let-down: vitex (chaste-tree berries), hollyhock, sow-thistle, lettuce, basil, garden fennel, wild fennel, anise, dill, black seed (Nigella sativa), white briony, black swallowwort, echion.

Vitex Agnus-castus. Chaste-tree berries. Dioscorides says: the fruit of it, being drunk, "brings down the milk."

Today there is some debate about chaste-tree's effect on milk production.

No studies, however, have been done on the freshly pressed juice of the berries, as prescribed by Dioscorides.

For more information, see *A Lactogenic Herbal*, in Part Four.

Malve. **Hollyhock**. Malva silvertips. Alcea rosea. The broth of the plant, cooked together with the roots, "brings out milk." The hollyhock is the marshmallow's cultivated cousin. Marshmallow is traditionally used by Native Americans as a galactagogue. It is widely used in the US as a galactagogue today, often in combination with fenugreek, blessed thistle, or red clover flowers. For more information, see *A Lactogenic Herbal* in Part Four.

Sow's thistle. Sonchus arvensis, Sonchus oleraceus. Also known as 'hare's lettuce.' The juice "draws down the milk." This common 'weed' was brought over to the US by the pilgrims, along with other lactogenic plants such as the dandelion and a variety of thistles. In South America it was immediately lifted to the status of a holy plant, said to give stamina to those who chewed on its leaves. Today, sow's thistle is still used as a galactagogue in the Mediterranean, where it is eaten as salad. Sow's Thistle is also recommended by Nicholas Culpeper, who included most of Dioscorides' galactagogues in his herbal from the early 17th century.

Lettuce. Lactuca Sativa (BK. II, 165.) Dioscorides writes that lettuce, when eaten, "draws down of milk," but that cooked lettuce is more nourishing. Culpeper, the British physician of the early 17th century, writes that wet-nurses took boiled lettuce to increase their supply.

Native Americans use several species of wild lettuce to support milk production. Lettuce is used as a galactagogue in China as well.

Basil. Ocymum basilicum. Being eaten, basil "calls out the milk." Basil has been used throughout Europe as a galactagogue into recent times. It is estrogenic and relaxing. Both the dried and the fresh herb are delicious in salads and in tomato sauce.

Garden fennel. Foeniculum vulgare. "The herb itself (whole plant), if eaten, is of force to draw down milk, as is the seed being drank, or cooked together with barley-water."

Tall, **wild fennel**. Prangos ferulacea. "The decoction of the leaves brings out milk, and cleanses women after childbirth."

Anise. Pimpinella Anisum. "The seeds, being drunk, draw down the milk."

Dill. Anethum graveolens. "*Decoction* of the seeds and 'hair' (fine leaves), draws down the milk." The same preparation is used today in India for difficult milk-supply problems.

Black Seed. **Nigella sativa**. "Being drunk for many days together, it drives out the menses, the urine and the milk."

Black Swallowwort. "**Kirkaia**," Cynancum nigrum, (BK. III, 134.) "The seed, taken in liquors to be supt, draws down the milk."

White Bryony. Bruonia Ampelos Leuke. "The fruit of it being juiced, and supped up with sodden wheat, does draw out milk."

Echium. Echium rubrum. The root, leaves and flowers of the echion, taken with wine, draws down the milk. (This is a relative of borage, also used as a galactagogue.)

Soothing the Symptoms of Engorgement

Dioscorides gives us six medicinals for engorgement, or milk-clots: lentils, celery, castor oil plant, ocean-water, "Trux."

Lentils. Ervum Lens. "Being sod in sea-water, and so applied, does help swollen breasts, and the curdling of milk in women's breasts." One would probably apply it warm, as specified in the sea-water remedy below.

Garden celery. Ranunculus repens, Apium graveolens. "The herb of it, (leaves), being applied with flour of barley, slacks breasts swollen with *clotted* milk." It is not clear if Dioscorides means to prepare a decoction of celery leaves, and add barley-flour to get a paste that can be applied to the breasts, or if he means to actually use the leaves. (Today, we use leaves of cabbage to relieve breast swelling.)

Castor oil plant. Ricinus communis. "The leaves, bruised with the flour of barley, assuage edema and do abate milk-swollen breasts, when laid on by itself or with vinegar." Castor oil preparations are still used today, externally, to treat breast inflammation.

Sea-water. "Mixed with barley flour, being fomented on warm (applied as a poultice), it draws to, and dissolves, being good for... breasts swollen with milk...."

Trux (dregs at the bottom of wine). "Being anointed on with vinegar, it slacks swollen breasts that run out with milk."

Peppermint: A poultice with barley flour, laid on the breasts, soothes swollen or engorged breasts.

Keeping Milk Fresh (in the breasts of wet-nurses)

Beeswax: ten portions, each the size of a barley grain, are taken to prevent the milk in the breasts of wet-nurses from curdling. In other words, milk that is not emptied in a timely manner may change its taste. This remedy is supposed to prevent that. (No idea if it works!)

Soothing Inflammation

Dioscorides provides three medicinals for inflammation and breast infection:

Walnut, Greek Bean, Grapes

Walnut. Juglans regia (BK. 1, 178.) "The nuts, laid, with a little honey and rue, upon inflamed breasts."

Greek bean. Vicia Faba (Bk. II, 127.) "The flour of the dried bean, applied as a cataplasm, "helps swelling and inflamed ducts, and extinguishes milk." Similar bean preparations are used in India. Rarely, in extreme cases of mastitis, it is necessary to "extinguish" milk production temporarily. Dioscorides also provides a remedy for re-lactation.

Grapes. The refuse after pressing (for wine-making), is applied with salt for inflammations, and hardnesses, and swelling of the ducts."

Suppressing Milk Production

Dioscorides gives us one remedy specifically to suppress milk-production. It is made with hemlock. The remedy is applied externally only—it could be fatal if taken internally.

Hemlock. Conium maculatum. "The herb and hair (leaves), being beaten small and smeared on, does drive away milk and forbids the breasts to grow great in time of virginity." This remedy suggests that the Greeks had breast-growth inhibiting drugs, to help girls meet the small-breasted standard of Greek beauty, just as today we have breast-growth enhancing herbal products (which are comprised of galactagogues), to help girls meet our culture's large-breasted ideal.

Re-lactation

Dioscorides also gives us a remedy with which to re-lactate after milk has been extinguished.

Astragalus glaux. "This being sodden with barley meal, and salt and oil, and supt up, does call back again the milk that was extinguished."

Species of astragalus are used in China to support milk production. A great tonic and immunity booster, astragalus brings a mother's body into balance and into full production. Dioscorides recommends that it be prepared as a thin gruel with barley flour, salt and oil.

FROM AN EGYPTIAN HERBAL

Lise Manniche, author of several books on Egyptian culture, studied an herbal from Egypt written at about the same period as Dioscorides work. Although written by Christian Copts living in Egypt, she believes it contains medical traditions common to the geographical area.

Galactagogues from this herbal are: sesame seed, chickpea, garlic, cucumber plant leaves.

Sesame seeds, to increase milk production, the seeds are boiled and eaten – a lactogenic recipe still used in India today. (Boiling makes the minerals in sesame seed more easily accessible for digestion.)

Chickpea. "For the breasts so that they give milk: Take 'falcon's eye' and cook it. The patients are to drink the liquid first, and then eat the rest."

Garlic. "Take dried garlic; boil it in wine. The patient is to drink of it for three days in the bath."

The leaves of the **cucumber plant**. "Take the leaves, sprinkle with salt and place on the breasts. They will become full of milk."

TRADITIONS IN TURKEY

Turkey has a rich history of herbal medicine that reflects the traditions of the greater Mediterranean region. Prof. Dr. Iclal Saracoglu from Istanbul kindly looked into the traditional galactagogues. She found galactagogues recorded in herbals, and also recorded in the memory of her mother and her mother's friends. Her findings confirm that lactogenic traditions were varied and strong up until her mother's generation—women who gave birth in the 1940s and 1950s.

Foods: barley-water, Jerusalem artichoke, malt-syrup, tahini (sesame paste), lettuce (plant and seeds), garlic, and salad made of the leaves of the sow's thistle.

Herbals: common milkwort (decoctions of the roots), black seed (Nigella sativa), goat's rue, caraway, anise, dill, and fennel seeds.

A special remedy, (recalled by the women of her mother's generation), *if the milk does not arrive*, eat one raw, white bulb of a spring onion per day for a week[*].

---

[*] Onions in southern Europe are juicy and sweet.

CHAPTER TWELVE

Classical Medical Traditions of Asia

Ayurvedic Wisdom from India

Ayurvedic medicine has its beginnings in an oral tradition of healing and ritual that is thousands of years old. At about 900 BC, university doctors in major Indus cities were conducting empirical experiments in surgery and herbal medicine. These doctors are widely believed to have written textbooks that documented their discoveries. While these original books are lost to history, their future revisions became the foundation of Ayurvedic medicine in India.

The earliest extant revision was written by a doctor named Caraka in the first century BC. Caraka provided a system that divided herbs into fifty closely defined therapeutic effects. Two of these are for lactation: to increase milk production, and to cleanse the milk.

To increase milk supply, Caraka suggests herbals that are digestive tonics and estrogenic: "Satavari," fennel and dill. (Satavari is the folk-name for "Asparagus Racemosus.")

To clean the milk, Caraka suggests herbs that flush out toxins from a mother's body by dilating blood vessels, stimulating the kidneys and supporting the liver: "Guduci," ginger, and dandelion. (Guduci is the folk-name for "lotus stalk.")

Three Personality Types and Their Breastfeeding Problems

Ayurveda describes three basic types or "constitutions" for all people: airy, *vatta*; fiery, *pitta,* and earthy, *kapha.*

The airy, *vatta*-constitution woman (intellectual, artistic, creative) is the least 'vital' of the three. She tends to suffer from mood swings and is prone to nervous exhaustion. Vatta-women are said to most commonly have low milk supply, but it's also said that all women tend to become 'vatta,' or prone to nervous exhaustion, after birth. That's why Ayurveda prescribes a vatta-strengthening diet for all women in the postpartum.

Briefly, a vatta diet favors cooked food over raw, and sweet, sour and salty foods, over pungent and astringent foods.

The fiery pitta-woman can also have breastfeeding difficulties. She leads a highly-active life, and enjoys spicy food and alcohol. She may wear down her digestive organs and liver leading to 'ama,' or toxins in the blood—a condition that Ayurveda links to milk-insufficiency as well as to colic in the baby.

The kapha-woman does not have breastfeeding problems. Calm and down to earth with large, sweet eyes, her body-chemistry is even keel. However, in the West, the kapha type may be prone to lethargy, apathy, or depression when she finds herself isolated at home. Depression makes everything, including breastfeeding, seem like it's just too much to bear, sometimes causing kapha-imbalanced women to stop nursing.

Finally, most of us don't fit into one 'type,' but are a mixture of two or even all three types. It's best to think of the types as serving to broadly define a scope of potential health issues: nervous problems, digestive problems, and emotional problems. If that 'side' of us is out of balance, we suffer problems in that area. If a woman does tend strongly to be one particular type, she is most likely to have the health issues defined by that type, according to Ayurveda.

Suggestions from Ayurvedic wisdom:

- To avoid 'vatta-imbalance,' all women after birth should eat a 'vatta-balancing' diet, favoring naturally sweet and salty foods and avoiding pungent (sharply spiced) and astringent (drying) foods.

- Massages with oil, given to mothers and their babies, can help overcome the stress from birth.

- To avoid 'pitta-imbalance,' women should have household help that they can rely on. They should let go of as many responsibilities as possible and learn to relax and rest. Pitta women should not overdo spicy foods.

- To avoid 'kapha-imbalance' women after birth should be able to count on company and emotional support. They should not overdo sweets.

Ayurvedic Explanations for Low Milk Supply

Ayurveda sees milk production and milk quality as being dependent upon the quality of the blood. The blood is purified by 'agni,' the digestive fire, located in the liver. Hence, the proper functioning of intestines and the liver is essential to milk production (many galactagogues are good herbs for the intestines and liver). In my personal correspondence with Dr. Prof. Subhash Ranade, an international authority on Ayurveda, I learned that Ayurvedic doctors in India have observed that women who suffer from lack of breast milk after delivery also commonly suffer from dysfunction of the intestines or liver.

Broadly speaking then there are two main causes of milk-supply problems: nervous exhaustion, or vatta imbalance, and toxic conditions, 'ama,' or pitta imbalance. For the first, tonifying and relaxing herbs are prescribed, such as Satavari, fennel, or dill; for the second, herbs to detoxify the blood and support the liver are prescribed, such as the lotus stalk, ginger and dandelion.

Ayurvedic wisdom suggests that all women after birth drink warm beverages made with warming herbs, and eat warm meals, avoiding foods that tend to aggravate coldness, such as cold beverages, ice-cream, astringent foods, and raw vegetables.

Ayurveda also stresses detoxification after birth, both for a mother's health and for her ability to produce milk. Oil massage is used to pull toxins out of the body. Self-massage in the morning with sesame oil, followed by a warm shower that removes the oil (and the toxins in the oil) is prescribed for the mother during the first months after birth. Mothers may receive intensive oil-massages for several weeks after birth. (Massage, in itself, is a great support for milk production.)

Ayurvedic Remedies in the Postpartum

For reducing gas and constipation (and supporting milk production):

Put 1/2 teaspoon whole fennel seeds and 1/2 teaspoon whole fenugreek seeds in two quarts of water. Boil for five to ten minutes. Drink warm throughout the day.

Promoting healthy, rich breast milk:

Snack on almonds, coconut and sesame seeds.

Have one to two cups daily of boiled milk (or milk substitute) with a pinch of saffron, one-eighth teaspoon cardamom, one-eighth teaspoon ginger, and add brown sugar to taste. Also add one-half teaspoon ghee (clarified butter) if desired.

To increase milk production:

Foods to favor: rice; warm rice pudding with milk and sugar; pumpkin; sunflower seeds; black seeds (Nigella sativa) and sesame seeds.

A half-cup of boiled sesame seeds, once a day.

I would like here to thank Dr. Vinod Verma, the woman's Ayurvedic expert, who has provided the following remedies.

To support milk production:

50 grams each of: cress seeds, fenugreek seeds, black seed (Nigella sativa), lovage seed, cumin, and asparagus racemosus. Pulverize, and mix with honey into a paste. Take 1 – 1 1/2 teaspoons three times a day. Or add 1- 1 1/2 teaspoons to mung-bean flour and cook into a thin gruel.

To increase a mother's sexual energy after birth:

A pinch of saffron added to warm milk, or to a thin gruel made with flour and milk. Take twice a day, the first 40 days after birth.

The baby is upset:

If the baby cries and appears not to like the milk, the mother should take herbs that gently clean the blood and support digestion: fenugreek, cumin, dill, Nigella sativa. Pulverize 50 grams each and mix with honey into a paste. Take 1/2 teaspoon 3 times a day.

Traditional Chinese Medicine

Traditional Chinese Medicine (TCM) has a written tradition that is 2,000 years old and an oral tradition that is said to be thousands of years older.

Ancient doctors of TCM observed that the body functions within a dynamic system of opposites: hot and cold, active and restful, storing and dispersing. They explored 'energy systems' within the body, and they charted the flow of *qi,* thought to be a kind of biological energy that travels on the skin along invisible lines called 'meridians.' The chart of meridians provides the basis for acupuncture—a healing method that has received recognition in the West.

Chinese doctors named different energy systems after bodily organs, so that when doctors of TCM talk about "organs," they are referring to an energy system and to its corresponding meridian, and not solely to the organ itself. For instance, the meridian of the lung, or "lung energy," refers to the system of the lung and the skin. Both the lung and the skin interact with the environment, and both are organs of elimination. But 'lung energy' also includes a person's capacity for happiness. Weak lung energy (unable to breathe freely) goes hand in hand with sadness or depression. Liver energy relates to how we deal with anger. A person who harbors a lot of anger will weaken their liver energy and become physically and emotionally toxic.

A doctor of TCM will focus on the energy system that has become weak, blocked, or misdirected—and not on the physical illness. If the energy system is strengthened—so the theory—the corresponding organs and emotions will regain their healthy function as well.

I would like here to thank Christiane Husi-Simonis, a TCM nutritionist, and the founder of the school of holistic lactation consulting in Switzerland, both for exploring TCM's complex but fascinating view of breastfeeding, and for her patience in explaining it to me. Now let's look at what Traditional Chinese Medicine says about the postpartum and lactation.

The Ancient Chinese Key to Lactation Success

In Traditional Chinese Medicine (TCM), foods that help women produce milk are said to strengthen the 'center.' This refers both to a woman's physical center—the digestive organs—and to that elusive 'center' of her person. When the body and mind are in balance, the chemistry of lactation should be at its best.

Two energy systems are said to be responsible for milk production. One energy system regulates heat and vitality, and the other regulates fluids in the body. These are the energies of the liver/kidney and the spleen respectively.

Liver and Kidney Energy

Whereas liver energy is said to provide the heat necessary for milk production, kidney energy represents the bone-deep, primary vitality of a mother. Both heat and vitality are important to lactation.

These energies are strengthened when a mother takes foods that strengthen her 'center' (see below). Special remedies for kidney energy are chicken soup or sea-weed soup (recipes below). Chicken soup should not be taken more than once a week—otherwise the baby may become too alert and not sleep well.

Heat Regulation

Like Ayurveda, TCM aspires to a balance between 'hot' and 'cold.' The terms *hot* or *cold* have specific meanings within the language-system of TCM. Generally speaking, when talking about organs in the body, *hot* or *cold* indicates whether the organ or energy is under- or over-functioning.

Mothers can be a mixture of both hot and cold, in different organs and systems of their body. For instance, a woman can have cold feet (a condition of coldness), but also have red eyes and/or dry skin, (a condition of heat). Because diagnosis is complex it is always advisable to seek the guidance of a TCM practitioner.

Many galactagogues are *warming herbs and spices*, including anise, fennel, dill, cumin, caraway, and ginger. This is appropriate because women after birth are usually *cold*, meaning that many organs are slightly underfunctioning as women recover from the stress of pregnancy and birth.

However, for women who are naturally *warm*, these herbs are not appropriate. Taking them every day can generate a build-up of heat in the body, and may lead to diarrhea and to an increased risk of breast infection. According to TCM, women who already have enough *warmth* in their bodies may see a decrease in milk-production if they over-use these warming herbs, whereas women who always tend to feel cold, or who are tired all the time, or who recently took antibiotics (generates cold), may benefit by using these warming herbs every day.

According to TCM, the two best galactagogues are nettle tea and fenugreek seed tea, as neither herb leads to congesting heat. Nettle is neutral (not warming or cooling) and can be used every day. Fenugreek seeds are warming but do not lead to the congestion of heat. Fenugreek can also be used every day.

The Spleen and 'Qi'

The spleen is said to be the seat of *chi*, *qi*, or life-energy. This energy is directly responsible for pregnancy and lactation. If qi energy is depleted during pregnancy or birth, there will not be enough left for lactation. A mother may then feel exhausted, empty, or ill, and she may not have enough breastmilk.

Naturally sweet foods, such as grains, legumes, sweet vegetables, honey, and sesame seed, build up the energy of the spleen. But food made with white sugar and refined flour depletes the energy of the spleen.

Spleen energy can be depleted through a stressful life-style as well. To maintain and replenish spleen energy we need quiet, happy, contemplative activities to balance an active life. Chronic stress depletes qi.

Finally, spleen energy is depleted through loss of blood during birth.

Fluid Regulation

The spleen energy also regulates fluids in the body. According to TCM, women who do not have their spleen energy in balance will feel discomfort when fluid leaves their body, for instance, they feel exhausted by menstruation, or they may be incontinent.

Mothers with weak spleen energy are at risk to feel physically and/or emotionally drained or ill during a milk-ejection reflex, or while breast-feeding their baby. Symptoms include breaking out in a sweat, sudden weakness or nausea while nursing, and being unable to have a milk ejection reflex or maintain good milk flow.

These symptoms can signal a long standing spleen energy imbalance, though they may also result from loss of blood during or after birth, or from stress due to a difficult birth.

Foods that restore balance to the spleen and to fluid regulation are grains and legumes, especially *rice* and *millet*. In China, the herb dong quai is routinely given to women after birth to strengthen spleen energy, to restore blood, to build milk supply, and to prevent depression—especially if the mother experienced a significant loss of blood during birth.

Blood Loss During Birth

Women usually aren't told how much blood they lost during birth, but a phone call to the hospital may provide an answer. Losing more than 600 grams for an average sized woman is enough to cause the spleen imbalance described in the section above.

In the case of blood loss, mothers should take dong quai (angelica sinensis) to rebuild blood, support milk production and prevent depression. Dosage: 3x 1 – 2 capsules of dried herb (250 milligram per capsule) per day. Look for a good quality herb. *As with all herbs, it's a good idea to build up slowly, beginning with one capsule a day, to be sure that you don't have an allergy to the herb.*

Dong quai, one of our best women's herbs, can be added to sauces and taken with meals throughout a woman's life to bring hormonal balance and stability to the immune system.

If a woman lost a lot of blood during or after birth, *ginger should be avoided*, both as a spice and as an herbal remedy. Ginger expands the blood vessels and speeds blood circulation. If there is too little blood, this may lead to the body drying out even more. Verbena and fennel are two more 'drying' herbs that should be used cautiously if there was blood loss.

Foods that Strengthen the Center and Support Milk Supply

Lactogenic foods are said in TCM to strengthen the center, regulate body warmth, and help regulate fluids. A plethora of traditional remedies exist, geared to specific imbalances. However, I have been advised not to include these here, as applying them without adequate diagnosis could lead to health problems.

This is because TCM remedies are geared to the specific metabolic imbalances of the mother. A skilled doctor in TCM would prescribe different remedies to different women who have the same problem, depending on their underlying imbalances. This makes TCM different from western medicine, which commonly prescribes the same treatment for the same problem.

The following three lactogenic remedies are well-known and widely used in Asia. They are: seaweed soup to build strength, prevent depression, and support milk production; chicken soup, after birth to build strength and blood, and for severe milk supply problems; and cooked papaya, to help the milk flow.

Chicken Soup

To increase a mother's strength and to build blood, and for severe milk supply problems, take one bowl in the week after birth, and once a week thereafter:

1. One portion of fresh chicken (if possible, organically kept), for instance, the leg, including the bone and skin.

2. Cover with water, and simmer for three hours.

3. Add 2- 3 slices of ginger root, if the mother did not lose blood during birth.

4. Add pepper and salt to taste.

5. Add one capsule of dong quai (250 mg).

6. When a layer of fat has formed on top of the soup, stir it into the water again.

7. Prepare with additional (pre-cooked) adzuki beans, if the mother is very weak.

According to TCM, mothers should not take this remedy more often than once a week. Otherwise the baby may become too alert and will not sleep well at night.

Seaweed soup

Miyoguk (Korean Seaweed Soup)

The brown seaweed called miyok is different from more well-known Japanese varieties, such as wakame and nori (for sushi). Most American health-food stores sell both types. But miyok, when soaked, actually looks like a flat ribbon of dark, slimy green curls floating in a sea of muddy-colored broth.

1 cup (or 8 ounces) of dried seaweed

1/2 pound beef (shoulder or flank steak)

3 scallions

2-3 cloves garlic

1 Tbsp. sesame oil

1 tsp. soy sauce

1 Tbsp. salt

4 cups water

(Makes 4 servings)

1. Soak the seaweed in warm water for half an hour. Rinse and wash carefully. Cut into two-inch strips. Set aside.

2. Cut the beef into 2-inch lengths. Slice the scallions into 2-inch lengths (using the white and green parts) and crush the garlic.

3. Heat the sesame oil in a heavy-bottomed pot. Brown the meat, then add scallions, garlic, soy sauce and salt. (Note: if you need more sesame oil, add another 2-3 tablespoons.)

4. Add the water and seaweed. Bring the soup to a boil, reduce the heat and cover the pot. Simmer for at least 10 minutes. If you're not in a rush, let the soup sit for several hours to blend the flavors.

5. Sprinkle with pepper, if desired. Garnish with toasted sesame seeds. (Roast white sesame seeds in a dry skillet until brown. Crush with mortar and pestle to release the flavor.)

6. Serve with rice on the side. Very often, Koreans will shovel spoonfuls of rice into the soup as they eat it.[*]

⇨ Seaweed soup is taken after birth in Korea for convalescence, to prevent depression, and to increase milk production. The following recipe is by Brenda Paik Sunoo, owner of the website, www.compassionatwork.com. Brenda has written a moving account of how seaweed soup—rich in minerals, folic acid, antioxidants, and omega 3s (to stave off depression)—is exchanged as an expression of community between mothers, both in shared joy and grief. You can read her article at salon.com.

Green Papaya

Place a few slices of peeled papaya and ginger root into a small pot of water. Add a dash of organic apple vinegar and simmer 10 minutes on low heat. Sieve, and drink slowly. This remedy clears the milk-ducts and helps the milk to flow. *It is not to be taken with ginger if there was significant blood loss at birth.*

Other foods used in China to promote milk production

Millet and **rice**—balance fluid regulation. By eating a small dish of millet or rice in the evening, a mother's milk is richer during the night and her baby will sleep more soundly.

---

[*] This article (plus recipe) first appeared in Salon.com, at *http://www.Salon.com*. An online version remains in the Salon archives. Reprinted with permission.

Sesame—(roasted with salt, as 'gomasio' in Japan). An excellent milk-builder. In China, the black sesame is preferred, but its energy may be too potent for westerners.

Lettuce—improves the flow of the milk.

Prickly lettuce—prevents mastitis, cools.

Champignon mushrooms—supports milk flow. Its amino acids help to stabilize mood. (Do not take if you have a yeast infection of any kind.)

Figs—strengthen the center and support milk production.

Green papaya—eat as prepared above, or take as powder in capsules. Supports milk production.

Dandelion—Taraxacum japonicum, an Asian form of the dandelion, is commonly used as a galactagogue. The roots are cut and roasted and used in coffee in place of chicory. The leaves are eaten boiled, like spinach.

Pounded rice cakes called *moshi* are given to mothers in Japan after birth to improve their milk production. They are nutrient-rich and easy to digest. Moshi can be found in Asian stores or can be purchased online.

Anti-lactogenic foods—barley, used in moderate amounts, supports milk production. The Chinese have found however that when barley is eaten in large amounts it can reduce milk production. The same holds true for barley sprouts. Barley-water appears to be the safest dosage.

Two TCM Herbal Recipes

TCM herbal tea remedies are complex. I would like to thank here Dr. Long Chun-lin from the Kunming Institute of Botany, who kindly contacted traditional doctors in China and provided the following detailed recipes.

For those who are physically exhausted through giving birth many times, or through excessive loss of blood during childbirth, or who are weak of physique.

15 grams of roots of Astragalus membranaceus Bunge (or A. mongholicus), 15 grams of roots of Codonopsis pilosula Nannf. (or C. tangshen / C. nervosa / C. clematidea /C. subglobosa /C. canescens /C. cordiphylla /C. subscoposa /C. micrantha /C. tubulosa /C. ovata /C. tsinlingensis /C. macrocalyx), 10 grams of tuber roots of Atractylodes macrocephala Koidz., 10 grams of sclerotium of Poria cocos Wolf, 10 grams of roots of Angelica sinensis Diels, 6 grams of roots of Paeonia lactiflora Pall., 4.5 grams of rhizone of Ligusticum wallichii Granch., 15 grams of processed tubers of Rehmannia glutinosa Libosch. (especially f. hueichingensis Hsiao and var. lutea f. purpurea Makino), 6 grams of fruits of Citrus aurantium L. (or C. aurantium var. amara Engl. /C. wilsonii Tanaka /C. medica L.), 10 grams of fruits of Liquidambar formosa Hance, and 6 grams of fruits of pith of Tetrapanax papyriferus K. Koch.

To mix – the above combination of herbs in the amounts given is one dosage. Put the mixed herbs into a stainless steel pot, add one liter of drinking water, and soak for about 2 hours. Cook on a high heat first, later on low heat to keep the water boiling until it decreases to 200 ml, or one fifth the amount; it takes about 90 minutes. Switch off the heat, filter and eliminate herbs.

Take 100 ml (half the amount, or one/tenth of a liter) before a meal. After 4 – 6 hours, take the second 100 ml again before a meal.

Prepare one dosage a day. 7 days is one course of treatment. Low milk supply can usually be corrected in 1-2 courses of treatment. If it does not work after 2 courses (two weeks), stop it soon.

For those with strong health but depressed, or with a load on her mind.

6 grams of plant of Bupleurum chinese DC. (or B. scorzoneraefolium Willd.), 10 grams of rhizomes of Curcuma aromatica Salisb. (or C. domestica Salisb. /C. zedoaria Rosc.), 10 grams of bark of Acacia farnesiana Willd., 6 grams of fruits of Citrus aurantium L. (or C. aurantium var. amara Engl. /C. wilsonii Tanaka /C. medica L.), 10 grams of roots of Trichosanthes kirilowii Maxim. (or T. uniflora Hao), 10 grams of tubers of Ophiopogon japonica Ker.-Gawl. (or Liriope

spicata Lour.), 10 grams of seeds of Vaccaria segetalis Garcke), and 6 grams of thorns of Gleditsia sinenis Lam.

To mix, the assigned amounts of herbs listed above are one dosage.

The treatment method is the same as in Recipe 1.

The earlier the treatment begins, the easier is the cure.

Also, the more often a mother breastfeeds her baby, the better for the mother's milk-production."

Acupressure

Mothers with milk supply problems sometimes see improvement through treatment with acupuncture or acupressure.

The acupressurist treats the health issues, or energy systems, that underlie low milk supply.

Two acupressure points are specific to lactation. I include them here to show how compassionately the needs of breastfeeding mothers have been integrated into Chinese medicine: they have acupuncture points for low-supply moms. These are:

● The Absolute Yin-Meridian of the Arm – point 1. Too little milk after birth.

● The Meridian of the Spleen – point 12. Too little milk.

CHAPTER THIRTEEN

Milk Supply Difficulties Today

New Problems, Rare Problems, New Solutions

In the last chapter, we looked at ancient traditions of medicine and their views on breastfeeding. We saw that doctors from India emphasize the health of the intestine and liver, as well as a mother's nervous stability. Doctors from China emphasize the same issues but call them other names. Digestive strength is governed by "liver energy," and nervous stability is governed by "spleen energy," which is also responsible for regulating fluids in the body.

While mothers today share these same health issues, we also have new difficulties that ancient doctors could not have predicted: the effects of medical intervention. Pitocin, given to mothers to induce birth, and magnesium sulfate, to lower blood pressure during labor, have been observed to delay the onset of milk production. IV transfusions that cause edema (swelling in arms and legs) have also been observed to suppress milk production until the kidneys remove the extra fluid from the body. *If mothers are not aware that medical procedures have impacted their supply, they may give up breastfeeding when their milk production appears to be insufficient the first week after birth.* With proper information and support, however, these mothers go on to develop a full milk supply.

Cesarean sections may lead to supply problems if mothers are separated from their babies after birth, or if they do not feel physically comfortable breastfeeding and so do not breastfeed frequently, or if they were traumatized by the experience and are finding it difficult to relax and bond with their babies. Mothers after a cesarean section require extra support from the hospital staff for breastfeeding.

Babies may be born with issues of their own: a very high palate, a tight frenulum, or sensorial immaturity. Babies who are weak or underweight may have more difficulties suckling and removing milk from the breast.

One rare complication is when tiny pieces of the placenta remain in the womb, producing hormones that interfere with the chemistry of lactation and lead to insufficient milk supply. This can delay milk production for up to several weeks. Surprisingly, this complication can also happen after birthing by cesarean section.

Increasing numbers of women today have hormonal imbalances that can lead to low milk supply. These conditions may be hereditary, but they can develop or become exacerbated through a stressful life-style or inadequate diet. (Read below for information on treatment.)

If the mother is separated from the baby for medical reasons, a mother will require extra support from the hospital staff in pumping milk for her baby. (One study showed that domperidone is helpful for building supply in the mothers of premature babies. However, it is no longer legal to use domperidone in the USA due to a ruling in June 2004 by the FDA.) Using a supplemental nursing device can help the baby learn to finger feed. It also helps the baby bond at the breast while the mother builds up her supply.

Incompetent feeding practices in the hospital, such as giving fluids to a baby with a bottle, or forcing the baby onto the breast when he doesn't want to drink, can undermine a mother's breastfeeding efforts. Inadequate guidance from poorly trained lactation consultants can lead to problems when a baby's poor latch, weak suck, or tongue-tie are not properly diagnosed and treated.

If you feel that you are not receiving adequate breastfeeding support, please consult your healthcare provider, pediatrician, doula or La Leche League Leader for a referral to an international board certified lactation consultant (IBCLC). If you have a complex problem, and your IBCLC doesn't know how to help you, you may need to seek a more experienced, 'veteran' IBCLC. Some mothers see two or more IBCLCs before finding one who is able to assist them.

The reward is worth the effort. A few weeks or months later, the breastfeeding team may show no signs of their early difficulties.

Hormonal Imbalances and Breastfeeding Problems:

Breast Hypoplasia

When girls develop into women, they may experience hormonal imbalances. Occasionally, their breasts do not receive sufficient hormonal stimulation to develop abundant glandular tissue and/or hormone receptors. This is called breast hypoplasia. Women with hormonal imbalances such as the Polycystic Ovarian Syndrome (PCOS) may have breast hypoplasia, though the majority do not. Other imbalances, such as the Metabolic Syndrome, or hormonal imbalances caused by eating disorders such as anorexia nervosa may also lead to some degree of breast hypoplasia. It is important to note that there are varying degrees of breast hypoplasia. While many women have somewhat less glandular tissue than usual, very few have so little that they cannot build at least some milk supply.

Is hypoplasia rare? Considering that rates of eating disorders, PCOS, and the Metabolic Syndrome are increasing in the general population in the US and around the world (largely due to a poor diet and unhealthy lifestyle in childhood), it is likely that the rate of breast hypoplasia is also increasing.

Recognizing Hypoplasia

Hypoplasia can most easily be recognized during puberty, when, instead of developing perky breasts, the breasts—or one of the breasts in particular—seem to be empty and hanging.

Hypoplastic breasts in adults can be any size. Typically, their shape is conical or tubular, they are widely spaced, and the area where they attach to the chest wall is narrow rather than round. They frequently have stretch marks. The absence of glandular tissue gives a lack of fullness, and the areolas may seem unusually large compared to the width of the breasts. Finally, while it is normal and common for women's breasts to have slightly different shapes and sizes, women with hypoplastic breasts tend to have markedly different shaped and sized breasts. Even with all these indications, however, hypoplasia may not always be obvious or easy to diagnose.

Hypoplasia is not the end of breastfeeding!

Women with hypoplasia may see minimal or no breast changes in pregnancy: their areolas may not darken, their breasts may not enlarge, and they may not produce drops of colostrum. Nonetheless, Dr. Kathleen Huggins, an expert on insufficient glandular tissue, has found that approximately 40% of these mothers can go on to develop glandular tissue and a full milk supply with pumping, herbs, but also with patience: developing a full supply can take a few weeks or months. In the meantime, it is necessary to supplement-feed so that the baby is properly nourished. The good news is that even those mothers who cannot build their supply can still breastbond if they are able to keep their babies at their breasts with a supplemental feeding device.

Preparation during Pregnancy

Mothers can contribute to the development of milk-producing tissue during pregnancy by observing four things: *medical evaluation and treatment of hormonal issues, stress management, a balanced diet and sufficient intake of calories, and an herbal medicinal program.*

Medical Evaluation and Treatment

Metformin (Glucophage®), which improves the body's sensitivity to insulin, appears to increase the development of glandular tissue in some but not all mothers. Recommendations during pregnancy are not yet uniform. Studies are showing that mothers with PCOS who conceived using metformin have overall positive results on metformin throughout pregnancy. Mothers without prior use of metformin should speak to their doctors about using it during last third of pregnancy, due to a slight risk of miscarriage. It can be taken again after birth, where it has also been seen to improve lactation.

Natural, micronized progesterone (made from soy, it must be natural, not synthetic), prescribed to mothers in pregnancy who have low levels of progesterone and who are at risk of miscarriage, has also been observed to increase the development of glandular tissue.

Stress Management

- If at all possible, **eat three healthy meals a day and snacks in-between**. The body requires nutrition for the breasts to properly develop. Feelings of hunger lead the body to produce hormones of stress—and these exacerbate underlying hormonal imbalances.

- **Don't overdo caffeine**, as caffeine triggers adrenaline, a stress hormone.
- **Get** as much **rest** as is possible and enjoy activities in which you **breathe deeply**. Deep breathing will help you produce oxytocin, the hormone of the milk-ejection reflex.
- **Learn a relaxation technique** and practice it – if not during the day, then before sleeping at night. Deep relaxation increases the production of prolactin, the hormone of milk production.

A Balanced Diet

Eat a variety of foods to provide yourself and your growing baby with a wide range of fresh nutrients. Follow the guidelines in this book to improve your diet. If you are experiencing extreme nausea, eat whatever you can tolerate in tiny portions but get the calories you need.

Herbal Medicinal Program

Alfalfa leaf (not the sprout) is safe for most people to take during pregnancy as a nutritious supplement. It has been noted to greatly increase milk supply in mothers who take it during pregnancy, even leading to over-supply in mothers with normal breast tissue. Other herbs that prepare for lactation during pregnancy include red raspberry leaf, nettle, oat-straw, dandelion leaf, and red clover. These nutritious herbs support the liver and kidneys; they are rich in folic acid, minerals, and vitamins. Goat's rue increases glandular tissue *after birth* when taken at high dosage in concentrated tincture form. See the next section for more information on goat's rue.

Red raspberry leaf tea—famous for its tonic effect on the uterus— contains substances that, theoretically, could trigger miscarriage (this 'side effect' has never been observed, however). To be on the safe side, mothers should gradually increase their daily dosage. Take one cup per day the first week, two cups the second, and so on, up to four cups a day.

⇨ For these herbs to be effective, they should be taken every day for several months. However, mothers with normal milk supply should beware: they may develop over-supply if they regularly take these herbs, particularly alfalfa, up to their due date. These women should stop 2 weeks prior to birth. Nettle is beneficial up to due date and the first week after birth.

We Can Develop Glandular Tissue

Eating well during pregnancy supports the healthy development of the baby but also the development of mammary tissue. Learning to relax and breathe deeply promotes the production of prolactin and oxytocin. If, in addition, we take safe, nutritious herbs during pregnancy (see above), and treat underlying medical conditions (see page 184), we ensure the greatest possible glandular tissue growth. Studies on animals have shown that some herbs and foods do indeed promote the development of glandular tissue. The herb that appears to most reliably promote glandular growth in women is goat's rue. Goat's rue contains a substance, galegin, that is similar to metformin, (Glucophage®) medication for insulin resistance that also promotes glandular growth. It is erring on the side of caution to avoid therapeutic dosage of goat's rue during pregnancy. After birth, goat's rue is best taken as tincture, to easily reach therapeutic dosage.

About PCOS

The polycystic ovarian syndrome (PCOS) affects up to fifteen percent of women today in countries where children eat a lot of snack food, fast food, and sweets in their formative years. PCOS is a hormonal imbalance characterized by a tendency to gain weight around the middle (insulin resistance), by irregular menstrual cycles or infertility (estrogen dominance), and by the tendency to have acne, hair growth on the face and other 'unfeminine' places, as well thinning hair on the head (testosterone imbalance). These hormonal imbalances may interfere with the development of the breasts during puberty, pregnancy, and after birth.[58] About one third of women with PCOS have mild milk supply difficulties. Far fewer have severe problems.

⇨ PCOS is associated with inadequate growth of breast tissue during puberty (hypoplastic breasts) in a small percentage of those who have it.

When women have their first baby, symptoms of *mild* PCOS may not yet have become evident. It is not necessary to have facial hair, to be obese, infertile, or to have cysts on one's ovaries to have a mild form of the syndrome. Some mothers may therefore have lactation difficulties without realizing that an underlying hormonal imbalance is to blame. Now, although PCOS is a naturally occurring and genetic imbalance, *it can also be triggered or made considerably worse by* poor diet (white sugar and refined flour, stimulants and alcohol), lack of exercise, and a stressful lifestyle with irregular sleep habits. The rising number of women with PCOS and the Metabolic Syndrome doubtless reflects our deteriorating diet and lifestyle.

Preparedness after Birth

Mothers who have hormonal imbalances such as hypo- or hyperthyroidism, PCOS, who have a past history of low supply, or whose breasts show signs of insufficient glandular tissue (hypoplasia, see above) should prepare for possible breastfeeding difficulties well ahead of birth. Besides the measures described in this chapter, they should rent a hospital grade pump to have at hand if necessary, and acquire or make a supplemental feeding device. That way, should it be necessary to supplement after birth, she will not have to resort to a bottle. It is also wise for these mothers to eat lactogenically and to take herbs after birth. Two herbs recommended in the week after birth are nettle and dong quai. The latter is given in China if the mother lost considerable blood during birth.

Taking foods such as steamed fennel and carrots, millet, rice, hummus, dark green leafy vegetables, plus breakfasting on oatmeal, will further help establish the chemistry of lactation.

Prolactin Receptors and Time Limits

In recent years, lactation experts have come to believe that there is a small window of time in which to build an abundant milk supply. It is believed that prolactin receptors develop in breast tissue only during the first two months after birth. After that time, an adequate milk supply can supposedly no longer be established. This is not always the case, however. Many low-supply mothers who had a terrible start are able to build a full supply, months down the line. It is important not to generalize, or to lose hope, because we are indeed individuals when it comes to milk production.

Over-Production and an Overactive Milk-Ejection Reflex

Women with PCOS (and some who do not have PCOS) frequently have over-production of milk[59]. Ironically, over-production can lead to low milk supply. This happens when a baby feels overwhelmed by her mother's strong let-down reflex and rapid milk flow. Babies are clever and find ways to control the flow, such as clamping down on the nipple, or using a soft, inefficient suck. What the baby does not know is that in reducing the milk flow she is suppressing her mother's milk supply as well. Mothers can go from high supply to low supply within a matter of days—a confusing predicament.

When these mothers pump, or use herbs and foods, their supply rebounds. Unfortunately, the milk-ejection reflex and milk flow may again be strong, and the cycle repeats itself.

Mothers with an over-active milk ejection reflex (strong let-down) often find it helpful to hand express or pump off some milk before feeding. This reduces the initial force of their milk flow. They may also find it helpful to nurse on only one breast at a feeding—or on only one side for *two or more* feedings in extreme cases—to help bring down their supply to their baby's needs.

⇨ Some over-production mothers use sage tea, up to six cups a day, or parsley capsules, up to 12 a day, to reduce their supply. Use with care: you want to reduce supply, not wean.

It is important to note that each baby experiences milk flow differently. Whereas some babies deal well with a strong milk flow, others find moderate milk flow difficult to deal with. A baby usually learns to cope with her mother's flow as she matures.

Changes in feeding position can help babies control the flow of the milk. Some babies do well with the foot-ball hold. Some prefer lying on top of their mother's stomach while she lies on her back. Even the traditional cradle hold can be altered to help these babies: they may feel better if they sit or lie with their bottom lower than their heads while breastfeeding, and with their belly turned somewhat away from the mother, while their head is naturally turned inward toward the breast—rather than holding the baby's belly against the mother's belly. Mothers may also experiment with the 'scissors hold' on the breast (one or two fingers above the areola, the others below) rather than the C-hold. This enables them to press their fingers against their milk ducts to regulate (hold back) the flow. Be careful though: the scissors hold can contribute to the development of plugged milk ducts. *Massage any hard or tender areas after feeding, and hand-express to help prevent plugged ducts.*

A nipple shield may also help these babies be more comfortable with the flow: they can control it more easily. As the baby grows older and stronger she will no longer need the nipple shield and hopefully reject it, accepting the breast.

⇨ These strategies are best coordinated under the supervision of an IBCLC.

The Goal and the Good News

The hope for mothers with low milk supply, whatever the cause, is to keep their baby at the breast while building their supply. If, however, a baby refuses to feed at the breast, a mother may decide to pump milk and feed her baby her breastmilk with a bottle or cup. The baby may still return to the breast at a later time—sometimes very suddenly and unexpectedly.

When a baby becomes old enough that solid foods are his main source of calories and nutrients, a persistently low-supply mother who kept her baby at her breast will finally be able to relax and enjoy breastfeeding. She can then go on to breastfeed for as long as she and her baby choose. Do not introduce solids early, however, in an attempt to hurry this on. Follow your baby's individual clues for introducing solids, as is described in many baby books.

The good news is that any amount of breastmilk will give a baby immune benefits, even a few drops. As an extra bonus, suckling at the breast is thought to help develop a mother's milk supply for 'next time.' Mothers tend to have more milk with second and third babies— and this includes mothers who had severe milk supply problems. It is not uncommon for mothers with insufficient glandular tissue to go on to fully nurse their next baby.

Part Three

Recipes

About This Section

Mothers are smart about getting lactogenic foods and spices into their favorite dishes. For instance, they:

- sprinkle split or slivered almonds over lunch and dinner

- eat hummus or tahini as a side dish

- cut dandelion leaves into salad

- recall their grandmother's recipe for chicken soup or garlic dip

- make spaghetti sauce with basil and virgin olive oil

- add flaxseed oil to salad dressing

- drink fresh vegetable juices

- put oatmeal into everything, including meatloaf and smoothies

- splurge on old-fashioned oatmeal cookies

For mothers who would like more inspiration and insights into *mother food*, I have provided simple, lactogenic, whole-food recipes.

Where appropriate, I have mentioned connections between food, eating habits, health issues, and the possibility of triggering or aggravating colic in a baby.

CHAPTER FOURTEEN

Lactogenic Beverages

Grain-Drinks

Grain-drinks, flavored with lactogenic spices, are used by mothers around the world to support lactation. They are subtly sweet, low in calories, and high in nutrients and lactation-promoting substances that are easy to digest and absorb: minerals, vitamins, proteins, saponins, phyto-estrogens, and special polysaccharides (sugars) that favorably influence lactation.

In ancient Greece, women cooked the flour of barley into a thin gruel, adding fennel seeds or astragalus root. In ancient Egypt, a drink was made with chickpea-water. In Africa today, mothers drink millet-flake tea—reputed to restore milk to the breasts of grandmothers. Native Americans prepare white corn flour as a gruel spiced with lactogenic herbs. In Peru, the water is taken off of cooked quinoa or amaranth, and spiced with cinnamon.*

Mothers can test whether a particular grain boosts their supply by drinking that grain's *water* for a week. Some mothers may find it necessary to alternate grains, each for the duration of three or four days, for a sustained effect.

MILLET-FLAKE TEA

This delicious tea is famous in Africa, where it is reputed to bring back milk to a grandmother's breast and to improve milk flow. In Africa, red millet is used—a variety that is especially rich in calcium. Yellow millet can also be used.

Put 1 – 2 teaspoons of millet-flake and a dash of anise seed into a cup and add boiling water. Stir in honey to taste if desired, and steep for a few minutes. The millet and anise seed will sink to the bottom of the cup. Filter off the liquid, or drink as is.

---

* These cultures also prepare fermented grain drinks to support milk production. Their preparation is not quick and simple, however. For more information, see Sally Fallon's *Nourishing Traditions*.

CORNMEAL-TEA

Cornmeal-tea is used in Native American medicine to support lactation. Pour boiling water onto 1 heaping teaspoon of finely ground corn-meal in a small-holed sieve, or place the corn-meal directly in the cup, as in the recipe above.

OATMEAL-TEA

Pour boiling water onto 1 heaping teaspoon of oatmeal flakes in a cup. Add a pinch of powdered cinnamon and ginger, or other spices (such as powdered fennel, anise or fenugreek seed) and sweeten with honey, malt-syrup, blackstrap molasses or other natural sweetener if desired. The grain and spice will sink to the bottom of the cup. If you would rather not have them in your cup while you drink, strain the liquid off.

CHICKPEA-WATER (GARBANZO)

Chickpea water is mentioned in an ancient Egyptian herbal as a remedy to increase milk production. Thoroughly rinse, and then soak 1 handful of chickpea for at least 1 1/2 hours in plenty of water, and drain. On a low heat, simmer the chickpea in 1 quart of water for at least 1 1/2 hours, adding water if necessary. Add a pinch of sea salt if desired, and a dash of thyme, basil, or marjoram. Drink the chickpea-water throughout the day. Use the chickpea in a meal.

QUINOA-WATER

Quinoa is the ancient grain-like seed of Peru, where it is traditionally used by breastfeeding mothers to support lactation. Quinoa contains a good balance of all eight essential amino acids, and many vitamins and minerals. Thoroughly rinse, and then soak a half cup of quinoa for at least 1 1/2 hours, and drain.[*] Place the quinoa in a quart of water and simmer for twenty minutes, adding water if necessary. Strain the water off, add cinnamon (or other spices) and sweeten. Use the quinoa in soup or salad.

---

[*] Quinoa does not have to be soaked to become soft, but soaking improves its digestibility.

⇨ An alternative: 1 teaspoon of the *flour of any lactogenic grain* is added to a cup of water and stirred while heating. Add lactogenic spices (and natural sweetener) after the water has simmered for a few minutes, and allow to steep 3 – 5 minutes before drinking.

BARLEY-WATER

Barley-water is used medicinally to treat colds, intestinal problems and liver disorders, and was recorded in Greek medicine two thousand years ago as a galactagogue. (See beta glucan on page 135.) Taken regularly for a week or two, it often helps mothers with chronic low milk supply. Make a pot in the morning and drink throughout the day, warming each cup and sweetening with natural sweetener as desired.

Barley-water can be made with whole grain or pearl barley. Barley flakes can also be used, though these have been processed and are possibly less potent than the whole or pearled grain.

Preparation:

- Quick-and-easy: 1/2 cup of flakes can be simmered in 1 quart of water for twenty minutes.
- Long-and-intensive: 1 cup of whole barley is soaked overnight (optional), and then simmered on a low heat in 3 quarts of water for up to 2 hours. About half the liquid should cook off. (Some recipes call for only 1/2 hour cooking time. However, the longer the barley simmers and the more purple the water becomes, the more of the 'cream' will enter the water, and the stronger the medicinal effect will be.)
- Recipes from Italy and Africa call for adding a fig to barley-water while it is simmering. Figs are lactogenic, nutritious, and improve the taste of barley-water. A dried fig will also do.
- When finished, remove from the stove and filter the water from the grain (and fig). The grain is now tasteless and can be thrown out. Add 1 tablespoon of fennel powder or steep 2 – 3 teaspoons of fennel seeds for ten minutes in the barley-water.
- The traditional recipe calls for fennel seed. I personally find that powdered fenugreek seed is tastier than fennel in barley-water.

BARLEY-ASTRAGALUS GRUEL

The ancient Greek doctor, Dioscorides, suggested that astragalus be added to barley gruel in order to "bring back milk that was extinguished." (For more information on astragalus see page 263.) This recipe was probably made by cooking dried astragalus root with barley flour. I have never tried this recipe and would be very interested in feed-back from mothers who use it while re-lactating.

Preparation:

On a low heat, simmer 15 grams of astragalus root, or astragalus powder, in a quart of water for 20 - 30 minutes. Strain out the root. Combine barley flour with cold water and stir until it forms a thick paste. Stir in this paste until the mixture thickens to a gruel.

Juicing

Some mothers see both their milk supply and their energy increase when they drink freshly pressed vegetable juice, or juice made from vegetable extracts that can be purchased in health-food stores.

Carrot Juice

Carrots contain large amounts of beta-carotene (the yellow-orange pigment) which support the detoxifying action of the liver. Carrot juice often benefits mothers suffering from postpartum exhaustion, boosting their mood and stabilizing their energy. Some mothers, and also the clinical herbalist, Karen Vaughan, say that it supports and increases their milk supply.

Carrot and organic grown beet are sweet vegetables; together they blend into a darkly rich juice that can help satisfy a mother's sweet tooth.

A vegetable juicer is required to make juice from root vegetables such as carrots and beets. Affordable juicers (such as Juiceman®) will do. Juicers are available second-hand on ebay.com. Don't buy a citrus juicer by mistake!

⇨ Mothers suffering from **hypoglycemia** may dilute sweet vegetable juices with water, and add a dash of cream, coconut-milk, or sesame oil to prolong the digestion of the juice and avoid a sharp drop in their blood sugar.

Favorite Combinations

- Carrot and celery. For a sweeter taste, use fennel with or instead of celery.
- Carrot and beet juice. Carrot sweetens up the beet. Additional fennel makes it still more palatable. (Beet is protective against cancer.)
- Carrot juice combines well with raw garlic.
- Carrot juice with dandelion leaves and garlic may appeal to mothers accustomed to the taste of bitter greens; it requires a special juicer to juice leaves.
- Carrot, beet, fennel, dandelion and garlic are all lactogenic.

Green Juice

Freshly made green-juices are rich in minerals, vitamins, enzymes, folic acid and beta-carotene—all needed in extra supply while breastfeeding. They supply energy boost the immune system. They are reported to help with depression, fatigue, allergies, overweight, environmental sensitivities.

Green juice promotes milk production, often considerably so. Be careful though—some mothers experience uncomfortable symptoms of stark detoxification when they drink fresh green juices—raw emotions, congestion, flu-like symptoms. If this happens to you, reduce your use of fresh juices. Stark detoxification is not desirable during lactation.

For more information, see page 197.

Juicing with a Blender[*]

It is possible to make green juices using a home blender. The following tips will help.

- Prepare a variety of green vegetables such as celery sticks, kale, dandelion leaves, fennel root, cucumber, dark green salads, chard, and zucchini.

- With a home blender, add only 1 – 1 1/2 cups of bulk at a time to the blender, just covering with water.

- Start the blender on low and work up to high. Do not let the liquid become hot.

- Add more liquid and bulk while the blender is running, turn the blender off to add more ingredients.

- Adding fresh lemon juice, or raw apple or pear juice, may improve the taste. (Store-bought juice that is truly raw will probably have a warning label that it "may cause sickness especially in children & the elderly.") You can also add a peeled and sliced fresh apple or pear to the blender.

- After blending, sieve off the juice to remove the vegetable fiber. Otherwise, be sure to 'chew' the drink, to aid in the digestion of the fiber.

- Add a few drops of oil (flaxseed, sesame, or virgin olive), coconut-milk or cream, to help with the digestion of the fat-soluble vitamins and the minerals in the juice.

- For additional protein and calcium, mix in almond butter. Or, if you have a good, trusted source for organic-eggs, mix in raw egg-yolk. This used to be routinely given for convalescence-but be careful, salmonella may be present.)

- Save the moist vegetable fiber from your juices to make soup. Cover with water or broth, add 1/4 cups of quinoa or amaranth (for their excellent protein), simmer for twenty minutes and top with cream or butter. Optional: fresh pressed garlic, sea salt or

---

[*] These instructions were kindly provided by Sara Johnson, raw-foods chef and lifestyle consultant in Portland, Oregon.

seasoned salt, pepper, and the lactogenic spices of basil, marjoram and thyme.

- Or mix the vegetable fiber with eggs and oatmeal to make veggie-burger patties.

"Drinking green-juice enables me to pump about five additional ounces of milk per day." Sara Johnson

---

SARA'S RECIPE FOR A DAY'S SUPPLY OF JUICE:
1 bunch of kale, 1 bunch of flat leaf parsley, 1 bunch of celery, 1 beet or 1 burdock root, and 2 cucumbers. For a sweeter juice replace cucumbers with 2 apples, 2 pears or 5-6 carrots.

Commercial Green Drinks

Commercial green drinks contain powdered vegetable and fruit extracts and are rich in chlorophyll, enzymes, minerals and vitamins. Some ingredients are lactogenic: astragalus, kelp, alfalfa leaf, oat-straw. Others, such as spirulina, wheat-grass and barley-grass, are immune system stimulants and balancers, particularly the mushrooms maitake, reishi, and shiitake.

Lactation consultants have observed that green drinks often lead to an increase in milk supply *and also in the fat-content of breastmilk.* As a bonus, mothers (and fathers) have more energy. Green drink powder is also available in capsule form.

Caution: Do not take more than 1.25 grams of chlorella per day if you have or have had silver fillings in your teeth. If you have removed and replaced your silver fillings, you must chelate heavy metals from your body under the guidance of an expert before eating larger quantities of chlorella or cilantro, as both plants mobilize heavy metals in body tissues, possibly bringing them into the bloodstream where they may enter your milk. AIM Barleygreen ™: barley grass, barley juice and kelp does not contain chlorella or cilantro. This warning also pertains to pregnancy.

Homemade Green Drink*

Mix 1 cup of juice and a fruit of your choice in a blender. Open one dosage of green herbal supplements, such as alfalfa leaf, oat-straw, red raspberry leaf, blessed thistle, nettle leaf, spirulina and dandelion leaf. Blend well, adding natural sweetener if desired.

Almond-Milk

Nut-milk can be used over cereal, with fruit, or in recipes.

Almond-milk is commonly used for its natural sweetness and high levels of calcium, which is further improved by adding sesame seeds. Both *almond and sesame are used to support milk production,* and soaking renders their nutrients more accessible.

Recipe
- Soak whole almonds 12 – 24 hours in 2x as much water. Rinse the almonds. If they have their skins on, blanch by dipping them in boiling water. The skins will now easily come off. (Some people prefer to leave the skins on.)

- In a blender, puree the almonds just covered with water, slowly adding twice the amount of pure water while blending—regulate the amount of water depending on how thin or creamy the milk should be. Pour through a fine strainer.

- Optional: blend in raw honey, vanilla, and fruit such as banana, fig, or frozen or fresh berries.

- This recipe can also be made using a mixture of almonds and hulled sesame seeds. Soak equal amounts of both and proceed as above.

- Stored in the refrigerator, nut milk will keep about three days.

---

* This recipe is adapted with permission from the website and online store for pregnant and breastfeeding mothers, www.birthandbreastfeeding.com, whose owner, Michel Turner, is an IBCLC and certified herbalist.

Spiced Milk

Mothers may find that a cup of warm milk before or after nursing helps maintain their energy and their supply. Mothers who are sensitive to dairy can try rice-milk or almond-milk.

For a creamier, more lactogenic beverage, sweeten with malt syrup, blackstrap molasses, maple syrup, honey, or other natural sweetener, and stir in a teaspoon of almond butter.

For further benefit, add one or more of the spices recommended below. These spices are used traditionally in the postpartum in India, to prevent inflammation, address intestinal problems, and to increase milk production.

- Warm the milk in a pan and add 1/4 – 1/2 teaspoons of one or more of the following in powder form: turmeric, ginger, cinnamon, cumin. Top off with a natural sweetener to taste.

- Turmeric is a natural antibiotic and anti-inflammatory. Mothers who frequently ingest turmeric during pregnancy and the postpartum may boost their resistance to mastitis. Some sources list turmeric as a galactagogue.

- Ginger is also anti-inflammatory, and is taken together with turmeric in the treatment of rheumatoid-arthritis. Ginger is also taken to 'clean the milk' (prevent colic) in India.

- Cinnamon is strongly antifungal and supports the liver. It reduces insulin resistance. It is taken to support milk production in Asia. It is estrogenic.

- Cumin supports digestion and helps reduce flatulence. It is a galactagogue.

Chai Tea

If a mother in India doesn't have enough milk, she may drink chai tea, also called "yogi tea." Chai tea is black tea (also a galactagogue) that is steeped in a decoction of piquant spices (most of which are galactagogues). Its flavor is mild and pleasing due to the addition of warm milk and a sweetener.

There are countless chai tea recipes. This one is tasty and lactogenic. You can make it more or less potent by using more or fewer spices.

Preparation: In 4 cups of water, add a combination of the following and simmer for 5 – 20 minutes:

½ teaspoon fennel or anise seeds
4 whole black pepper corns
3 cloves
2 cardamom pods (or several seeds if pods are not available)
¼ inch cinnamon stick
1/4 inch ginger root, sliced thinly

Turn off the heat. Add 4 teaspoons of black tea leaves or 4 teabags and steep for five minutes.

Add sweetener to taste (for instance, brown sugar or honey)

Warm ½ cup milk (or more if desired) and add it to the Chai after straining off the tea from the spices.

Kefir – A Homemade Probiotic Beverage

Kefir, a sour, slightly alcoholic, and refreshing drink, is made using live kefir "grains" that are a combination of yeast and bacteria. These grains transform pasteurized milk into a beverage brimming with living, healthful probiotic bacteria. (See pages 37 and 64-65 for more information on probiotics and breastfeeding.)

Kefir-grains digest lactose (milk sugar) and break down casein (milk protein), making dairy more tolerable for the breastfeeding mother. Kefir-grains grow and multiply. They will not die if used carefully, and can be given to friends and family so that all can benefit. Many people now send kefir-grains to others for only the cost of postage[*].

How to Make Kefir

To make kefir take two large jars, quart-size, for instance, large pickle jars. Wash them with mild soap—not in the dishwasher. The screw-on top should be plastic or plastic coated on the inside. Kefir should not come into contact with metal, except stainless steel, as ions from metal will damage the culture. Have plastic or wooden spoons available for stirring and tasting, and a plastic or stainless steel large-holed sieve for straining.

Place milk into the jar. (I use milk cold from the fridge, though the first time the kefir is used after it arrives through the mail, milk that is room temperature will be more gentle.) Add kefir grains, close the jar, and place it in a dark cupboard. Shake the jar gently one or two times a day, so that the grains come into contact with fresh 'food' (the milk).

Measurements: Per half liter or two cups of milk, a walnut-sized clump of kefir-grains. This is an approximate measurement. The more grains that you use, the shorter the fermentation time will be. On warm days, kefir ferments more quickly.

The kefir is ready to drink 16 - 24 hours later, though it can be left to ferment for up to 48 hours. Gently shake the jar to re-combine the kefir-curds with the whey. If you would like, add a bit of water to make the kefir thinner and easier to strain. Gently shake the kefir in the sieve or colander, or stir and press with a spoon, to separate the fluid from the grains. Put the kefir into a storage jar. Refrigerate the kefir, or leave it out at room temperature if preferred. It will continue to thicken.

Rinse the jar. Refill with milk, put the grains into the jar, close and shake gently. A good place to ferment kefir is in a dark cupboard. The next batch of kefir will be ready in 16 - 24 hours.

Dosage: 1 – 2 cups a day.

---

[*] Do an internet search for "kefir" and you'll be sure to find donors.

Warning: rarely, overdosing on strongly acidic fermented products such as kefir and kombucha is suspected of causing or contributing to lactic acidosis, which is harmful to the liver.

Coffee Substitute

Herbal coffee substitute is a gentle galactagogue and a fabulous pick-me-up. It is made of an assortment of lactogenic ingredients that can include roasted barley, roasted chicory and/or dandelion roots, malt, nuts, figs, rye, and beet root. It should not contain coffee or caffeine.

Herbal coffee can be found at health food stores, ordered online, and can even be found in some supermarkets.

Increase the lactogenic effect of imitation coffee (and enrich the taste) by adding approximately one teaspoon of any or all of the following: blackstrap molasses, malt, almond butter, whole-milk or milk substitute. Almond butter will blend in when milk is added. If desired, spice with cinnamon, anise, ginger, or other lactogenic spices.

One mother excitedly told me that the combination of all these ingredients produced "coffee" that could compare with expensive coffee blends in New York restaurants.

⇨ Mothers of very young babies (in their first to third month) should be careful when taking any drink or food that contains a high concentration of natural sugar, as many babies react to sugar with colic.

Molasses Coffee

Molasses is a rich source of minerals, including calcium.

- Stir a heaping teaspoon of organic black strap molasses into a cup of boiled, steaming water. Add milk or milk-substitute to taste.

- Some mothers also add malt, coffee substitute, or a teaspoon of organic apple cider vinegar to the molasses.

Fruit-Nut Shake

- In a blender, mix together milk, butter-milk or milk substitute, with fruit and almond puree, and, if desired, add brewer's or nutritional yeast.

- Sweeten with malt syrup, honey or blackstrap molasses. Spice with powdered cinnamon, aniseed or a tiny amount of nutmeg.

- If you know your egg source and are sure that they are quite fresh, add one or two raw egg yolks to your shake. Raw egg yolks used to be routinely given to persons in convalescence—and they are delicious in shakes or juice.

Do not use raw egg whites, as they are difficult to digest.

Alcohol

Breastfeeding mothers sometimes drink alcohol to relax. For more information, see *Alcohol—Set Your Limit* in chapter three

- Microbreweries have become popular in the US. They usually produce beers with no additives.

- Mothers who enjoy wine should look for organic wine that does not contain pesticides, herbicides, fungicides, and chemical fertilizers.

Ginger Ale / Ginger Beer

Many brands of ginger ale are made with real ginger, as is ginger beer. If so, one 8 ounce glass will contain about a gram of ginger. One mother saw that she pumped significantly more milk if she drank ginger ale beforehand. That's good news for mothers who enjoy the taste of ginger ale.

Ginger dilates the tiny blood vessels, the capillaries, and improves circulation in the breast. I recommend ginger to mothers who have an impaired let-down due to stress, as the hormones of stress constrict the capillaries, reducing the level of oxytocin that reaches the breast.

Ginger Tea

Ginger tea has the same effect as ginger ale or beer. It is made both with powdered or fresh ginger root.

- Fresh root: simmer a few thin slices of ginger root in 2 cups of water for 10 minutes. Toward the end, stir in unrefined sugar or honey. This tea recipe tastes milder than commercial ginger tea.

- Powdered root: stir 1/2 teaspoon into a cup of boiled water, and sweeten.

- It is important to sweeten ginger tea with raw sugar or honey, according to TCM.

A Selection of Teas as Beverages

The following teas are chosen for their palatability; prepared as a mildly steeped tea, each has a special, unusual, but enjoyable taste that mothers appreciate.

More teas and herbals are described in *A Lactogenic Herbal,* Part Four, where you can also read about the preparation and dosage of these teas *as a beverage.*

Borage
Commercial "Lactation Tea"
Dandelion Root and Leaf
Dill Seed
Elder flower
Fenugreek seed
Hollyhock
Lemon balm
Nettle
Red raspberry leaf
Umbel seeds:
      anise; fennel;
      dill; cumin; caraway
Verbena

CHAPTER FIFTEEN

Breakfast

"...eating a good breakfast not only provides needed energy... but will lead to the consumption of about 600 fewer calories at dinner." — James Braly, M.D., *"Dr. Braly's Food Allergy and Nutrition Revolution"*

This chapter looks at breakfast, at its impact on a mother's health, and at how it can provide clues to a baby's food sensitivities. The recipe section includes traditional breakfast recipes.

A substantial breakfast, one that includes a complex carbohydrate, healthy fat, and protein, is important for breastfeeding mothers. A good breakfast will stabilize a mother's blood sugar (and her mood), provide calories for milk production, balance the thyroid's activity, and prevent overeating later on in the day. Taking a hearty breakfast also helps prevent weightgain.

Mothers who produce a lot of milk are usually hungry, and will instinctively make time to eat in the morning. Mothers with low milk supply, however, may not feel inclined to eat in the morning. If you recognize yourself here, you may discover that forcing yourself to eat breakfast will improve your eating habits, increase your energy, and build your supply.

⇨ Eat a hearty breakfast to break through the vicious cycle of *no hunger and low milk supply.*

Food sensitivities cause some mothers to avoid eating breakfast altogether. These mothers feel over-full and sluggish after eating, so they prefer to live on coffee, soft drinks, smoothies, and fruit during the day. Eating a large meal in the late evening is more comfortable for these mothers, because then they can sleep off the sluggishness. However, eating a large meal in the evening may leave mothers feeling full in the morning, undermining their good intentions to have an ample breakfast. Overeating in the evening will also lead to weightgain, regardless of how few calories are taken during the day. Calories from an evening meal are turned into fat during the night, whereas calories taken during the morning and afternoon can be burned off by normal activities.

⇨ It is best to eat both breakfast and lunch, using foods that do not make you feel sluggish (it may take some detective work to discover what works).

⇨ If nothing works, try using a food combination diet, such as that found in "Fit for Life" by Harvey Diamond. This diet may not be regarded as a diet for life, in my opinion, but allergists agree that it can help people with food sensitivities regain their vitality. If you do the combination diet, *do not* only have fruit for breakfast, and *do* get in extra portions of lactogenic grains.

⇨ If you are not up to a hearty breakfast you might try a *grain-drink*, described in *Beverages*, or have a piece of toast with a hard-boiled egg, an instant oatmeal recipe, or a bowl of good quality commercial cereal made with oats such as Quaker Oat's Life® Cereal, or Malt-o- Meal®.

• Breakfast is important in the postpartum period.

• Breakfast can stabilize your energy and mood for that day.

• Skipping breakfast sets a mother up for blood-sugar highs and lows and mood swings.

• Sensitivity to low blood sugar is stronger in the postpartum, (as it is also premenstrually), so that low blood sugar is more likely to lead to exhaustion and irritability.

• Meal-skipping tends to lower the thyroid's activity and may set a mother up for weightgain. Indeed, women with hypothyroidism say that they feel better and lose weight more easily if they eat meals and snacks regularly throughout the day.

- Meal skipping, and living off caffeine, causes the body to produce stress hormones. In some women, this may inhibit the let-down reflex and contribute to milk supply problems.

⇨ If you find yourself on a blood-sugar roller coaster (craving coffee and sugar), see information on pages 99-117.

Indigestion, Breakfast and a Baby's Colic

In the weeks that follow birth, mothers frequently suffer from flatulence and indigestion. This is often because their intestines are adjusting to a new position within the abdomen, compounded by hormonal changes affecting digestion—but it may also be linked to digestive weaknesses that were exacerbated by pregnancy and birth, and possibly by medication or antibiotics.

Lactation consultants have observed that mothers with chronic flatulence or other signs of indigestion often have babies who are fussy or who have colic. This is not surprising. As discussed in Chapter Four, mothers and babies usually share food sensitivities. On the positive side, this means that when a mother identifies foods that trigger her baby's fussiness or colic, she also identifies foods that are causing *her* to be fatigued, have flatulence, or other symptoms. So a food-sensitive baby can act as a barometer for the mother, helping her to implement dietary changes that will lead to improved health.

Sometimes, however, it is not a specific food that is the culprit, but a combination of foods. One problematic combination for all people to digest is starch, fat, and sugar. This combination is typically found at breakfast: toast, butter, and honey; oatmeal, milk, and dried fruit; packaged sugary cereal, and milk.

By watching her digestive response to breakfast (does she have flatulence, does she feel suddenly fatigued), a mother may gain clues as to why her baby becomes fussy or starts to cry a few hours later. Solving this problem may be as simple as taking away one of the three foods, for instance, bread with honey or jam, but *without butter*, or bread with butter or cheese, *but without anything sugary*. Oatmeal with butter and salt, but without sugar is surprisingly tasty; oatmeal with honey, but without fat (milk or butter) also works. Sometimes, though, a mother may have to do detective work to discover the culprit. See Chapter Four for more information.

Grains and Spices for Breakfast

The combination of a lactogenic grain and lactogenic spices is widely used to increase milk production. In India, breastfeeding mothers cook 1/2 teaspoon of powdered fenugreek and other spices into mung-flour, rice-, or cracked-wheat porridge. To increase milk production in Brazil, mothers cook white corn flour in milk with sugar and cinnamon. This traditional Native American galactagogue is called 'canjica.' In Peru, quinoa or oats and cinnamon are taken: the grain is prepared with a lot of water; the grain-water is taken as a beverage, and the grain is eaten for a meal.

Preparing Oatmeal and Other Breakfast Cereals

In the US, oatmeal is the number one food used to increase milk supply. Oat is one of the most nutritious of all foods, including substances that relax and nourish the nerves. Oat's beta glucan, its saponins, and its phytoestrogen support lactation, whether taken as long-cooking oatmeal, as quick-cooking, pre-flavored oatmeal, as oatmeal cookies, oatmeal bread, or oatmeal cake.

Oats are, of course, more healthful if organically grown, and if pre-soaked, gently cooked, and taken with natural sugar and healthy fats. The good news however is that no matter how you take oats, you get a wealth of nutrients and a lactogenic boost.

Basics of Oatmeal
- Oatmeal can be prepared with water or milk. I prefer water.
- Gently simmer oatmeal, stirring occasionally.
- Steel cut grains require more water, and may simmer gently for more than a half hour, until the grain is tender and the water is absorbed. However, if it has been pre-soaked, (see below), the cooking time may be less than 10 minutes.
- Depending on the type of oatmeal you use, adjust the amount of fluid and cooking time.
- Thick, rolled flakes require more cooking time than finely cut flakes.
- Pre-soaked oats require the same amount of fluid that was used for soaking to be added again for cooking, i.e., double the amount of fluid.

Thin, Cool, and Sweeten Your Cereal

After preparing oats, stir in milk, milk substitute, butter, or cream to thin the oatmeal and to cool it down more quickly. Oatmeal can also be thinned by using a natural sweetener such as honey, molasses, maple syrup, or apple butter.

Spice Up Your Cereal

- Add raisins, split almonds, coconut flakes, flaxseed, sesame or sunflower seeds.

- Sesame, flaxseed, and almonds are particularly lactogenic. Crush the seeds to improve their digestibility.

- Add a natural sweetener such as honey, maple syrup, malt syrup, pear syrup, apple butter, or blackstrap molasses.

- Almond-milk, rice-milk, or coconut-milk can be substituted for cow's milk, should a mother or the baby be sensitive to dairy products.

- Soymilk should be used sparingly. Its strong phytoestrogen could possibly be anti-lactogenic if taken in large amounts. Soymilk also suppresses thyroid function, frequently giving sensitive women symptoms of hypothyroidism.

- Cinnamon, aniseed, powdered fennel seed, and powdered fenugreek[*] seed, taste fine with oats, millet, and barley.

- Oatmeal and barley-meal are also delicious prepared with butter and salt.

---

[*] Powdered spices can be found at super-markets and Asian food stores, or can be bought online.

About flaxseed

Use fresh flaxseed for its essential fatty acids and regulating effect on the bowels. Flaxseed oil can become rancid, even in the refrigerator; it should be used within about six weeks. Grinding 1 tbsp. of whole flaxseed immediately before adding it to a breakfast cereal ensures highest quality, fresh flaxseed oil. Soaked overnight, the whole soft seed can be added to a breakfast cereal as a laxative.

⇨ If you use a mini-grinder to grind flaxseed, clean it often, as the oil will become rancid.

Quick Recipe for Finely Flaked Grains

Organic oats, millet, and barley can be bought in healthfood stores as *finely ground flakes*. Place the flakes in a cereal bowl, add boiled water (1–2 times water to flakes), stir, and soak for 3 – 5 minutes. The cereal will fluff up and thicken. Add more water as necessary.

Options: add water, milk, milk-substitute, cream, butter, and natural sweeteners to thin and cool the cereal, plus a combination of spices, nuts, seeds, and dried fruit mentioned above.

A Healthier Way to Prepare Breakfast Cereal

Oats and barley are traditionally pre-soaked in water, along with an acidic substance, such as yogurt or vinegar, for at least 7 and up to 24 hours before cooking. Soaking breaks down phytic acid and turns off enzyme inhibitors in the grain, rendering it more digestible.

Women who experiment with pre-soaking find that they can tell the difference between cereal that has been soaked and cereal that has not. Cereal that has *not* been soaked has a raw, unfinished taste compared to soaked cereal.

Pre-soaked oatmeal has an old-world taste, and is slightly sour and thick. It is invigorating while calming the nerves. Oat porridge was prized by farmers, fishers, and by people who performed hard physical work. It was routinely given to mothers convalescing from birth.

Traditional American Oatmeal
3 - 4 portions:

Ingredients for soaking:
1 cup rolled or cracked oats
1 cup of warm water
2 tablespoons of acidic substance: unflavored yogurt, kefir.
⇨ For mothers avoiding dairy, add lemon juice or organic vinegar.

Additional ingredients for cooking:
1 cup of water
1/4 – 1/2 teaspoon salt (optional)

Soak overnight, or from morning to morning in a warm place. (To avoid spoilage in warm weather, soak in the refrigerator.)

Next morning, bring the cooking water and optional salt to a boil. Add the pre-soaked mixture and simmer on a low heat for up to five minutes. Add more water if necessary. Remove from the heat and stir in spices, seeds, nuts and other ingredients listed above in *Spice Up Your Breakfast Cereal.* Thin and cool the cereal with butter, cream, milk, or milk substitute, and with a natural sweetener.

Traditional Irish Cut Oatmeal: Non-Slimy
Irish Oatmeal is steel cut rather than rolled, and is less slimy than American brands. Irish Oatmeal can be made by grinding whole oats in the bowl of a food processor, using the blade fixture. If you bake the whole oats on a baking sheet at 350 degrees until they turn light brown before you steel cut them, the oatmeal will have a nuttier texture.

Steel cut oats contain both coarsely cut pieces, and pieces so finely cut that they are powder. More water is absorbed, both in soaking and in cooking.

Serves 4 – 6

Ingredients for soaking – overnight or from morning to morning.

1 cup steel cut oatmeal
2 cups warm water
4 tablespoons of acidic substance:
unflavored yogurt, kefir.

(For mothers avoiding dairy, add
lemon juice or organic vinegar.)
Additional ingredients for cooking:

2 cups of water
1/2 – 1 teaspoon salt (optional)

Soak the covered steel-cut oats in warm water, plus an acidic substance (see above) in a warm place, either overnight or from one morning to the next. (To avoid spoilage during warm weather, soak in the refrigerator.)

Next morning bring the cooking water and optional salt to a boil, add the pre-soaked mixture and simmer on a low heat for up to 10 minutes, stirring frequently and adding water if necessary. Remove from the heat and stir in spices, seeds, nuts and other ingredients listed above in *Spice Up Your Breakfast Cereal*. Thin and cool the cereal with butter, cream, milk or milk substitute, and with a natural sweetener.

Alternatives to Oatmeal Porridge

Oatmeal is not the only grain that can be used for porridge. Cracked wheat or rice, mungbean flour, buckwheat, millet and barley (as flakes), quinoa and amaranth are lactogenic alternatives to oatmeal.

Women with chronic low milk supply frequently say that foods and herbs lose their effect with time. They see better results if they alternate, reaping the benefits of each and preventing their bodies from becoming insensitive to any one food or herb.

Finely ground flakes of oatmeal, barley or millet, and also amaranth and quinoa, can be quickly prepared (described above in *Quick Recipe for Rolled and Ground Grains)*. Rolled or cracked grains can be pre-soaked for up to 24 hours and then prepared as with traditional oatmeal. Flour of any kind can be roasted in butter or oil with lactogenic seeds and spices, and then cooked into gruel by adding water and stirring frequently. Flour can also be pre-soaked to improve digestibility (see below).

⇨ See page 170 for Dr. Vinod Verma's special mixture of spices to mix into cereal or mungbean gruel.

Pancakes

Making pancakes from scratch is easy: one egg, one cup of milk, one cup of flour and a pinch of salt will produce a pancake that fills the bottom of a medium-sized frying pan, and just about covers a dinner plate. Spread it with butter and honey, cut into bite-sized pieces, and this children's favorite can be eaten without making too much mess.

Over the years, I have learned different ways to make pancakes. Add oil, subtract flour and, voila, French crepes! Add egg and subtract flour for a European-style omelet. Add baking powder and sugar for American pancakes.

⇨ Pancakes are more nutritious if made from whole-grain flour, or from half white flour and half whole-grain.

⇨ Pancake batter can be left to soak up to 24 hours to reduce the phytic acids. Add buttermilk, kefir, or yogurt instead of pasteurized milk.

⇨ Dairy allergies: pre-soak with water and one tablespoon of lemon juice or vinegar. After soaking, thin with a milk substitute.

⇨ Pancakes can be cooked in butter or coconut oil.

Recipe 1: Plain Pancake

Serves 1 –2

Combine well:	1 egg
	1 cup milk
	1 cup flour
	1 pinch of salt

Spread the warm bottom of a pan with very little butter; heat but don't brown. With a soup ladle, pour the pancake onto the pan, from the center outwards. Once the pancake is firm, toss it to briefly cook the other side.

Place on plate, sprinkle with sugar or honey, cut into bite-sized pieces for a child.

Recipe 2: American pancakes

Serves 1 – 2

Combine well:	1 cup of flour
	1 1/2 teaspoons of baking powder
	2 tablespoons of sugar
	1/4 teaspoon of salt

| Add, blend until smooth: | 1 egg |
| | 1 cup of milk *or* 2/3 cup of milk, 1 tablespoon of melted butter |

If desired, stir in 1 tablespoon of oat flakes, coconut flakes, ground almond or sesame seeds, raisins or berries.

Let the batter stand for a half hour—it will become bubbly. With a sauce ladle, spoon the batter onto a thin layer of hot butter to make several pancakes that can be served with maple syrup, honey, butter and whipped cream. They can also be frozen, and popped into the toaster for a quick snack.

Muffins

Muffins are as easy to make as pancakes. They are a delicious addition to breakfast, and can be taken as a snack.

Basic Recipe

Mix well together:	2 cups all purpose flour, or half whole grain flour
	1/8 teaspoon salt
	1 tablespoon baking soda
	1/2 cup sugar, finely ground raw sugar honey or maple syrup[*]

---

[*] If you choose to use honey or maple syrup, mix it together with the melted butter in the pan.

Gently heat in a pan: 3 – 5 tablespoons butter
1 2/3 cup of fluid, (apple juice, water, milk or milk substitute)

Combine all ingredients and mix until you have slimy, thick, wet dough. Pour into well-buttered muffin tins, 3/4 full.

Bake at 325 degrees for about 20 minutes.

Options: Additional ingredients such as raisins, seeds, nuts, chopped dry figs, dates, apricots, should be added to the dry ingredients and thoroughly mixed in before adding the wet ingredients.

Suggestions:

Raisin-Aniseed: 1/2 cup of raisins, 1/2 teaspoon of aniseed.
Raisin-Cinnamon: 1/2 cup of raisins, 1/2 teaspoon of cinnamon.
Date-ginger: 1/2 cup of chopped date, 1 teaspoon of ground ginger.

Chickpea (Garbanzo) Ayurvedic Breakfast

The chickpea is recorded as a galactagogue in Greek and Egyptian herbals. They are rich in saponins and phytoestrogen, and are an easy way to get solid nutrition into your menu. Sprouted, they can be eaten throughout the day as a snack. They can be added to salad, stew or soup. Refrigerated, they remain fresh for about four days—though they lose their delightful crunchiness after two days.

Sprouted chickpea no longer cause flatulence—so common with legumes. In India, sprouted chickpeas are prescribed for pregnant women for breakfast, either raw, or sautéed in butter with yogurt sauce. (Try spicing yogurt with curry powder and seasoned salt, or with dill seed, fresh garlic and seasoned salt.)

To sprout, wash a handful of dried chickpeas under flowing water in a strainer. Place them in a bowl covered with at least double the amount of water and soak for one hour or longer. Pour off the water, cover the bowl, and allow it to stand for 24 hours. If you live in a hot, humid area, rinse off the chickpeas occasionally throughout the day. Rinse again before eating.

- If you enjoy chickpea, set up a handful each morning for use next day. Along with being one of our healthiest foods, chickpea is one of our least expensive.

- A tasty dish based on chickpea is hummus. Another is falafel. You'll find a recipe for hummus in *Snacks*.

- Canned chickpea can also be used in chickpea recipes. Be sure to use the liquid from the can.

Nut and Fruit Blender Breakfast

You will need 1/3 cup of raw, unsalted nuts and seeds. Make almonds the main ingredient and add lesser amounts of the others. Choose between almonds, hazel nut, pumpkin seeds, sesame seeds, sunflower seeds, and flax seeds.

Soak the nuts and seeds in 1 cup of water for 12 – 24 hours. Rinse, put into blender, and liquefy while slowly pouring in 1 – 2 cups of water. Blend in 1 – 2 teaspoons of a natural sweetener such as honey or maple syrup, and 1 – 1 1/2 cups of fruit such as banana, berries, raisins, figs or dates.

Optional: 1/2 – 1 teaspoon of nutritional yeast; 2 tablespoons of quick-cooking oat flakes.

⇨ Colic and allergy concern: nuts and seeds are common triggers for food sensitivities, so keep an eye on your baby's response to this meal.

Egg

If there's one great food that almost everyone knows how to prepare, it is the humble egg: hard or soft boiled, fried sunny side up or down, scrambled, as an omelet with delicious fillings, poached or Benedict.

Take advantage of the complete protein in egg white and the vitamins A, D, E, and B group in egg yolk, including B 12.

Add an ample pinch of dried marjoram leaves to your eggs. Marjoram is a mild anti-depressant as well as being lactogenic. Basil, another lactogenic, mood-boosting herb, blends well with marjoram, and both taste great with eggs.

⇨ If you are concerned about cholesterol in eggs, see the section *Eggs and Cholesterol* in Chapter 3.

⇨ If at all possible, buy eggs that are raised organically. They may be available in your local health food store, and are often not much more expensive than commercial eggs. In some areas in the US, families keep organic-raised hens in their gardens. Perhaps a neighbor will sell you eggs for as long as you are breastfeeding.

Virgin Olive Oil for Breakfast

In Mediterranean countries, people suffer from less heart disease than we in Europe or the US, partly because the fats they use—olive oil, sesame oil, fish oil, avocado and nuts all protect the heart.

In these countries, whole-grain bread is dunked into virgin olive oil mixed with spices, mashed olives, or honey for breakfast. I thought this was interesting, and that I would include it here for mothers who are having a difficult time incorporating healthy oils into their menu plans.

Simply pour out a thin layer of olive oil (or sesame oil—tastes sweeter) onto a plate. Sprinkle in lactogenic spices, such as marjoram or basil, or place a spoonful of honey in the center of the dish. Using bread or toast, mop up the oil, spices, and honey. As a side-dish, take a portion of hummus, tahini, or halvah.

Toast

Toast is a great way to get quick nutrition onto a dish. Try to find good-quality bread. Prepare lactogenic spreads for toast or crackers. For more information, see below, in *Snacks*.

Breakfast Beverages

- Look in the section on beverages to find one that suits you.

- If you have low blood pressure and depend upon a stimulating drink to get you going in the morning, read *Caffeine (coffee, tea, soda, chocolate) on pages 55-57*.

- Do not take a stimulating beverage *instead* of breakfast.

- If you usually take coffee or tea with sugar, you might consider learning to appreciate it plain, or with a dash of milk, cream or milk substitute. The two stimulants, caffeine and sugar, are particularly unhealthy when taken together as each depletes calcium and drains the nervous system[*].

- Dilute fruit juice with water to prevent a dip in your blood sugar levels.

- A cup of mild, lactogenic tea can be taken before and during breakfast. If you have digestive difficulties, try dill seed tea ten minutes before breakfast.

- A list of my favorite, most palatable teas is found in the beverage section.

---

[*] Just as there are "nervine tonics," or foods that relax and nourish the nerves, there are "nervine depleters," or foods that stimulate the nerves without however providing any of the nutrients necessary to maintain their healthy function. Coffee and sugar are such depleters.

CHAPTER SIXTEEN

Snacks

Toast or Sandwich

Bread, if not overused, is a wonderful food. Whole-grain bread is more nutritious than bread made from white flour, but some people find it hard to digest and do better with white bread, or with bread made from half white, half whole-grain flour. Sourdough bread, and bread made from bulgur flour may also be easier to digest, and toasting bread makes it easier to digest as well.

If you feel fatigued after eating bread, be sure that you are combining it with protein and fat so that your meal is digested more slowly and doesn't lead to a dip in your blood sugar levels.

If you still feel fatigued, and if you suspect an allergy to gluten in wheat, look for gluten-free bread and flour in your health food store. For more information on gluten, see *Gluten Sensitivity* on page 137.

Crackers: look for the large, thick kinds used in Europe as a substitute for bread. Your healthfood store may carry crackers that are made with organic whole grain flour and other organic ingredients. Because they do not contain yeast, they are useful for mothers who are sensitive to yeast.

Pumpernickel bread is another useful food for persons who are sensitive to yeast, i.e., mothers who have chronic, recurring thrush or vaginal yeast infections. As far as I know, no studies have been done on colicky babies and yeast sensitivity. Because yeast is a common allergy with children, however, eliminating yeast from the mother's diet may be worth an experiment if unknown food sensitivities are suspected in the baby[*].

---

[*] Yeast is found in bread, fermented dairy products, (cheese, yogurt, kefir), in vinegar, ketchup and salad dressing, and in foods made with vinegar. Yeast sensitivity and allergy is thought to correspond to fungal overgrowth in the intestine and body. For more information, see page 64.

Mayonnaise

Mayonnaise found in supermarkets is made with vegetable oil that has been refined at high temperatures. It contains trans-fatty acids that are counterproductive if you are trying to integrate healthier fats into your diet or increase your milk supply. Fortunately, it is fairly easy to make mayonnaise from fresh ingredients. Mayonnaise is a good substitute for butter if you are avoiding dairy.

You will need:

1 fresh egg
4 – 5 teaspoons of fresh lemon juice
1 – 2 teaspoon of mustard
1/2 teaspoon of sea salt or seasoned salt

Briefly mix these ingredients in your blender. While blending at a medium speed, slowly dribble in 1 cup of unrefined, cold-pressed sunflower seed oil, safflower oil, or walnut oil. To better balance your EFAs, take 3/4 cup of any combination of the above oils, and add 1/4 cup flaxseed oil.

If you don't mind the unusual taste, try making mayonnaise with virgin olive oil. Homemade mayonnaise remains fresh for about two weeks in the refrigerator.

Various Toppings

Make a quick lactogenic snack by spreading any of the toppings and spreads described in this section onto buttered (or *mayonnaised*) toast or crackers.

Nut butters: look for almond butter, cashew butter, sunflower seed butter and sesame seed paste (tahini) at a healthfood store or online.

Almond butter and *sesame seed paste* (tahini, gomasio) are widely used to support milk production.

Miso: a thick paste made out of fermented soy beans. Miso—a good source of protein—is usually added as flavoring to vegetables and grains, but it can also be used as a very thin spread. It is very salty.

Basil Pesto: made of lactogenic fresh basil leaves, virgin olive oil, parmesan cheese, garlic, lemon juice and pine nuts. This sauce is usually reserved for pasta—but in the postpartum we are allowed to cheat and spread it thinly onto toast when we crave a piquant taste.

Vegemite®: contains yeast and is taken to improve milk supply. Though it is bitter, it tastes fine spread thinly on buttered toast.

Seasoned salt and **herbs** (marjoram, thyme, caraway seed). Sprinkle on organic seasoned sea salt (available in health food stores) onto buttered toast or cracker, and cover with a pinch of marjoram, basil, dill, or caraway seeds.

Blackstrap molasses. True mineral-rich blackstrap molasses is somewhat bitter but delicious as a topping.

Leftover spaghetti sauce. Leftover sauce is a tasty topping.

Avocado slices, sprinkled with seasoned salt, topped with alfalfa sprouts or lettuce, and dappled with hulled sesame seeds, are a luxurious snack for a tired mother.

Cheese and cottage cheese are less allergenic than straight milk. Mix seasoned salt and one lactogenic spice, such as dill seed or caraway seed, into cottage cheese. Leave the cottage cheese in the refrigerator for several hours so that the flavor of the spice can permeate the cheese. Use it as a spread on bread or crackers, or as filling for an omelet.

Hard boiled eggs are useful when you feel the need for protein but don't have time to cook (yes, in theory they can be taken every day, except in case of allergy to egg). Layer toast with mayonnaise, seasoned salt, lettuce and possibly tomato.

Slices of leftover poultry or meat. Save slices of meat in your fridge and don't forget to use them promptly! Prepare toast as above with eggs.

Hummus

Hummus is tasty, filling, and it provides a complete protein if combined (as in the traditional recipe) with sesame seed paste.

Canned chickpea can be used for this recipe. Otherwise, soak for at least 1 1/2 hours, and simmer for at least 1 1/2 hours (not in the soaking water) and allow it to cool before using.

One low-supply mother was very enthusiastic about hummus. She found that it supported her supply just as well as barley water or oatmeal. If she took it to work with her, she could pump more milk. Here is her 'quick' recipe:

"Put drained chickpeas in a food processor with 2 – 3 garlic cloves, a little lemon juice (up to 1/2 cup), and some dill weed. Add about ½ cup liquid from the can, process until smooth, and then add a bit more liquid, about 3/4 cup in all. Process again until smooth. If you use 2 cans you have lots of hummus. It travels well, for instance, to work for lunch."

Extras: add any combination of the following:

- 1 tablespoon of flaxseed oil

- 2 tablespoons of sesame paste (tahini)

- Olive oil to make it smoother

- For more taste, add coriander and cumin seeds, and a pinch of cayenne pepper.

- If you have severe supply problems, try leaving out the lemon juice and adding more of the liquid from the can.

Baked Garlic Clove Spread

Garlic is a well-known galactagogue, for mothers who tolerate it. It encourages babies to drink longer and more eagerly, leading to a stronger milk supply. Here is one mother's recipe.

"Us Italians just cut off the top third of a cluster of cloves and pour olive oil over the top. Put the cluster of cloves in aluminum foil (skins and all), bake at 350 for about 1 hour. When done, just squeeze each clove and the roasted garlic will slide out. To make it really sinful, mash it up and add freshly grated cheese and a little more oil. I then spread it on Italian bread and YUMMY! Everyone I serve it to loves it!"

Butter Spread

Spiced butter offers a simple way for time-pressed mothers to get healthful herbs into their diets.

Allow a stick of butter to become soft at room temperature. Mash the ingredients below into the butter. Scoop into a container with a cover and keep it in the refrigerator.

Combinations:
Sea-salt to taste and fresh, finely diced basil and/or marjoram leaves.
Same recipe, but using dried leaves.
Sea-salt to taste and dill weed, dried or fresh.

Coconut Spread

Coconut oil can be used to make spreads, too. Virgin coconut oil (non-processed) tastes best and has the most health benefits, but it is more expensive.

Add turmeric to coconut oil. Turmeric, a powerful antioxidant, fights inflammation all over the body including the inflammation caused by auto-immune diseases. In India, it is said to prevent mastitis.

Preparation: Into 1/2 cup of coconut oil, mash 2 – 4 teaspoons of powdered turmeric. Add in powdered anise, ginger and cinnamon and mash together until you have a thick paste. Mix in honey until the spread is smooth and easy to spread.

Refrigerate the spread; take it out an hour or so before using so that it becomes soft. Careful—this spread is delicious and you may be tempted to eat it like candy[*].

Raw Veggies and Nut-Butter Snack

Celery sticks, carrot sticks, and slices of beet, fennel, or apples can be spread with nut-butter made from calcium-rich almonds or sesame seeds—both of which are widely used to support milk production. Sunflower-seed butter does not share the lactogenic reputation of almonds and sesame, but it can be used for variety.

Preparation: Wash and separate the layers of fennel. Cut into one inch wide slices. Peel or scrub carrot and cut lengthwise into fourths. Scrub beet root, cut in half, and cut the halves into 1/4 inch wide half-circle shaped slices.

With a knife, place a small pat of nut-butter onto the veggie before biting off that piece.

⇨ Colic concern: it is possible that you or your baby could have digestive problems from raw veggies (and possibly raw fruit as well). If so, you may have to restrict yourself to cooked vegetables (and fruit) for a while.

⇨ If you are eating mainly raw vegetables and food, and if you are also suffering from supply problems, please read *Strike a Balance between Hot and Cold Food* in chapter three.

⇨ Naturopaths recommend that people with digestive difficulties take salad and raw vegetables before 2 p.m., to allow plenty of time to digest them before sleep.

---

[*] If you use a lot of spices in your foods you can quickly approach a daily dosage. Don't overdo it. As with any food, gradually build up your usage and test your tolerance to the herb or spice.

Snack on Raw Veggies

Use the same vegetables described above as a snack. Celery is good for the kidneys, carrot for the liver, fennel is strongly lactogenic, and beet root is perhaps our most nutritious vegetable, with strong anti-tumor properties.

⇨ If you feel fatigued after eating these sweet vegetables, this may signal that your blood sugar is responding ultra-sensitively to your diet. Taking protein and/or fat (such as nut butter spread) with these sweet veggies may help.

Snack on Sliced Beet-Root

Root vegetables, such as beet and carrot, are said to be particularly lactogenic. I am giving beet root its own section because most people do not know how delicious and satisfying beet root can be. It is a mess to prepare though. Here is the easiest way I've found to date.

Brush off the vegetable under flowing lukewarm water. On a *plastic cutting board that can be washed off*, slice off the upper and lower ends of the beet. Halve the beet from top to bottom and place the exposed sides down on the cutting board. Halve again, lengthwise, and then slice in 1/4 to 1/2 inch slices, down the width of the beet root.

Beet root, if not absolutely fresh, contains an acidic substance that will burn the back of your throat and make you wish to never eat beet root again. The *trick* is to separate the slices in a bowl, and allow the beet root to air out for about ten minutes. The acidic substance will evaporate, and the beet will be delicious. Through oxidation, the pores of the beet will close tight so that it is no longer as messy when you hold a slice in your fingers—though you still have to wipe off your pink fingertips occasionally.

My whole family eats raw beet root. Something about the taste communicates to the brain that it is a great food, so that it can be hard not to binge on beet. Fortunately, it is so healthy that it is okay to binge. Beet root is my favorite 'dieting to lose weight food' because its nutrients truly satisfy my hunger. However, you do have to be sure that you and your baby can tolerate raw veggies before indulging in raw beet. (Beet sliced in cubes cooks quickly, too.)

⇨ Iron: if we eat beet root regularly, my children and I test for very high levels of iron in our blood.

⇨ If beet root is not allowed time to ripen, it will taste bitter. Look for home-gardened or biologically grown beet.

Trail-Mix

Raw nuts are more healthful than roasted or salted nuts, as well as being a pleasure for the palate. The bad news is that nuts do contain phytates and enzyme inhibitors, so that eating a lot of them could make you feel sluggish and heavy. Knowing this, it is easier to resist overeating delicious nuts.

Because many people aren't used to eating raw nuts they may taste plain at first. If you feel inclined to eat chocolate covered nuts, and if they don't cause you and your baby digestive problems—by all means do. Generally though, we should eat plain raw nuts and seeds.

Trail Mix Recipe
Combine any or all of the following:

Nuts and seeds: raw almonds (without skin is easier to digest), cashews, pecans, macadamias, hazelnuts, pinenuts, sunflower and pumpkin seeds.

Dried fruit: raisins, figs, apricot, date, papaya, mango, pineapple. Look for unsulfured products.

⇨ Colic concern: the concentrated sugar in dried fruit can lead to digestive problems. Introduce them gradually to your diet and observe your baby's reaction.

Popcorn

I make popcorn from scratch. First, cover the bottom of the pan with a film of virgin olive oil—not too much though, you don't' want to smother the corn. Add just enough corn to cover the bottom of the pan. Heat the pan at a high temperature. When the corn begins to pop, turn down the heat somewhat and shake the pan occasionally.

I don't add butter or other fat to my popcorn. Instead, I sprinkle on an organic seasoned salt, such as Trocomare. My kids and I have come to love this snack, even though it doesn't have much in common with popcorn at the movies.

Leftovers

Plan for leftovers when you prepare meals. Poultry can be sliced and shredded for sandwiches or salad; and vegetables can be stored with their sauce, and taken on toast.

Leftover pancakes can be frozen and toasted for a snack.

Even oatmeal can be mixed with egg and turned into an oatmeal-burger.

CHAPTER SEVENTEEN

Lunch and Dinner

The Main Meal of the Day

In the US, we snack for lunch and splurge for dinner. Enormous dinners contribute *in a big way* to the fact that the US has so many more overweight persons than countries in Europe, where lunch is still the main meal of the day. If being overweight is one of your issues, try to have a hearty breakfast and a satisfying lunch so that you can use the rest of the day to burn calories. Snack between meals, and keep dinner a reasonable size.

In this Chapter, I do not always provide exact measurements for ingredients, especially when describing recipes for vegetables and soup. Mothers tend to get a *feel* for how much their family can eat. When you make these recipes, keep the hunger and the taste preferences of your family in mind, and let yourself be intuitive when it comes to just how much of this or that goes into the pot.

Make Lunch and Dinner more Lactogenic

Remember to include lactogenic veggies, complex carbohydrates, spices, condiments, and fats in your meals. For more information on these ingredients, see *The Lactogenic Foods* in Chapter Nine.

Grains and Legumes

Preparing Grains

Grains can be cooked without pre-soaking, but their nutrients are more available if they have been soaked overnight or longer. Soak in the fridge if the weather is hot and humid.

Salt: add 1/2 to 1 teaspoon of salt per cup of grain. Use only a small amount of salt while cooking, and allow your family members to add seasoned salt, each to his or her taste.

Liquid: use water, or chicken, meat or vegetable stock. After cooking, add butter or virgin olive oil.

- The easiest way to prepare grain works especially well with soft grains: brown rice, oats, barley and millet. Place the rinsed grain in a pot together with the amount of necessary liquid and salt. Bring to a rolling boil for ten minutes, turn off the heat, cover the pot, and leave in a warm place for at least two hours. Cover the pot with a warm towel or blanket to reduce heat loss. The grain will be perfect by lunchtime.

- The *next* easiest way is to first boil the liquid and salt, add the rinsed grain, bring to a boil again, then cover the pot and continue to cook at the lowest possible heat for the time indicated in the chart below.

- Pilaf method: while stirring, toast the rinsed grain, together with minced onions and spices, in a pan until dry. Add just enough butter and/or olive oil to coat each kernel, and toast until golden. Add double the amount of boiling liquid to grain, and cook for approximately the time in the chart below. This works well with: brown rice, wild rice, barley, bulgur, and millet. For buckwheat, you may want to roast the grain in a dry skillet with a beaten egg to harden and separate the grains before boiling.

- Soft grains that absorb water quickly, such as millet, buckwheat, quinoa and amaranth, need to be checked often to prevent scorching the pan; or use a double boiler.

- The most time-intensive cooking method is to rinse the grain in cold water, soak for 8 – 12 hours, and rinse again before cooking. Add enough liquid to more than cover the grain, plus salt, bring to a boil, cover, and allow to cook at the lowest possible temperature until the water has been absorbed and the grain is soft. The longer it has been soaked, the shorter the cooking time.

● Another method is to bring the rinsed grain to a boil for ten minutes, soak for 8 hours, change the liquid, (do not cook in the soaking liquid), add salt, bring to a boil again, cover and simmer at a low heat for twenty minutes.

Add extra water to have lactogenic 'grain-water' as a   beverage.

Add extra spices about ten minutes before the grains are finished.

1 cup of:	liquid	cooking time	yield
Amaranth	3 cups	25–30 min.	2 1/2 cups
Barley	1 cup	20–30 min.	4 cups
Buckwheat	4 - 5 cups	20 min.	3 cups
Bulgur	2 cups	15 min.	2 1/2
Cornmeal	4 - 5 cups	30–40 min.	4 - 5 cups
Millet[*]	4 cups	25–30 min.	4 cups
Oats	3 cups	30–40 min.	3 1/2 cups
Quinoa	3 cups	20–30 min.	2 1/2 cups
Rice-Brown	2 - 2 1/2 cups	35–45 min.	2 1/2 cups
Rice-Wild	4 cups	40–50 min.	3 - 3 1/2 cups

Preparing Legumes

Legumes should be soaked between 12 – 24 hours, depending on the size of the bean, in three times their volume of water. *Lentils* are the exception. They only need to be soaked a few hours; they can also be prepared without being soaked, though they are a bit less digestible.

---

[*] Millet does not need to be pre-soaked.

Discard the soaking water. Add plenty of fresh water, more than necessary to cover the legumes, so that you can drink the extra, lactogenic "legume-water" later on.

Grain-legume combinations provide a complete protein. Grains and legumes that share the same cooking time can easily be combined together. Examples include: rice and lentils; rice and split peas; or rice and split mung beans.

1 cup of:	cooking time
Adzuki beans	1 1/2 – 2 hours
Chickpea	1 1/2 – 6 hours
Fava beans	1 1/2 – 2 hours
Kidney beans	1 1/2 – 2 hours
Lentils	1 hour
Lima beans (baby)	1 1/2 – 2 hours
Lima beans (big)	1 hour
Mung beans	1- 1 1/2 hours
Split mung bean[*]	45 min
Dried Peas	1- 1 1/2 hours
Split peas	45 m. – 1 hour
Pinto beans	1 1/2 – 2 hours

---

[*] Split mung bean without the shell does not have to be presoaked.

Variations on a Vegetable Theme

Women around the world think nothing of heaping ingredients into one pot and serving their families stew or thick soup that is hearty enough to be called a meal on its own. Dr. Vinod Verma, an authority on Ayurvedic traditions for women, suggests that mothers combine several vegetables into a meal so that the body is given a wide variety of vitamins and minerals from which to pick and choose.

Cooking this way is easy, except that we are not used to doing it. In this section, I explore ways to get as much nutrition as possible into one pot. Use small amounts of several vegetables and cut them into large pieces to shorten preparation time.

Shopping

Buy medium amounts of a variety of vegetables. If you combine several vegetables in your meals, medium amounts should last several days. Of course, if you are cooking for children and for your husband as well you'll have to adjust your shopping to account for more 'mouths.'

Keep stocked up with frozen vegetables as well. Frozen vegetables require less preparation time, and are nearly as nutritious as fresh vegetables. Choose combinations that contain naturally sweet, lactogenic veggies such as corn, peas, green beans and carrots.

Choosing Combinations: Sweet and Bitter

Vegetables combine sweet and bitter tastes. For instance, the inner core of a carrot is sweet, whereas the outside is somewhat bitter. By playing with different combinations, and by experimenting with lactogenic condiments and spices, vegetables become an interesting and satisfying food.

- **Sweet veggies** such as **peas**, **carrots**, and **fennel** blend well together.

- **Mushrooms** blend well with most sweet vegetables and tend to make them taste 'interesting.'

- **Onions** blend well with all vegetables, though onions are actually rather sweet themselves.

- **Potato** blends well with both sweet and bitter veggies.

- **Yam** and **sweet potato** blend well with other sweet vegetables, and taste 'interesting' with bitter veggies.

- **Chinese cabbage** is sweeter than usual cabbage; it can be cooked or used raw in salad.

- **Yam** does well in the same dish with potatoes. One would ordinarily never think of cooking yams, potatoes and carrots together, or beets, potatoes and carrots, though this is commonly done in other parts of the world. Sweet, starchy veggies satisfy our need for natural sugars.

- A few **bitter vegetables**, such as **green beans, broccoli** and **Swiss chard**, have such a distinct taste that they demand to be the main veggie in a mix. While they don't do very well with each other, each does blend well with potato, carrots, and onion.

- **Asparagus** has such a distinct flavor that it begs to be eaten alone, as does **kale** and **artichoke**.

Sample combinations (see next section for more cooking explanation):

- Carrots, sweet potato, potato, (red beet if you don't mind your meal turning red), beet greens, marjoram. Suggestion: steam all together with butter and seasoned salt, and then add olive oil.

- Onions, potatoes, mushrooms, carrots (or zucchini), Swiss chard. Suggestion: Sauté onions in butter, add other ingredients and steam together with butter in the pan.

- Green beans, carrots, onions, potato, mushrooms. Suggestion: Sauté onions until they are transparent, then add other ingredients and steam together with butter in pan.

- Fennel, potato or sweet potato, carrot, Chinese cabbage, kale, or Swiss chard. Suggestion: Steam all together with butter and seasoned salt.

Methods of Preparation

Estimate the Quantity

Take into consideration how many people will be eating, and also, remember that you may want leftovers to snack on, or extra portions to freeze.

Washing Vegetables

To wash, hold the veggie under lukewarm flowing tap water, rub with your fingers or scrub with a veggie brush, making sure that all parts of the vegetable are exposed to the water. Some experts recommend soaking veggies in lukewarm, salted water, (salad should be soaked in cold water so that it doesn't wilt), or in diluted soap (there is soap especially for vegetables available in healthfood stores), in order to remove all residues of pesticide. Organically grown vegetables have fewer pesticide residues and are preferable—though not all mothers do have access to fresh, organically grown food.

Washing Tips

Choose your veggie combination and wash (as above). Here are some extra preparation tips:

- Scrape off **carrot** skin because it may contain residues of pesticide.

- Scrub **potatoes** with a veggie-brush—but keep on the saponin-rich skin.

- If you use **onion** (can cause gas in some mothers and babies), cut it into large pieces (to save preparation time).

- For **fennel** root, cut off the thick bottom and the top upper 1/2 inch, separate the wedges and wash under flowing water.

- A pod or two of **peas** can be cut open, and the peas pressed out, rinsed and added to the mix. **Corn** can be rinsed and cut from the cob directly into the pan.

- **Green beans**—rinse, remove their tips, and cut into bite-sized pieces. You may find it faster to snap of their ends, and snap the beans into smaller pieces. (This may sound like a lot of work, but because you are doing a veggie-mix, you'll only need a few.)

- **Swiss chard** should be rinsed under flowing water, and then the stalk cut into large bite-size pieces, and the leaves into strips. You'll only be using one or two leaves (unless you are cooking for several people as well as yourself), so this isn't really very much work.

- **Asparagus** should be rinsed and the base cut off. Depending upon the kind of asparagus (how tough the skin is), you may want to peel the outer skin. Thinner, dark green asparagus does not need to be peeled

Paring Tips

For quicker preparation time, cut veggies into large pieces. For instance, halve a carrot lengthwise, then quarter (as if making carrot sticks), and divide into approximately two-inch long pieces. Potatoes can be halved lengthwise, halved again, and sliced into bite-size pieces. The same goes for yam and sweet potato. Fennel wedges can also be cut lengthwise and halved again if necessary. Chinese cabbage and other leafy greens can be cut into thin strips and added to the veggie mix.

Peeling an onion: Cut off the very top and bottom. Cut the skin from top to bottom of the onion, and then again, at the middle, all the way around the onion. Now the skin is in two halves that can be lifted off. (Sometimes it is necessary to cut into and remove the uppermost layer of the onion.) Easy!

Cooking Procedures

About salt: Not all vegetables require salt to be tasty, but some do become softer more quickly if cooked in salt. Green beans may remain tough if not cooked in salted water, and whole potatoes also do better if salt is added to the cooking water.

- With fat: Sauté vegetables in butter or olive oil (keep the temperature low enough to protect the oil from damage—it should not smoke). Begin with onions, and once they are transparent, add remaining vegetables (those that are denser and take longer to cook are added first). After a few minutes, add enough water to half-cover the veggies, cover the pot, and simmer until the veggies are as soft as you want them.

- Without fat: Place veggies in a pot, add water and simmer until the veggies are soft. If you have a steamer net, steam the veggies. Use the extra cooking water to make a sauce or stew. After cooking, add as much virgin olive oil, butter or other healthful fat as you like.

⇨ Small children will eat any veggie-mix with tomato sauce.

Variations:

- Stew: add stock or pureed tomato, water and oil to produce a vegetable stew.

- Chili: combine kidney beans and tomato puree, plus enough water to dilute the tomato puree into a smooth sauce. Spice mildly with cumin and pepper, and top with grated cheese.

- An Italian note: add tomato puree, water and a dash of milk. Spice heavily with dried or fresh basil, marjoram, plus seasoned salt. Dribble olive oil onto the veggies. Optional: fresh garlic and grated cheese.

- Florentine Soup: in the green countryside that envelops Florence, Italy, the locals love 'bread soup.' Prepare a vegetable stew in water and virgin olive oil (see above). When the vegetables are soft, add enough bread that has been cut into large chunks (with the crust) to soak up the broth. Mash them into the vegetables. Hold a bottle of fresh virgin olive oil above the pan and pour profusely, stirring until the 'soup' is a bit thinner (Italians take it with puddles of olive oil). Enjoy! Optional: press fresh garlic into the soup, and garnish with parmesan cheese.

In the US, we are literally starved for healthy fats. I've seen normally well-mannered people wolf down Florentine soup, tomato sauce, or salad into which I've poured generous amounts of virgin olive oil. It's as if the body recognizes a food that it direly needs.

Sauce

The secret behind a delicious sauce that blends perfectly with the meal is to use the water off the vegetables, and/or the stock off the meat, in making the sauce.

White Sauce
Proportions: 1 tablespoon of butter or oil, and 1 tablespoons of flour for 1 cup of sauce.

- Melt the butter in the sauce pan; careful not to brown the butter. Add all-purpose or non-gluten flour, and blend well into a paste.

- Add milk, almond-milk, or other milk substitute, and blend well, adding enough to thin the paste.

- Add warm water, or better, add the broth off your vegetables or meat, until you reach the consistency you desire. Careful: if you let the sauce sit for a few minutes, it may thicken again, in which case you'll want to mix in more broth before serving.

- Add seasoned salt and other spices if desired. Optional: garlic.

Cheese Sauce
Add grated or thinly sliced cheese to the above sauce. While stirring, allow the cheese time to melt while simmering on a very low heat. Optional: garlic.

Onion Sauce
Sauté diced onion in the butter, until the onion is transparent. Proceed as above (the paste will be clumpy with onions at first). Add dillweed and thyme; optional: garlic.

Meat Sauce or Mushroom Sauce
Leaving the broth of the meat in the pan, add a dash of real cream, and perhaps a dash of freshly ground or crushed pepper, or other spices of your choice. The same method works for mushroom sauce. This is a very delicate, very European sauce.

Thickened Broth Sauce
If your vegetables are swimming in their own broth, you can put 1 tablespoon of flour (per estimated cup of broth) in a cup and add just

enough cold water, while stirring, to make a very thick paste. Stir this into the warm vegetable mix and broth. While stirring, the paste will expand and thicken. If you were to put the flour directly into the hot broth, it would clump.

Spaghetti Sauce

Recipes for spaghetti sauce travel in families, and mothers may prefer to stick by their grandmother's secret formula. I do wish to share this easy, fast sauce that children love.

Put a portion of tomato puree into a sauce pan. Add enough milk, rice-milk or other milk substitute to make a medium-thick, orange sauce. The milk will actually curdle, giving the sauce cheese-like tanginess. For richer flavor, add butter or meat broth. Throw in generous amounts of spices (marjoram, basil), black pepper and seasoned salt. Close your eyes and pour in virgin olive oil (so that you don't stop yourself from using a lot), and press in fresh garlic.

Variation: sauté vegetables such as diced onions, paprika, thinly sliced carrots and mushrooms in butter before adding tomato puree.

Salad

Salad can be made from a variety of raw vegetables—not only lettuce and dark green leafy vegetables. However, since mothers need the folic acid in green foods, it is a good idea to concentrate on these in the postpartum. (Avocado is also rich in folic acid.)

Simple garden leaf lettuce has a huge lactogenic reputation. Mothers frequently find that eating lettuce every day increases their supply. This is probably because lettuce contains a milky substance (lactucarium) with sedating properties. This explains why lettuce has been used as a sleeping aid since ancient times. Lettuce has also been used in traditional medicine to 'build blood,' and this may contribute to its lactogenic effect.

Nutritionists recommend that people with digestive difficulties only take salad and raw vegetables before 2 p.m., giving their body plenty of time to digest them before sleep.

When shopping for salad, look for richly colored leaves. Lighter green sorts, such as iceberg or crisp head salad, contain fewer minerals. Supermarkets often carry a variety of salad greens, including butterhead, Romaine, rocket, water cress, dandelion, mustard and beet greens. If you would like, enjoy a selection of delectable greens. Typical green lettuce, however, remains a powerful choice.

You may be lucky and have a source for organic or homegrown salad greens. Sometimes these can be found in supermarkets, freshly packaged. Rinse before using. Packaged salad mixes are best used within two days as they spoil quickly.

There are ways to quickly prepare salad. For instance, cut off a portion of leaves from each sort and toss them into a colander; let cold water flow over the leaves while you separate them with your fingers, allowing the water to wash all surfaces. (Centrifugal salad spinners in which we can first soak and then spin dry salad leaves are not very expensive and do the trick.)

Extras
If you and your baby tolerate raw veggies, don't hesitate to add ingredients such as diced onion, grated beet root, carrot and fennel to salad. Thinly sliced mushrooms in salad are an acquired taste—you may not be able to enthuse your children, but do try as children often surprise us. A few spoon-scoops of avocado enrich the taste of salad and most children like it.

Sprouts
True salad buffs add varieties of sprouts to their salads, for their taste, enzymes and concentrated nutrients. Sprouts also contain very high levels of plant-estrogen. Whereas moderate amounts of plant-estrogen support breastfeeding, too many sprouts—too much plant-estrogen—could potentially have the opposite effect. If you love sprouts, try chick-pea, mung bean and alfalfa sprouts in moderate amounts.

Easy Salad Dressing
Dribble virgin olive oil over your salad. Toss the salad to coat all the leaves. Sprinkle on seasoned salt, and add either a dash of tamari soy sauce, lemon juice, or organic vinegar. Toss again. The proportion of oil to vinegar, lemon juice or soy sauce is approximately 3 to 1, or three times the amount of oil to vinegar. Instead of olive oil, try a mixture of flaxseed oil and sesame oil, for a balance of EFAs (see *Get Your Fats Right, in Chapter Three*).

Basic Salad Dressing Proportions

- 4 – 6 tablespoons of oil, cream, yogurt or milk
- 1 – 3 tablespoons of organic vinegar or lemon juice
- 1 – 3 pinches of salt,
- optional: 1/4 teaspoon mustard, or tamari sauce, tabasco sauce, or horseradish.
- optional: 1 pinch of pepper, 1 pinch of sugar
- optional: 1/4 – 1/2 onion, minced or finely chopped
- optional: 1 – 2 tablespoons of chopped chives or fresh herbs (see below)
- optional: 1 – 3 teaspoons of brewer's or nutritional yeast; mix the yeast with the vinegar or lemon juice first, so that it dissolves. It will clump if added to oil first.
- optional: for Italian flavor, add 1 tablespoon of dried herbs such as marjoram, basil, thyme
- optional: for a sharper sauce, add: 1/2 teaspoon dill seed, 1/4 – 1/2 teaspoon dry mustard

Egg Dressing for Salad

1 – 2 hard boiled eggs.
Mash the egg yolks together with dry herbs.
Mix in well to salad dressing (above)
Cut egg white into cubes, and add to salad dressing.

Probiotic Yogurt Dressing

Mix together:
1 1/2 cups probiotic yogurt
2 teaspoons tamari soy sauce, or virgin olive oil (or water)
1 teaspoon seasoned salt
1/2 tsp onion, garlic powder; or freshly minced onion and garlic.

Mild Cream Dressing for Grated Veggie Salads

1 – 3 tablespoons of lemon juice
4 – 6 tablespoons of cream, yogurt or mixture of both
1 – 3 pinches of salt
1 pinch sugar

Soup

A hearty soup can serve as lunch or dinner. Follow the European tradition, and dunk a thick cut of bread in your soup. (Some children who would never take soup alone, relish it as a warm topping for buttered bread.) Below are three easy cooking procedures for soup.

1. Sauté veggies in butter or olive oil, then add water (or stock) and allow to simmer for 15 minutes or until all the veggies are soft. Top off with virgin olive oil, butter or cream.

2. Add veggies to water (or stock), bring to a boil, and simmer for 15 minutes. Add a good helping of dried herbs such as seasoned salt, marjoram and basil (a tablespoon of each for a four-person pot of soup), and continue to simmer for 5 minutes. Top off with virgin olive oil, butter or cream.

3. To make a creamed-soup: you can put all, or only part, of your soup into a blender. Add butter, cream, milk, rice-milk or soy-milk.

⇨ Garlic: garlic should be pressed into the soup when it has finished cooking—or press garlic into the individual soup bowls of those who dare.

⇨ Carbohydrates and extras to add into the soup while cooking: quick cooking grains such as quinoa, millet, rolled oats, instant rice. A few leftover or canned beans, such as pinto or lima. Noodles of various shapes and sizes.

Homemade soup almost always tastes better the next day. Store in the fridge, or freeze in portions for a later date.

A few typical hearty soup combinations.
- **Potato Soup**: onions or leek, potato. Spice with salt, pepper and a curry powder or dill seed to taste. Stir in fresh pressed garlic or add garlic powder to the bowl and garnish with extra butter or cream.

- **Potato-Carrot soup**: onions or leek, potato and carrots. Spice with salt, pepper and a bit of curry powder to taste. Stir in fresh pressed garlic or add garlic powder to the bowl and garnish with extra butter or cream.

- **Pumpkin Soup**: pumpkin, carrots, potato. Spice with salt, pepper and a *quite a bit* of curry powder to taste. Stir in fresh pressed garlic or add garlic powder to the bowl and garnish with extra butter or cream.

- **Lentil Soup**: onions or leek, potato and carrots. Prepare lentils first with water, tomato juice or stock. Add vegetables and spices about twenty minutes before the soup is finished. Spicing with considerable fennel or cumin powder will improve digestibility and make the soup more lactogenic. Add quinoa or other grain for a complete protein.

- **Spicy Split Mung-Bean Soup**: thinly cover bottom of pan with olive oil; add mustard seed or powder, plus considerable cumin powder; wait a minute for the mustard seed to pop. Sauté optional vegetables such as onion, carrot, potato. Add pre-soaked mung-bean to the sautéed veggies, plus salt and pepper, and simmer for an hour, or until the mung-bean falls apart. Add quinoa or other grain for a complete protein. Mung-bean soup should be creamy. Blend a portion of the soup to increase the creaminess if desired. Additional spices include bay leaf, ginger, turmeric, and coriander.

CHAPTER EIGHTEEN

Sweets

Breastfeeding mothers tend to crave sweet food, and mothers also find that sweet food supports their milk supply. Young babies, however, may react to even small amounts of concentrated, refined sugar with fussiness or colic.

Refined sugar is hidden in many foods (including catsup and store-bought salad dressing). Finding a source of sugar that satisfies the mother without causing her baby to become fussy can be tricky. Naturally sweet foods such as fruit, nuts, seeds and grains are a healthy source of sugar, but babies may, when they are young, also react to these sugars. Gradually introduce sweet foods into your diet after birth, to help prevent colic from developing. Read the sections on sugar in Part One and keep an eye on your use of sugar and on your baby's reaction.

The following sweet foods are made of concentrated lactogenic ingredients. If your baby tolerates them, enjoy!

Barley Malt

Malt, made from barley, contains beta-glucan that raises prolactin levels. For a lactogenic effect, it is necessary to take several large spoonfuls at one time, and possibly to repeat several times a day.

Buy true malt syrup or powder online at brewery shops (stretched with wheat-malt or oat-malt is fine, but not with corn syrup), or experiment with quality commercial products such as Carnation Brand Malted Milk. See also page 59.

Malt can be added to milk or dairy substitute for a malted shake. It can be used as a topping for ice cream, or added as a sweetener to coffee substitute or to warm, spiced milk. It can be used to sweeten oatmeal, and it can be spread on bread and butter. It can also be eaten plain, by the spoonful, before meals.

Halvah – sesame and honey

Halvah is a Mideastern candy made of crushed sesame seeds and honey. It is the only candy my grandmother snacked on, and she lived to 94 with never a broken bone or hip joint (sesame is a good source for calcium)! Look for an organic product; they can be ordered online.

Marzipan – almonds, organic raw cane sugar, organic vanilla

This almond-based candy also has Mideastern origins. It is commonly used to make decorations for cakes but it can also be eaten plain. Just cut into small pieces, and roll in coconut flakes if desired. Look for an organic product; they can be ordered online.

Sliced Beet

Sliced beet can reduce the urge for sweets. A recipe is in *Snacks* on page 225-226. A recipe for beet-carrot juice, another combination that satisfies a sweet-tooth, can be found in *Beverages* on page 195.

Fig-Ginger Topping For Natural Probiotic Yogurt or for on Toast

In a pot place two handfuls of chopped dried figs, (optional: also/or dates) and 1 – 2 teaspoons of peeled, diced ginger root. Add approximately the same volume of honey or raw cane sugar, twice as much water, and simmer on a low heat, stirring, until thick. Add anise seeds while simmering for a stronger lactogenic effect.

Crunch-Balls

In India, chickpea flour is commonly used to make this recipe. Barley and oat flour are also very lactogenic.

2 cups of flour

1/2 teaspoon aniseed or anise powder

1/2 cup ground almond

2 tablespoons of raw, hulled sesame seed (or desiccated coconut)

1/2 cup finely ground cane sugar

Optional: 2 tablespoons finely chopped dried fig, date or black currents.

175 grams of butter

Desiccated coconut meat or roasted sesame seed in a bowl.

Preparation: at medium heat and while stirring, roast flour, ground nuts, anise seed (or powder) and sesame seed in a dry skillet pan, until golden. Stir in sugar and optional chopped dried fruit. Put mixture into large bowl and allow it to cool. Cut cold butter into small pieces, add to the dry ingredients. With your fingers, knead into thick dough. Form small balls from the dough, and roll in roasted sesame seed or roasted desiccated coconut. Store in the refrigerator.

*Oatmeal-Sesame Cookies**
Mix together:

2 cups oatmeal

1 cup raisins, or chopped almond, dried fig or dates

2 teaspoons cinnamon or powdered aniseed

1/2 cup honey

2/3 cup sesame paste (tahini)

Drop by spoonfuls onto non-greased cookie sheet.

Bake at 350 for 10 to 12 minutes.

Let cool on the cookie sheet.

Makes about 25 cookies.

Oatmeal Banana Nut Bread
An IBCLC and RN, Theresa Johnson, discovered the meaning of *mother food* in a very personal way after the birth of her first daughter, when her midwife gave her a recipe for oatmeal banana bread.

Her daughter was two weeks old, and was not gaining weight. Another person might have suggested that she supplement with

---

* This recipe is from a large file on oatmeal recipes found at "pumpmoms," an email list that is an precious resource for mothers doing extended or exclusive pumping. (Many mothers on this list take oatmeal to support their supply.) To join pumpmoms, register with Yahoogroups and sign up at http://groups.yahoo.com/group/pumpmoms. If you have any questions, contact one of the moderators at: listowner@pumpingmoms.org.

formula. But this wise midwife asked a few simple questions that helped her understand the cause of the low milk supply. She asked how clean Theresa's house was, if she got enough rest, and whether she was eating properly. Theresa answered that her house was sparkling (of course!) and how could she possibly get rest if it meant not having a clean house, and that she had absolutely no time to eat.

Her midwife gave her husband a recipe for oatmeal banana nut bread (below), suggested that he make 2 loaves and that Theresa should eat 2 – 3 slices a day. She was told to take the baby to bed with her and to let the house go for the rest of the week. Her daughter gained 12 ounces in one week! Theresa Johnson says, "This midwife changed my life, and now I help others likewise."

1/2 cup shortening

1   cup sugar

2   eggs

1   cup banana's (about 3- dark ripe ones are better than yellow new ones)

1 1/2 cup flour

1 tsp baking soda

1/4 tsp salt

1/2 cup oatmeal (I use a little more like 1 cup)

3/4 cup chopped nuts (pecans are great)

1 tsp butter or vanilla flavoring

Cream shortening and sugar together. Add egg 1 at a time mixing thoroughly after each addition. Add banana's and mix well. Add flour, soda, and salt and mix well. Add oatmeal to creamed mixture.

Stir in nuts and flavoring. Pour into greased 9 x 5 loaf pan and bake at 350 for 50-55 minutes until bread tests done. (knife inserted in center comes out clean)

Part Four

Mother Food and Herbs: supporting breastfeeding and a mother's health

CHAPTER NINETEEN

Indications, Recommendations

This chapter looks at a few common health problems—those that I am most often asked about—especially autoimmune illnesses, and provides suggestions for augmenting medical treatment under the guidance of your doctor with time-honored home treatments, with herbal and other nutritive supplements, and with immune-boosting herbs. If you have a health condition, talk to your doctor about breastfeeding-friendly treatment. It is almost always available. If your doctor advises you to stop breastfeeding due to a medical condition or because of your need for a specific medication, get a second opinion. Be sure to ask your lactation expert as well.

Cold or Flu

If you come down with a cold or flu, drink plenty of fluids, and including lactogenic tea. Allow your fever to rise significantly before using natural or medical means to reduce it. Allowing fever to develop is healthy. It teaches the immune system to recognize and respond to viruses, and strengthens its ability to respond appropriately.

Lactogenic teas helpful in fighting viral infection:

- **Elder flower**, **vervain**, and **fenugreek** increase sweating during fever to speed the healing process. Elder flower tea is traditionally used in the treatment of colds and flu.
- **Elder berry** extract or syrup is a potent antiviral and speeds recovery.
- **Ginger tea**: opens the bronchia and sinuses, helps expectorate congestion from the lungs.
- **Thyme, fenugreek, and marshmallow**: these herbs loosen and draw out congestion from the lungs.
- **Chicken soup** has potent anti-inflammatory properties. (See page 176 for a recipe.)
- For stomach flu, take **barley-water** to sooth the intestine. Another tip: boiled water with a squirt of lemon juice is helpful and refreshing. Chew on raw fennel if you feel too ill to eat.
- When the illness is nearly over, and for the next several days, take **verbena** tea to overcome or prevent lingering exhaustion.

Steam inhalations loosen congestion in the sinuses and lungs and help keep them free of infection. Boil a pot of water and add a pinch of salt or a pinch of thyme or ginger powder. Place the pot on a pot holder on the table. Lean over the pot, loosely covering your head and the pot with a towel. Inhale as best you can through your nose and/or mouth—this should not be painful! Repeat as necessary.

If your baby has a stuffy nose, and is uncomfortable swallowing, place a drop of breastmilk into his nostrils to help free his sinuses. Because his stuffy nose may lead to his drinking less, it may be helpful to increase your use of herbs and foods, and to pump or hand express to keep up your supply.

"If you need to take cold or sinus meds, drink a lot of extra water along with them. I drink at least two extra 8 ounce glasses per pill taken. I know that sounds like a lot but it helps keep my supply up. A few times I haven't drunk the water and it took 2 – 3 days for my supply to go back up."

Colic

See the sections in this book that deal with colic and food allergies. Treatment can include:

- The mother taking digestive teas (umbel seeds) or gripe water
- Giving her baby 1 teaspoon of very mild, lukewarm digestive tea before a feeding
- The mother taking digestive enzymes, lactobacilli and probiotic products
- The mother taking astragalus
- See in particular the remedies for "Promoting Healthy Breast Milk" and "The Baby is Upset" in the Ayurvedic section

Colic can be caused by food allergies or GERD, and treatment for one or both may be necessary. If problems persist, and if your doctor is not able to help you, look for a pediatric allergist, preferably with training in environmental medicine, or a NAET specialist.

Allergies

Allergies should be treated under the direction of your allergy specialist. In the treatment of any allergy, it is wise to supplement with vitamins that are essential to immune system: vitamins E, C, B-complex, essential fatty acids (EFAs), calcium, magnesium, and zinc[60]. Look for non-allergenic formulas.

- Helpful herbs in the treatment of allergies include: turmeric, mushrooms, dong quai, red clover, astragalus, milk thistle, nettle, Nigella sativa.
- Read *Get Your Fats Right* and the various sections on allergy throughout Part One of this book.
- Some experts believe that fungal infection in the intestine contributes to allergies—it makes the intestines more permeable, burdening and wearing down the immune system with undigested food molecules in the bloodstream. For more information see *Leaky Gut* on pages 63-64.

- Identify problem foods. Foods commonly involved in allergy include: cow's milk protein, beef, egg, wheat, fish, peanuts, nuts, wheat, corn, fish, and sometimes tomato, berries, citrus fruits, currants, and seldom: chicken, pork and potato—as well as any other food frequently eaten. For information on identifying problem foods, see page 69.
- Read the sections below to learn more ways that lactogenic medicinals can assist allergy treatment.

Asthma

Asthma is a serious disease and requires your doctor's direction in treatment. In the treatment of any allergy, it's wise to supplement with the nutrients that are essential to the health of the immune system (see above).

Check the label of your decongestant to be sure that it does not contain pseudoephedrine—a substance that can reduce supply. Ask your doctor or lactation consultant about breastfeeding-friendly medication, and observe the reaction of your baby to any medication that you take. Does he become overly alert, nervous or have sleeping difficulties? If so, discuss a change in medication with your doctor.

Herbs:

- **Ginger** expands the capillaries and improves blood flow to the lungs.
- **Nettle** is a natural antihistamine, as is chamomile, though some people react allergically to chamomile. The renowned botanist, James Duke, Ph.D., suggests using the fresh juice of nettle root for the full antihistamine effect.
- **Nigella sativa** oil is a natural bronchial dilator—helpful in mild cases of asthma.
- **Turmeric** is a superb anti-inflammatory and antioxidant, and is used in India against asthma.
- **Essential fatty acids** reduce inflammation. It's important that your EFAs be in balance in order for your immune system to properly function.
- Avoid trans-fatty acids in margarine and processed oils as these promote inflammation. Reduce your intake of saturated fats *if* these have been the main source of your fats and take

more monounsaturated fats and essential fatty acids instead. See *Get Your Fats Right in Part One* for more information.

- Astragalus and other Chinese tonic herbs are used in the treatment of allergic disease.

Respiratory disease is a reaction to an air-borne allergen, often compounded by underlying food sensitivities—most commonly to dairy. See *Dairy* in Part One for more information.

As with any allergy, it is important to keep your home completely mold-free and as dust-free and dust mite-free as possible. Also, restrict your use of chemicals such as furniture polish, paint, strong detergents, pesticides and herbicides. Chemical additives in foods and even electro-smog in the home and car can compromise the immune system.

Read the following two sections for more tips on dealing with allergies.

Hay-fever

Follow the general advice on allergy prevention in the section above on asthma.

Check your decongestant to be sure that it does not contain pseudoephedrine—a substance that can reduce supply. Ask your doctor or lactation consultant about breastfeeding-friendly medication.

- **Lactobacilli** are proving to be helpful against allergy— perhaps because they enable dairy products to be better digested, so that the underlying dairy sensitivity is not as acute. Lactobacilli also improve intestinal health—the first guard against allergy.
- In any case, a Californian study showed that eating yogurt every day (lactobacilli) reduced the incidence of hay fever attacks, especially those caused by grass pollens. A recent study also showed that mothers with eczema were less likely to pass it to their infants if they took lactobacilli.
- **Magnesium** is also helpful. A study from Germany showed that 3 bananas were enough to quell a hay fever attack, as they contain a lot of magnesium. If this works for you, look into

changing your diet to include more nuts, seeds, grains and legumes, or into supplementing with magnesium.

- **Showering frequently** (especially after being outside) and changing clothes; having a well-dusted, well-vacuumed house, frequently changing bedding; and if possible, having an air purifier in the room you are most often in, will help reduce the allergic load.

- **Drinking enough water** is important. Try to get 8 cups a day, a cup before meals, a cup or two between meals and snacks, and use sea salt on your meals so that your body absorbs and utilizes the water. Sometimes allergic symptoms signal dehydration, and they improve with improved drinking habits[61].

Eczema

Read the above two sections on asthma and hay-fever to learn how to clean up your environment, and to use supplements and herbs to nourish and strengthen the immune system.

Look for possible food sensitivities—allergies on the skin may be triggered by substances in the environment, but frequently underlying food-allergies conspire to weaken the immune system.

If your baby has eczema, the intake of EFAs by the mother is of particular importance in treatment, as your EFAs will reach him through your milk. It may be helpful to massage an EFA, such as evening primrose oil, directly onto the baby's and/or mother's eczema. For more information, read *Get Your Fats Right*, in Part One.

⇨ Egg white is a frequent trigger of eczema in adults.

⇨ The intake of lactobacilli was shown in a Finnish study to protect the infants of mothers with eczema from also getting eczema—usually a high risk factor.

⇨ Read the section on astragalus and mushrooms in *A Lactogenic Herbal*. These herbs help to hone your immune system to reduce allergies.

⇨ Finally, the long-term intake of nettle tea is helpful in healing eczema. Freeze-dried nettle products have the best effect.

Rheumatoid Arthritis

Read the sections above for general information pertaining to auto-immune diseases and allergies.

Herbs and supplements of particular importance are fish-oil or an algae-derived source of omega 3 EFAs; turmeric and ginger. These have potent anti-inflammatory and antioxidant effects and are used therapeutically to treat inflammation in the joints.

⇨ A study from 2002 showed that four or more cups of decaffeinated coffee per day increases the risk of rheumatoid arthritis, whereas black or green tea reduces the risk and normal coffee appears to have no influence. For more information see page 114.

Fatigue

Mothers commonly experience fatigue after birth. When you're too tired to wash your hair or prepare yourself a meal, it's time to take action. Read the section *Keep your Health the Best it Can Be* in Part One. Then peruse *A Lactogenic Herbal* below for herbs that address different causes of fatigue, for instance: alfalfa, astragalus, blessed thistle, milk thistle, chlorophyll, dandelion, dong quai, EFAs, garlic, valerian, and healing mushrooms.

As is explained in *Keep your Health the Best it Can Be,* profound exhaustion or depression in the postpartum can recur premenstrually, in a serious form of PMS. This is a good reason to take measures now to limit your fatigue.

Lack of Sleep

Chronic lack of sleep goes with the territory of parenting. A baby who wakes up during the night is following ancient patterns that are crucial to his development—he is affirming his sense of being alive, affirming his knowledge of being protected, and also seeking nourishment for his quickly growing body and brain.

Co-sleeping or having the crib next to your bed is usually the best solution for the baby and the parents.

Fathers are often surprised to discover that co-sleeping improves their quality of sleep as well. The baby's rooting movements wake up the mother so that she can latch on the baby before he begins to cry, and before he disturbs his father's sleep.

• Herb for sleep-deprived mothers, see: valerian.

Depression

Mothers after birth are at risk to develop depression, especially if the birth was difficult or if breastfeeding problems seem overwhelming. See the section on *Postpartum Illness and Depression* for more information, including breastfeeding-friendly treatment for depression.

Poor diet, lack of EFAs (especially omega 3s), vitamin B-complex, folic acid and zinc can lead to depression when the brain lacks the nutrients to make crucial neurochemicals. Improving one's diet can therefore be preventative of depression. See *Get Your Fats Right*, and *Keep Your Health The Best It Can* Be in Part One for more information.

As is explained in *Postpartum Illness and Depression,* profound exhaustion or depression in the postpartum can recur as a serious form of premenstrual syndrome (PMS). This is something to watch out for. PMS can be treated.

Forgetfulness, Lack of Concentration

Mothers complain of being generally forgetful, having difficulties remembering words and names, being unable to read complex books, and follow adult conversation. There are different opinions as to what causes this, and the hormones of pregnancy and lactation may be involved.

I mentioned this "mind fuzz" once in an online discussion group, only to be upbraided by the young men who thought I was taking a sexist view. Gradually a few veteran mothers joined in, confirming that although they could still do intellectual work, it took more effort.

A degree of "mind-fuzz" seems to be normal in the postpartum. It may be nature's way of getting us to think of nothing else but our baby. Still, it is to hope that dietary and life-style factors can improve clear-mindedness in the postpartum. One study showed that mothers who took DHA/EPA supplements during late pregnancy had better cognitive abilities in the postpartum. (A later study put these findings into question.) Another substance, choline, nourishes the brain and improves memory. Turmeric contains anti-inflammatory substances that reduce inflammation in the brain—this is more common than one would think, and leads to dementia or Alzheimer's in old age.

In Anthroposophic medicine, barley grain, beet root, and carrot are said to be strengthen mental abilities and concentration. Carrot juice helps mothers feel less fatigued and more focused.

Plugged Ducts and Stringy-Looking Milk

Lecithin helps chronically plugged milk ducts. There are different suggestions on dosage. Dr. Ruth Lawrence recommends 1 capsule (1200 mg) 3 – 4 times a day, or 1 tablespoon of liquid or granulated lecithin a day. Some lactation experts recommend up to twice this amount. Start with a low dosage, and work up; reduce the amount again for long-term prevention treatment.

If lecithin is not sufficient, add evening primrose oil. Equally important is to make adjustments to your intake of healthy fats. See Chapter Three, *Get Your Fats Right*, for more information.

⇨ Ask your lactation expert to show you how to massage the plug out of your breast.

Engorgement, Thrush, Mastitis

For information on engorgement and thrush, see *Prepare to Prevent Pain* in Chapter One, pages 15-17

Mastitis is usually a sign that a mother is not getting enough rest or nutritious food, and that she needs to slow down and get in touch with her needs. For more information, see *Prepare to Prevent Pain* in Chapter One, pages 15-17. Also, see *Echinacea*, pages 275-276, and *Turmeric*, pages 295-297.

Less Milk before Menstruation

Many mothers experience a drop in their supply during the second half of their menstrual cycle. Patricia Gima, IBCLC, was the first to observe that mothers can improve their supply by supplementing with calcium and magnesium throughout the two weeks before menstruation. For more information, see page 153.

Caffeine can change the taste of milk during the premenstrual phase, according to Maureen Minchin, and babies may refuse to drink, or may drink less, and may have colic during that time. Avoiding caffeine solves the problem.

CHAPTER TWENTY

A Lactogenic Herbal

Pregnancy Considerations

During pregnancy, mothers take herbs for their nutritional value, to tone the uterus for birth, and to promote an abundant milk supply. Of the herbs mentioned in this chapter, experts warn against taking large amounts of anise, basil, blessed thistle, chasteberry, fenugreek, thyme, and verbena during pregnancy, due to the slight risk of miscarriage associated with these herbs. Red raspberry leaf, widely used as a tonic for the uterus, should be introduced slowly for the same reason.

In addition, the medical tradition of India warns against all so-called *warming* herbs during pregnancy: anise, basil, caraway, cardamom, cinnamon, coriander, cumin, dill, fennel, fenugreek, garlic, ginger, black seed (Nigella sativa), and turmeric. In India, these spices are commonly used in large quantities. Women in the US and Europe, who use these herbs infrequently as spices, probably have little cause for concern. However, if you have a history of miscarriage, you may consider avoiding these herbs.

Concerning Allergy

Any person, even those with no previous history of allergy, can become allergic to any herb or food (though allergy usually develops when a person comes into excessive contact with a food or substance). In order to avoid a severe reaction, it is wise to initially take a new herb or food at minimum dosage. Observe your response: do you develop indigestion, skin changes, bright red ears, have difficulty swallowing, congestion, breathing problems, sudden fatigue, or involuntary movements such as nervous, twitching legs? If not, gradually increase the amount you take per day.

Sometimes mothers experience side effects with herbs, though these usually pass after a few days of taking the herb at reduced dosage. Potential allergies and side effects are listed in each herb's section. If no remark is made about allergy and side effects in an herb's section, that herb or spice is not generally considered allergenic, and has no particular known side effect.

Herbs for Pregnancy

The herbs recommended here for pregnancy are selected for their wealth of vitamins and minerals, their vitamin K, and their folic acid. Some support the mother's liver and kidneys, helping to keep her blood as toxin-free as possible. Others may maximize the development of glandular tissue.

To promote glandular tissue, take the herbs listed below regularly, beginning at mid-pregnancy. These herbs can be taken altogether or alternated as single teas every one or two weeks. Taking "singles" prevents the body from becoming insensitive, or from getting too much of any one herb, and is preferred by some herbalists. You can also combine different mixtures of two or three herbs, and alternate these every few weeks. Infuse one ounce, or two handfuls, of the herbal mixture in a quart jar for several hours or over night. Warm each cup and sweeten with a natural sweetener, if desired, before drinking. If you drink red raspberry leaf tea in addition to this program, introduce it slowly (see page 293). Unless you have a history of low milk supply with a younger baby, or have good reason to suspect that you will have low milk supply, reduce your intake of these herbs, especially alfalfa, about two weeks before due date to avoid developing an over-supply of milk.

alfalfa leaf • dandelion leaf • nettle • oat-straw • red clover

Herbs and Foods Following Birth

Eat at least one cooked, warm meal per day that includes a source of protein, a green salad, a grain such as millet or rice, and cooked vegetables such as yam, carrot, and fennel. Spice moderately, for instance with sea-salt or gomasio, with small amounts of umbel seeds, or basil and marjoram, and, if tolerated, with garlic. Avoid food that is hard to digest, such as fried or extremely fatty food. Take probiotic yogurt, preferably unsweetened and plain, or lactobacilli supplements, to protect your intestinal flora and to help prevent colic and allergy in your baby. Get healthy fats such as butter and olive oil. Drink to thirst, not too much or too little; your morning urine should be light-colored. It is best to avoid carbonated, caffeinated water and soft drinks as they impair milk supply in sensitive mothers.

Herbs useful after birth include stinging nettle to rebuild the blood lost during birth, turmeric, to help avoid mastitis, oatstraw, to nurture the nerves and to help prevent nervous exhaustion. These herbs also increase milk supply, so keep an eye on your supply and reduce or increase your dosage of these herbs if necessary. Avoid taking ginger for several weeks after birth if you lost a lot of blood during birth.

A traditional Chinese remedy in the early postpartum is homemade chicken soup, taken **only once a week**. It is reputed to prevent depression, to restore a mother's vitality, and to help develop an abundant milk supply.

Individual Dosage Requirements

Mothers have individual needs when it comes to lactogenic foods and herbs. Although most mothers produce milk well without having to consider their use at all, other mothers have to take a low to moderate dosage every day to keep their supply stable. To increase my milk supply, it was necessary that I take these foods and herbs at a high dosage for one to four days. Sheila Humphrey in "The Nursing Mother's Herbal" writes that lactation experts have observed mothers needing to take double or triple the usual dosage of herbs or tincture for one or two days in order to kick-start their milk production. Most mothers then have normal milk production and can reduce or stop their use of these herbs and foods altogether. Mothers with persistent milk supply difficulties however continue taking these herbs and foods at a normal dosage.

As a breastfeeding mother gathers experience about her unique reaction to herbs and foods, she will develop an understanding for the dosage that works best for her, both for building and for maintaining milk supply. Remember though, if you are trying an herb for the first time, to taper up your dosage gradually over several days in order to test for allergy and side effects, even if these are rare.

In addition, consider this: if you do not have low milk supply, and you take herbs and foods to increase your supply, you may create unnecessary difficulties for yourself such as over-supply, engorgement, plugged ducts, or mastitis. Your baby may develop colic due to *too much foremilk*, or sucking difficulties due to an *overly strong let-down reflex*, both of which are common with over-supply. Use these foods and herbs wisely, and reduce or stop their use if you notice such problems.

How to Prepare Tea

Water

If using tap water first thing in the morning, let the faucet run for several minutes to flush out the water that was standing in the pipe—especially if you have older pipes, if you suspect that they may contain lead, or that the water may have absorbed lead from solder that joins the pipes together. Before making tea at other times of the day, run the faucet for half a minute.

Heating Water

Connoisseurs recommend that tea water be heated just *prior to boiling;* they say that losing oxygen from boiling gives tea a flat taste. Obviously, mothers with a newborn do not have time to watch a pot—letting it boil is just fine. Most of us can't taste the difference anyway.

The Container

Use a container or cup made of glass or ceramic, not plastic, or metal. Cover the container tightly; for instance, use a canning jar with a screw on top. If using a cup, cover it while steeping so that the herb's volatile oils do not escape with the steam.

Measurement of Herb to Water

The amount of herb per cup may vary, depending on the herb used, the effect desired, one's sensitivity to the herb, and one's personal taste.

Per Cup: One teaspoon of dried herb, or one tablespoon of fresh herb, per cup of water. When taking lactogenic tea, stronger doses may be necessary—or double or triple this amount—especially at the beginning when building supply.

Per Quart: Two rounded tablespoons of dried herbs, or one handful of fresh herbs, to a quart of water. Double or triple this amount if you are starting an herbal program to increase milk supply.

Remember: new herbs are to be tried individually at low dosage in order to be sure that there are no allergic reactions or side effects. Be especially cautious with herbs that are noted to trigger allergic reactions or produce other side effects.

Steeping

Mild, or Medicinal Tea

Tea can be steeped for as little as a half minute, and for as long as 20 minutes. For a mild cup of tea, steep from 1/2 to 3 minutes. For a stronger, or 'therapeutic dosage,' steep between 5 to 20 minutes.

Note: Some mothers see therapeutic effects with low-dose, mildly steeped teas, i.e., mild borage leaf or lemon balm tea may be mood elevating, and mild hops may be relaxing. Different persons have different levels of sensitivity; each of us has to experiment to learn about our own sensitivities to different herbs.

Steeping Tea in a Cup

If you do not own a special herbal teacup with fitted strainer and top, improvise. Place the herb in a tea strainer. Steady the strainer on the rim of the cup. Pour boiling water into the cup until the herbs are submerged. Cover the cup and strainer with a small plate and steep. An alternative is to put the herbs directly into the cup, cover with boiling water, cover the cup with a plate, and, after steeping, to strain off the liquid into a new cup.

Steeping Tea in a Teapot

In a covered teapot, cover the herbs with boiling water, steep the tea and then strain the tea off into another pot, or, leave the herb in the pot and strain each individual cup when poured. If the herb remains in the pot, the tea will have a stronger, medicinal effect, but it will also taste more bitter.

Sweeteners

Honey, maple syrup, blackstrap molasses, barley malt, and other natural sweeteners are rich in minerals, whereas white sugar actually pulls minerals right out of the body. White sugar should therefore be avoided generally, and not be used to sweeten tea. **Stevia**, a sweet-tasting herb, has medicinal properties that may benefit the pregnant and breastfeeding mother. Stevia is an option if mothers are trying to reduce calories.

Dilution: If a therapeutic cup of tea is too bitter to drink, dilute it well and sweeten it with stevia or other natural sweetener. It is better to drink diluted, sweetened tea throughout the day than to be unable to drink even one bitter cup of tea.

Infusions and Decoctions

How to make an infusion

To make an infusion, you will need a container such as a heat-resistant quart canning jar with an airtight cover or screw-on top. Place the herbs in the quart jar—two to four rounded tablespoons of dried herbs, or one to two handfuls of fresh herbs, to a quart. Fill the jar with boiling water right up to the top and cover tightly. Infuse the herbs for between three and eight hours, or overnight. Then strain the liquid into another airtight container and discard the herbs.

Infusions will keep in the refrigerator for up to two days, though it is best to make them fresh each day. They can be taken cold, but for some mothers, herbal teas support milk supply better if warmed in a pot. Do not microwave herbal tea. Sweeten to taste with a natural sweetener.

How to make a decoction

Decoction uses continuous heat and water to extract substances from tough plant fiber, such as roots, bark, seeds, or thick, fibrous leaves. Decoctions can simmer for 10 – 30 minutes, or longer, and they become more concentrated, the more liquid has simmered off. The proportion of herbs to water is about the same as for an infusion, or two to four rounded tablespoons of dried herbs, or one to two handfuls of fresh herbs, to a quart. However, as with all herbal teas, some mothers are responsive to milder dosages.

Alfalfa Leaf (Medicago sativa L.)

Alfalfa leaf, one of our most nutritious herbs, has a wide range of therapeutic applications. It contains blood-cleansing chlorophyll, a host of minerals—calcium, magnesium, phosphorus, potassium, silicon, zinc—numerous vitamins—A, B1, B2, B3, B5, B6, C, D, E, and K—as well as essential and non-essential amino acids.

Alfalfa leaf is estrogenic and antifungal. It contains substances that nourish the liver, activate the kidneys, suppress inflammation, address digestive disorders, and balance blood sugar. It is also taken to promote the function of the pituitary gland, which is the source of lactation hormones.

Because the abundant minerals in alfalfa leaf are well balanced and easily absorbed, pregnant and lactating women frequently take alfalfa leaf as a mineral supplement. Alfalfa leaf also builds milk supply. Taken during pregnancy, it may help promote the development of glandular breast tissue.

Mothers with normal milk supply should reduce or discontinue alfalfa and other nutritious lactogenic herbs a few weeks before their due date. Mothers with a history of low milk supply should also be cautious, especially if their breasts showed signs of better development this pregnancy. Over-supply can develop in these mothers as well.

Pregnancy: Safe. Estrogenic. Although alfalfa can be taken to promote menstruation, there are no warnings regarding its use during pregnancy.

Allergy: Rare.

Side Effects: Diarrhea or loose stool in the mother or baby. Reduce the dosage for a few days.

Warning: Do not overeat alfalfa sprouts or seeds. These may trigger an auto-immune, Lupus-like condition in sensitive individuals. Indeed, the American Pharmaceutical Association warns that persons with systemic lupus erythematosus should avoid alfalfa products.

Sources: Health-food stores. Herbal pharmacies.

Dosage and Preparation:

- Tea: 1-2 teaspoons of dried herb per cup of water. Drink up to three cups per day. (To kick-start milk supply, double this dosage a few days. Increase is seen within two to four days.)
- Infuse 1-2 handfuls in a quart of water, steep overnight.
- Alfalfa Supplements: Up to 8 capsules per day.
- Dried juice powder: 1 tablespoon, two times per day.
- Homeopathy: X30 is used in combination with Lactuca virosa X30 for exhausted, nervous, stressed mothers.

Anise (Pimpinella anisum) see also Umbel Seeds

Anise seed tea was taken in ancient Greece to "bring down the milk." In China, both anise seed and star-anise are used as a galactagogue. It is best to avoid star-anise however, as commercial products may be contaminated with Japanese star-anise, which is toxic.

Pregnancy: The American Herbal Products Association lists anise as unsafe during pregnancy (class 2b). It has been used in traditional medicine to promote menstruation, suggesting that it could trigger miscarriage. Ayurveda also warns against anise during pregnancy.

Allergy: Anise seed occasionally triggers allergic reactions of the respiratory tract, gastrointestinal tract, and skin.

Sources: Spice sections of grocery stores and health food stores.

Dosage and Preparation: *see also* Umbel Seeds.

- Anise tea: Gently crush 1 - 2 teaspoons of anise seeds, and cover with one cup of boiling water. Cover and steep between 5 - 20 minutes. Sweeten to taste. Take 3 cups a day.
- Infusion: In Eastern Europe, umbel seeds such as anise that are given to breastfeeding mothers to promote milk production, are covered with boiling water and steeped for four hours.
- The usual dosage is 3 cups a day. To kick start milk production, take up to 6 cups of anise tea for two to four days, carefully observing your and your baby's reaction.

Asparagus, Wild (Asparagus racemosus; Shatavari)

Wild asparagus is the most widely used galactagogue in India. It is a tonic herb, used both to increase overall vitality and to address serious illness. Called *shatavari* in India, it is taken in Ayurveda medicine as a cleanser of the abdominal reproductive organs and also to treat menstrual disorders. It is used in the treatment of stomach, intestinal, and liver disorders—placing it in good company with many galactagogues that also focus on digestion. It is also estrogenic.

Warning: In India, shatavari is counterindicated for women who have massive fibrocystic breasts.

Sources: Health food stores.

Dosage: There is no toxic dosage, according to Ayurvedic tradition. Follow the recommendations of your doctor.

Astragalus (various species)

The sweet, yellow-white root of astragalus is valued as a food by the Chinese, who attribute to it much of their good health and try to eat it as often as possible. As a medical plant, astragalus is esteemed as one of the great tonic herbs and as a promoter of vitality. It has been under scientific scrutiny for its ability to boost the immune system. Studies have shown that it increases the activity of *interferon*, the body's defense against viruses, and it increases the number and the activity of antibodies, including increasing levels of *IgA*[62], the antibody in the intestine that prevents undigested molecules from being absorbed through the intestinal wall. For more information, see page 63.

Astragalus membranaceus is taken in China to promote milk production. Astragalus glaux L. was used in ancient Greek medicine as a powerful herb for re-lactation. Astragalus glycyphyllos, from the Ukraine, and Astragalus hamosus, from India, are also used as galactagogues.

Astragalus has other rather "interesting" attributes. In Chinese medicine, it is said to increase vitality, and to improve one's ability to stand or sit up straight—so if you find it hard to straighten up, this may be the herb for you. It is also said to make people less sensitive to temperature change and drafts, and to help people feel less emotionally vulnerable to the moods and actions of other people. So if you need 'thicker skin,' consider astragalus.

Astragalus is frequently taken together with another herb, dong quai. See the section on dong quai for more information.

Pregnancy: Safe.

Sources: Health-food stores. Bulk and capsules.

Warning: Although astragalus is considered safe, Chinese doctors warn that it should not be taken during the acute phase of a cold or flu.

Dosage and Preparation:

- Decoction: 10 – 30 grams of root (combine with 6 – 15 grams of dong quai root), in 1 to 2 quarts of water. Simmer at the lowest heat for 20 minutes. Strain the tea into a container and sweeten. Drink throughout the day, and chew on the fibrous roots. Dong quai is rather soft and can be eaten. Astragalus is more fibrous; chew off the soft flesh and dispose of the rest.

- Capsules: If you are taking concentrated extracts of the root, follow the dosage recommendations on the package or your doctor's recommendation.

Basil (Ocimum basilicum)

Basil comes from India. Today it flourishes as a potherb throughout the Mediterranean. Fresh, pungent basil imparts an invigorating quality to food and salad, and is an indispensable ingredient in Italian cooking, along with oregano and marjoram. Whereas, however, oregano is reputed to be anti-lactogenic, basil is specifically taken as a galactagogue throughout Eurasia, and going all the way back to ancient Greece.

Basil is a good source of carotene, niacin, thiamin, and iron. It is estrogenic, calms the nerves, and relieves stomach cramps. It strengthens digestion, increases appetite, and reduces flatulence. Medically, it has been used for inflammation of the stomach and intestines, for respiratory disease (was once used against tuberculosis), and for bladder and kidney infection.

Today, basil is officially restricted as a *therapeutic medicinal*. One of its chemicals, estragole, is mildly carcinogenic in extremely high dosages—hundreds of times higher than what we would ever use. Experts in herbal medicine are debating the restriction on basil, and someday, basil may be removed from the list of restricted herbs. Experts do agree that because estragole is easily eliminated from the body in normal dosages, basil may be used *as a spice*.

Together with marjoram (also a galactagogue), basil brings the sunny flavor of the south to our kitchen. I like a pinch of dried basil sprinkled on plain buttered toast or cracker.

Sources: Grocery stores.
Warning: Do not take at therapeutic dosage.

Black Pepper

Black pepper, or peppercorn, is listed as a galactagogue. It is antiseptic and antibacterial, and has a stimulating effect on the digestive tract and the circulatory system. Black peppercorn is a common kitchen spice. For additional benefit, add a few black peppercorns to a teaspoon of a lactogenic tea mixture. Include it as an ingredient in Chai tea.

Sources: Grocery stores, Asian food stores.

Black Seed, Black Cumin, (Nigella sativa)

This tiny seed of a blue, star-like flower has a biting taste. It was known as a galactagogue in ancient Greece and is used today to increase milk supply by mothers across Asia. Black seed—also called black cumin, black caraway seed, or blessed seed—is most reliably known by its botanical name *Nigella sativa*. Black seed is estrogenic. It contains amino acids that support lactation, essential fatty acids, calcium, iron, sodium, and potassium.

⇨ In an experiment with rats, black seed significantly increased the development of mammary tissue—even more so than diets containing umbel seeds.

Two of black seed's main components, nigellone and thymoquinone, relax and open the bronchial passages and loosen congestion in the lungs. Black seed oil is taken in Asia, the Mid-East, and Africa to treat respiratory problems such as chronic bronchitis, emphysema, whooping cough, as well as for flu and cold-like symptoms. It is frequently used as a natural bronchial dilator. (Consult your doctor if you wish to add black seed to your medical treatment.) Black seed is also taken for digestive complaints, to support the kidneys and liver, to boost the immune system, and to reduce allergic symptoms.

⇨ Unlike ephedra (a Chinese herbal for asthma that is anti-lactogenic), black seed is considered safe to use for breastfeeding mothers.

Pregnancy: Ayurvedic medicine from India warns that black seed should not be taken during pregnancy.
Side effect: Occasionally, people find black seed to be hard on the stomach. This usually disappears within a few days.
Sources: Health food stores; Asian food stores; online.
Dosage and Preparation:
• Seed: sprinkle onto salad.
• Tea as galactagogue: steep one teaspoon of the seeds in a cup of just-boiled water and drink 3 times per day.
• The oil in treating chronic bronchial conditions: 4 x 10 drops per day, or 2 x 20 drops. The oil is also available in capsules. Follow the dosage directions on the package.

Black Tea

Black tea is listed as a galactagogue, and mothers sometimes report that drinking black tea increases their milk production. Be careful however not to rely on tea, coffee, chocolate or sugar for energy throughout the day, as this can result in blood sugar issues and related insulin problems that are not only bad for your health in the long term, but also are not conducive to building a good milk supply in vulnerable mothers.

Blessed Thistle (Cnicus benedictus)

Blessed thistle increases the flow of gastric and bile secretion. It is used in the treatment of stomach, intestines, liver, and gall bladder disease. It increases appetite, and, as it heals the underlying condition, will reduce flatulence. Remember that bitter teas need to taste bitter in order to trigger the release of gastric juices and stimulate the production of bile, so do not over-sweeten this tea.

Blessed thistle is said to prevent or ease depression through its support of the liver—the major organ that detoxifies the body, and, apparently, the emotions as well in the body/mind health paradigm. Blessed thistle is thought by some herbalists to improve blood circulation to the breasts.

Pregnancy: Avoid use during pregnancy.

Allergy: Rare. People who are allergic to the daisy family, (Asteraceae), may be allergic to blessed thistle.

Caution: Stimulates gastric juices; persons with ulcers, hyperacidity or acute stomach inflammation may be advised not to take blessed thistle.

Side Effects: Rare. Diarrhea in the mother.

Sources: Health food stores.

Dosage and Preparation:

- Tea: Pour a cup of boiling water onto 1-2 teaspoons of the dried herb and steep for 5 - 10 minutes. Drink three cups a day, before meals or snacks. To kick-start lactation, take up to 6 cups a day.
- Capsules: Up to 3 capsules, 3 times a day in combination with other herbs such as fenugreek.

Borage (Borago officinalis)

Borage leaf tea has an interesting, cucumber-fresh taste. It contains hormonal precursors, and is a *euphoric* (borage leaf was traditionally added to wine to make parties jollier). Therapeutically, borage leaf has been used to improve mood, to nourish the adrenal glands, and to bring balance in times of stress. Like many galactagogues, borage can be used to induce sweat.

Borage has been widely used as a galactagogue in the US. At present, however, the American Herbal Products Association (AHPA) does not recommend borage for long-term use, or for pregnant or nursing women. This is due to an alkaloid in the leaves—*not equally present in all leaves*—that can damage the liver if taken *at therapeutic dosage over a long period of time*.

That said, dried borage leaf, if taken as one of many ingredients in a lactation tea mixture, should be considered as safe, as you would not be taking anywhere near therapeutic dosage.

If you have borage growing in your garden (it grows easily and multiplies from year to year), do not use it *every day* as a medicinal infusion or eat it every day as a vegetable. Do feel free to lightly steep the fresh leaves as a lactogenic beverage, or to drink it occasionally for a mood lift. Use the young leaves and blue flowers in salad now and then.

Borage seed oil, on the other hand, is considered safe and is widely used by breastfeeding mothers. Borage seed oil has the highest concentration of gamma linoleic acid of any seed. Occasionally, mothers find that borage oil boosts their supply, "even better than fenugreek," as one mother reported.

Warning: Borage leaf tea should not be taken at therapeutic dosage.

Borage Tea as Mild Beverage:

- 1 - 3 fresh small leaves, or 1/4 - 1/2 teaspoon or dried leaves, steeped for 1 - 3 minutes produce a palatable tea. Add stevia or other natural sweetener to taste.

Caraway (Carum Carvi)

Caraway is a tangy carminative spice. Use caraway when cooking vegetables that are difficult to digest, such as cabbage or cauliflower. These foods will then become easier to digest—important if your baby has colic or is fussy.

Umbel seeds, including caraway, share the following properties: they are estrogenic and relaxing (sedative); they support digestion, ease colic and flatulence (may ease a baby's colic through the mother's milk), and they aid in treating bronchitis and bronchial asthma (are anti-spasmodic)

Pregnancy: Ayurvedic medicine from India warns against taking large amounts of warming herbs, including caraway, during pregnancy.

Allergy: Occasional.

Caution: Mothers of lethargic babies should avoid taking large amounts of herbs that have sedative effects—such as hops and umbel seeds—as these could possibly make their baby sleepier. Lethargic babies should see their pediatrician as soon as possible.

Caution: Traditional Chinese Medicine warns that warming herbs, such as umbel seeds, should not be taken in large amounts by mothers who tend to develop breast infections.

Sources: Grocery stores. Health-food stores.

Dosage and Preparation: *see* Umbel Seeds.

Chasteberry (Vitex agnus castus)

In the 1st century A.D., the Greek doctor Dioscorides wrote, "the fruit of the chaste tree, being drunk, brings down the milk." Dioscorides' words suggest that chasteberry juice improves the let-down reflex: it brings down the milk. He may however have been referring to lactogenesis, or the onset of lactation after birth. In other words, he may have been advising this herb to speed the initial onset of milk production.

Indeed, the proper use of chasteberry as a galactagogue is unclear. One interesting study, from 1957 in Germany, tested chasteberry on mothers after birth with different medical conditions, and showed positive results with increased milk supply in all groups compared to controls. However, this study was never repeated, nor have any other studies been conducted on chasteberry and breastfeeding women. Today's studies show that chasteberry lowers prolactin in fertile women. Researchers assume that chasteberry will lower prolactin in lactating women as well. However, a study using homeopathic preparations showed that a lower dosage caused a *rise* in prolactin—however, this study was done on *men*[63].

Some herbalists advise that chasteberry be taken only a week or two before a mother's due date, to increase the strength of her contractions, and during the first ten days after birth, to enhance her milk supply. This advice is for all mothers, not specifically mothers who suspect that they may have low milk supply. Perhaps, however, chasteberry may be recommended in this specific dosage to mothers who experienced delayed lactogenesis with a previous birth. It's worth considering.

Some herbalists fear that if chasteberry is taken longer than a few weeks, it may initiate fertility, since chasteberry is used to promote and regulate ovulation in mothers with fertility issues. However, one woman I know who had PCOS, and who had her first menses five months after birth, began then to take chasteberry. Her milk supply rebounded within three weeks, and she did not have another menses for several months. In any case, because so little is known about chasteberry, it is probably wise for most mothers to select other galactagogues, reserving chasteberry as a galactagogue of last-resort, to be tried only if nothing else has helped. Then, it is said to take up to three weeks to fully enhance the milk supply.

Pregnancy: Avoid chasteberry during pregnancy, with the exception of the last two weeks.

Allergy: Rare. Skin, rash, itching.

Warning: There is a risk that chasteberry may reduce supply and initiate ovulation, especially if taken longer than one or two weeks at a time.

Sources: Tinctures available at some health food stores and online.

Dosage: Tincture: 15 drops, 3 times per day, before meals.

Chlorophyll (Green-drinks: Alfalfa, Spirulina, Barley Grass, Oatstraw)

Chlorophyll, the green color of plants, is reputed to have a lactogenic effect. Dark green leafy vegetables, eaten during the weeks after birth, are said to help ensure that an abundant milk supply is established. Green-drinks are another good source of chlorophyll. Their ingredients include barley-grass, alfalfa leaf, spirulina, chorella, kelp, oat-straw and other herbs with lactogenic and medicinal properties.

Mothers who drink chlorophyll mixtures notice an increase in their energy and in milk-supply. Some also report an increase in fatty part of the milk that they pump. Green-drinks are sold both in capsules and in powdered form, to be mixed into a drink just before use. They can be taken with carrot juice to improve their flavor. There is a recipe for homemade green-drinks on page 198.

Warning: A breastfeeding mother should not undergo a 'detox' because the toxins from her liver and fat will enter her milk. Use constraint with green-drinks or any detoxifying herb, and lower the dosage if you or your baby experience any sign of discomfort.

Warning: Chlorella, a common ingredient in commercial green-drinks, is used by medical specialists to chelate (remove) heavy metals from the body, especially mercury. If not taken at the correct, low dosage, chlorella can lead to an increase of mercury in the bloodstream and in a mother's milk. It is wise to choose green-drinks that only contain a low percent of chlorella, or that do not contain chlorella at all, such as Barley Green™ from AIM International.

Sources: Health food stores, and online.

Cinnamon (Cinnamomum zeylanicum)

Originally from Asia, cinnamon's scent has been prized in unguents and incense since ancient times. In China, cinnamon is taken to cause sweating (like many galactagogues) and the Chinese variety of cinnamon is used as a galactagogue. Although not commonly taken as a galactagogue in the west, in Brazil and Peru today, cinnamon is a spice for lactogenic foods.

Cinnamon has one especially unique and valuable property: it is helpful in keeping a mother's blood sugar levels steady by improving the body's sensitivity to insulin. Hypoglycemic patients report that taking cinnamon with or soon after a meal helps prevent a hypoglycemic reaction (a dip in blood sugar), whereas taking it once a day won't have the same effect. If you have blood sugar issues, take cinnamon as a spice in your meals, or stir cinnamon powder into cold or warm water, milk or milk substitute.

Cinnamon also acts as a potent antifungal in the intestine, which may possibly help curb allergies in the mother and her baby in the long term. Cinnamon is estrogenic, and a very mild sedative. As tea, it is tasty and calming. It is helpful for digestion, and to treat a sluggish intestine.

Pregnancy: Cinnamon should be used with caution during pregnancy. Very high dosages of cinnamon have been traditionally used to trigger abortion. Women with a history of miscarriage may avoid cinnamon and other 'warming' herbs altogether.

Allergy: Allergic reactions on the skin and mouth may occur in people allergic to cinnamon or Peruvian balsam, or who are prone to allergic dermatitis and react to toothpaste or mouthwash which contains cinnamaldehyde.

Caution: As a breastfeeding mother, stay on the low side of dosage. Carefully look for any reactions in your baby.

Sources: Grocery stores. Health-food stores. Asian stores. Online.

Dosage and Preparation:

- Up to 3 tablespoons per day have been used in the treatment of insulin resistance or diabetes. However, as little as only one teaspoon per day, or approximately ¼ teaspoon with meals, is sufficient to improve insulin resistance. Ask your certified herbalist or doctor for treatment guidelines.
- Take cinnamon as a spice in your meals, or stir cinnamon powder into cold or warm water, milk or milk substitute.

Commercial Lactation Teas and Tinctures

Health-food stores and super-markets often carry a mixture of herbs from local producers that support breastfeeding, known as *lactation tea*. A variety of brands and mixtures are available. Check to see whether the ingredients are fresh (should maintain some color, not look completely dried and faded, and should smell intensely), and whether at least some of the ingredients are organically grown.

Mother's Milk® Tea from Traditional Medicinals has an excellent reputation, though some mothers find it very bitter.

Quality tinctures to increase milk production are available from online sources such as motherlove.com, and birthandbreastfeeding.com.

Sources: Grocery stores. Health-food stores. Online stores.

Cumin (Cuminum cyminum)

Cumin gives curries and other traditional Asian and African dishes their zing. It is well known as a galactagogue. Like all the umbel seeds, cumin is added to food to make it easier to digest. This can be helpful if your baby has colic or any sign of digestive stress. One mother from Africa spoke of the women in her community eating small green lentils with plenty of cumin and tomatoes to increase their milk production.

Umbel seeds share the following properties: they are estrogenic and relaxing (sedative); they support digestion, ease colic and flatulence (may ease a baby's colic through the mother's milk), and they aid in treating bronchitis and bronchial asthma (are anti-spasmodic).

Pregnancy: Ayurvedic medicine from India warns against taking large amounts of warming herbs, including cumin, during pregnancy.

Allergy: Rare.

Caution: Mothers of lethargic babies should avoid taking large amounts of herbs that have sedative effects—such as hops and umbel seeds—as these could possibly make their baby sleepier. Lethargic babies should see their pediatrician as soon as possible.

Caution: Traditional Chinese Medicine warns that warming herbs, such as umbel seeds, should not be taken in large amounts by mothers who tend to develop breast infections.

Sources: Grocery stores. Health-food stores. Asian stores. Online.

Dosage and Preparation: *see* Umbel Seeds

Dandelion (Taraxicum officinale)

Many of our common weeds were brought over to the US by settlers who appreciated their nutritional and medicinal worth. Among these are varieties of thistle and dandelion that are still valued today in the Mideast and Asia as galactagogues.

The common dandelion is nutrient-rich with estrogenic properties. It contains calcium, iron, magnesium, manganese, phosphorus, potassium, selenium, zinc, vitamins B1, B2, B3 and high amounts of vitamin C. The dandelion cleanses the blood and the liver, increases bile production, reduces cholesterol and uric acid levels, and improves the functioning of the kidneys, spleen, pancreas and stomach. It is useful for fluid retention, anemia, constipation, abscesses, boils, cirrhosis of the liver, and rheumatism. It is also used in the treatment of hepatitis and jaundice.

In China, varieties of the dandelion have been used since ancient times to treat breast problems such as cancer and mastitis, and for increasing milk production. Native American quickly realized the value of dandelion and thistles; dandelions are recorded as a galactagogue in the Native American medicinal cornucopia.

Allergy: Rare. Persons allergic to the daisy family, (Asteraceae), may be allergic to dandelion.

Warning: Dandelion is an herbal diuretic, and should not be combined with prescription diuretics. It is not recommended for people with obstructed bile ducts, or gallbladder empyema. Use only under the guidance of your physician if you have gallstones.

Sources: Health food stores. Herbal stores. Online.

- For mastitis: An ounce of minced root is simmered in two to three cups of water until only half the liquid remains. Soak cloths in the lukewarm decoction to use as a compress for the infected breast[1].
- As a diuretic: The leaves of the dandelion can be safely used to relieve fluid retention. Its minerals, including potassium (4%), will replace the minerals that are otherwise leached from the body by its diuretic effect.
- It is thought that by drinking dandelion root and leaf tea after birth a mother can help prevent mastitis, can speed her convalescence, reduce fluid retention, support milk production and possibly prevent jaundice in her baby—the liver-strengthening properties of the root will reach her baby *through her milk*. However, the guidance of a physician is advised in the case of a prematurely born baby.
- For a baby with pronounced jaundice, the milder liver-herb, yarrow, may be the preferable herb, to be taken by the *mother*.

<u>Homemade dandelion root tea medicinal</u>: Pull dandelions from the garden, preferably, before the plant begins to flower, in early spring. Wash the roots, slice in half lengthwise, and chop into small pieces. Spread the pieces out in one layer and allow them to dry in a cool, dry, shady place for two to three weeks.

Dosage and Preparation:
- Tincture: 1 – 2 ml of the tincture, or 10 - 15 drops 3 times daily.
- Capsules: Follow directions on package.

[1] From James Duke's "Green Pharmacy".

- Infusion: Soak 1 tablespoon of roots in 3 cups of cold water overnight. Next morning, briefly boil and strain. Sip 1 cup 1/2 hour before meals.
- Decoction: Gently simmer 1 tablespoon of finely chopped fresh, dried or powdered root in 3 cups of water for 10 – 15 minutes.
- A tasty combination—approximately 1/4 teaspoon of dandelion root, fenugreek seeds, and marshmallow or hollyhock root. Prepare as the decoction above.
- *As food*: The leaves can be eaten whole, can be chopped and sautéed in virgin olive oil with onion and garlic, or cut into salad. The young root *melts on your tongue* if halved lengthwise and sautéed in olive oil for five minutes.
- Dandelion tea as beverage: Steep a 1/4 teaspoon of leaves in 1 cup of boiled water for 3 minutes.
- Dandelion root tea as beverage: Dandelion root is considered a bitter tasting tea. However, lightly prepared dandelion root tea tastes earthy-sweet. Simmer 1/4 – 1/2 teaspoon of root in 2 cups of water for 5 minutes for a gently sweet medicinal.

Dill (Anethum graveolens)

Dill, both the seed and the leaf, has a special reputation for treating flatulence and colic in a baby through her mother's milk. As a spice it is used to flavor salad dressing, sauces, bread, eggs, cottage cheese, minced meat, chicken, vegetables, in pickling, and fish and shellfish dishes.

Dill is an umbel seed and shares the following properties: estrogenic and relaxing (sedative); supports digestion, eases colic and flatulence (may ease a baby's colic through the mother's milk), and aids in treating bronchitis and bronchial asthma (anti-spasmodic).

Pregnancy: Ayurvedic medicine from India warns against taking large amounts of warming herbs, including dill, during pregnancy.

Allergy: Occasional.

Caution: Mothers of lethargic babies should avoid taking excessively large amounts of herbs that have sedative effects—such as hops and umbel seeds—as these could possibly make their baby sleepier. Lethargic babies should see their pediatrician as soon as possible.

Caution: Traditional Chinese Medicine warns that warming herbs, such as umbel seeds, should not be taken in large amounts by mothers who tend to develop breast infections.

Sources: Grocery stores. Health-food stores. Asian stores. Online.

Dosage and Preparation: *see* also Umbel Seeds.

- Tea: 3 – 6 cups a day. Steep 1 teaspoon of the crushed seeds in a cup of boiled water for 10 – 15 minutes. For flatulence in the mother, sip a cup of dill tea 10 minutes before meals. Sip throughout the day to treat colic in the baby through your milk, or as a galactagogue.

- Decoction: The ancient Greek doctor, Dioscorides, recommended a decoction of dill to "bring down the milk." He may have been referring to the letdown reflex, but he may also have been referring to a delay in full milk production several days after birth. Soak 3 tablespoons of dill seed in a quart of water overnight, and gently simmer until half or more of the liquid has evaporated off. Sip throughout the day.

- Dill seed tea as a beverage: Lightly steeped dill tea has the most satisfying flavor of all the umbel seeds, in my opinion: not too tangy or sweet, just right. Steep 1 teaspoon of the seeds in a cup of water for 3 minutes. Sweeten to taste.

⇨ Remember, some mothers respond well to mildly dosed herbals.

Dong quai (Angelica sinensis)

Dong quai root, a tonic herb from China, is best known in the US and Europe as a woman's medicinal, taken to promote fertility, to regulate menstrual cycles, to relieve the pain of menstruation, and to reduce symptoms of PMS.

In China, dong quai is revered as a major blood tonic and is used in the treatment of anemia and other blood related disorders. It is given in the early postpartum to mothers to address blood loss during birth, and is believed to prevent postpartum depression and to build milk supply.

Dong quai is also taken to boost the immune system, in the treatment of auto-immune disorders and allergy. Another Chinese herb, astragalus root, has a complimentary effect, and the combination of astragalus and dong quai is powerfully synergistic and one of China's best tonic formulas in the treatment of a wide range of disorders, and wonderful for mother's with *thin skins* or *frazzled nerves*, and for mothers who are so tired that they feel as though they cannot even sit up straight. Both dong quai and astragalus are traditionally taken to support milk production.

Pregnancy: Dong quai should not be taken during the first three months of pregnancy, or at any time during pregnancy if a mother is at risk of miscarriage.

Caution: Do not take during a cold or flu, or for diarrhea, due to the herb's laxative effect.

Warning: Due to its anti-coagulation effect, dang quai should not be combined with blood thinning medications, and should be avoided by people with bleeding disorders.

Sources: Drug stores. Health food stores. Herbal stores. Online.

Dosage and Preparation:

- Capsules: Follow the dosage directions on the package. Extracts of the herb can be toxic in high dosages.
- Tea: Per day, 6 – 14 g of the root. Simmer gently in 6 cups of water until 2 cups have evaporated. Sip the tea throughout the day. The roots can be eaten as food. (See *Astragalus* for more information.) Take with honey or raw sugar.

Echinacea (Echinacea angustifolia)

Breast infection / mastitis: Echinacea can help stave off inflammation of the breasts that might otherwise require antibiotics. Echinacea is thought to be most effective against breast infection if taken at the *first sign* of tenderness or redness on the breast. A quick response with echinacea almost always wards off infection. However, studies suggest that echinacea may have less effect, and may even weaken the immune system, if used on a regular basis to prevent infection.

⇨ Do not take echinacea unnecessarily as a so-called preventative measure.

Proceed normally to ward off mastitis: feed often and position your baby so that his chin is on the same side as the inflamed area to be sure that that area is well-drained. Contact your local LLL-leader or lactation consultant for information as to treating breast infection. Early response usually makes the use of antibiotics unnecessary.

Allergy: Persons who are allergic to the daisy family, (Asteraceae), may be allergic to echinacea (especially the leaf and flower) and should use it cautiously. Try to get a tinctured product made only with the root.

Warning: Echinacea is not to be used for a prolonged period of time (longer than eight weeks), because of concerns that it could exhaust the immune system through over-stimulation.

Warning: Echinacea is not to be used in treating: tuberculosis, leukosis, collagenosis, multiple sclerosis, AIDS, HIV infection, and other autoimmune diseases.

Warning: Echinacea must be taken under medical supervision if you have diabetes.

Sources: Health food stores. Drug stores. Herbal stores. Online.

Dosage:

- Capsules: Follow dosage directions on the package.
- Tincture: General dosage suggestions are to take 15 - 30 drops, 3 - 5 times the first day, and reduce to 3 times a day for following days.

Elder Flower and Berry (Sambucus nigra)

The elder flower is the traditional galactagogue of the traveling Romany in northern Europe, the people once called gypsies. It is also a traditional German galactagogue.

Elder flowers relieve fluid retention and promote sweating during fever, accelerating the healing process of a cold or flu. This places elder flowers in good company with other galactagogues that stimulate perspiration: fenugreek, goat's rue, borage, and vervain (it has been speculated that these herbs may stimulate mammary glands in a fashion similar to sweat glands).

Elderberries contain a potent antiviral substance that attaches to the surface of viruses and prevents them from infiltrating new cells. Elder berry speeds healing in colds and flu by reducing the number of potent viruses, and may be of help in treating chronic illness that involve viruses. Elderberry syrup is always available in my home, ready to be taken at the first sign of a flu or cold.

Sources: Health food stores; online.

Dosage and Preparation:

- Lactogenic tea: Pour one cup of boiling water onto 2 teaspoonfuls of dried or fresh flowers, cover, and steep for 5 - 10 minutes. Sweeten to taste.
- Elder Flower Tea as Beverage: A light tea is made by steeping 1/2 teaspoon of the dried flower for 3 minutes in a cup of just-boiled water. Take three cups a day. This tea tastes slightly lemony and sweet. Add stevia or other natural sweetener to taste.
- Medicinal syrup: 1 – 2 tablespoons of syrup per hot cup of water.

Essential Fatty Acids (EFAs)

Many mothers find that supplementing with EFAs, such as **borage seed oil**, **evening primrose seed oil**, **black currant seed oil**, or **flax seed oil**, increases their milk production. These oils contain hormonal precursors which may influence the chemistry of lactation.

Do not overdose on these oils, as this could prompt the body to absorb less of them. Follow the dosage directions on the package. After 3 – 4 weeks on the oil, reduce the dosage as your body now probably has regained healthy levels of the particular fatty acid(s) in each oil.

Sources: Drug stores, Health food stores. Some grocery stores. Online.

Fennel (Foeniculum vulgare)

Fennel is highly regarded as a galactagogue—both the vegetable, as food, and the seed as an herbal medicinal.

Taken at a high dosage for a few days, fennel seed can increase milk supply and improve the mother's digestion, and her baby's digestion as well through her mother's milk. However, in Traditional Chinese Medicine, fennel seed is said to have a *drying* quality that will reduce milk production if taken at a high dosage over a long period of time.

Fennel seed tea is frequently one ingredient in a lactation herbal mixture, or can be alternated with other lactogenic beverages.

Pregnancy: Ayurvedic medicine from India warns against taking large amounts of warming herbs, including fennel seed, during pregnancy.

Allergy: Occasional.

Caution: Mothers of lethargic babies should avoid taking large amounts of herbs that have sedative effects—such as hops and umbel seeds—as these could possibly make their baby sleepier. Lethargic babies should see their pediatrician as soon as possible.

Caution: Traditional Chinese Medicine warns that warming herbs, such as umbel seeds, should not be taken in large amounts by mothers who tend to develop breast infections.

Sources: Grocery stores, online.

Dosage and Preparation: *see* Umbel Seeds.

Fenugreek (Trigonella foenum-graecum)

The best known and most frequently taken galactagogue in the US today is fenugreek seed. Originally from Asia, fenugreek was not known in Europe and the west until recently, and, ironically, is not recorded in any traditional western herbal as a galactagogue.

Fenugreek has medicinal effects in common with other galactagogues. Fenugreek enhances perspiration, relaxes, supports the liver, and it also contains very high levels of phytoestrogen. Based on its century-old reputation for increasing breast-size, it is possible that its particular phytoestrogen specifically targets the breast. Fenugreek also loosens and discharges lung congestion. It soothes the intestine, and reduces flatulence. Fenugreek also lowers 'bad' cholesterol and relieves water retention.

Though most mothers with low milk production respond quickly to fenugreek seed tea, capsules, or tincture, not all do. Some mothers see more success when they take fenugreek in combination with other herbs. If you do not respond well to fenugreek, open a capsule to check the freshness and quality of the powdered herb. It should have a distinct color and smell. If not, the herb may be old and may have lost its therapeutic effect. Buying a fresher product may solve the problem.

Fenugreek usually increases milk production within one to three days, though for some mothers it may take four to five days to see an effect. If you do not see an effect, in spite of using a quality product and smelling like maple syrup, talk to your lactation specialist about alternatives, such as one of the herbal-combinations described on page 280.

Pregnancy: Do not take fenugreek seed during pregnancy.

Allergy: Mothers sometimes develop asthma or wheezing when they take fenugreek. This is an allergic reaction. Mothers who already have asthma may see it triggered if they take fenugreek. Women who are allergic to fenugreek may also be sensitive to chickpea and peanut.

Side effects: Occasionally, mothers experience nausea, faintness, diarrhea, or running sinuses from fenugreek, though these symptoms usually pass in a few days. Fenugreek seed occasionally triggers migraine headaches and high blood pressure.

Hypoglycemia: If you suffer from low blood sugar, you could possibly feel light-headed or fatigued while on fenugreek, though this is reported very rarely.

Baby: Babies may become fussy when the mother is on high-dose fenugreek. Some babies become gassy and have runny stool. This usually passes in a few days.

Diabetes: Only use fenugreek under the guidance of your doctor if you have diabetes.

Blood-thinning medication: Only use fenugreek under the guidance of your doctor if you are taking blood-thinning medication.

Sources: Health food stores. Some drug stores. Herbal stores. Online.

Dosage and Preparation:

- Capsules: Try one capsule the first day to see if you have an allergic reaction, then 3 capsules, and then 6 capsules a day, divided into three dosages, taken before meals. Add one additional capsule per day and build up to 9 per day. This is considered standard dosage, though some mothers take larger dosages. Gauge your reaction carefully, and ask your lactation expert and doctor for guidance if you are unsure about your individual optimal dosage.

- Although rare, a very low dosage of fenugreek does increase milk production in some sensitive women. One woman I spoke to saw significant improvement with only 2 capsules per day.

- Tincture: Follow the directions on the product you choose. The first day or two, taking a dose of tincture (approx. 30 drops) every two or three hours may kick-start your milk production.

- Lactation experts say that when a mother's perspiration and urine smell like maple syrup, an optimum dosage has probably been reached (in India, people eat fenugreek seed especially to achieve this 'perfume'). However, some mothers do not see improvement in their milk supply with fenugreek alone, and may need to try fenugreek as tincture, or as one herb in a mixture or combination of lactogenic herbs.

- Tea: Fenugreek seed can also be taken as tea—steeped, infused, or decocted, mild or bitter. Add a natural sweetener to taste.

- Sheila Humphrey in "The Nursing Mother's Herbal" recommends steeping 1 – 3 teaspoons of whole seed in 8 oz. of boiling water for 5 – 10 minutes, or longer.

- Infusion, cold: Like the umbel seeds, fenugreek can also be set in cold water and left to soak for several hours or over night. The liquid is then strained off, refrigerated, and each cup gently warmed before drinking.

- David Hoffmann in "Holistic Herbal" suggests that mothers decoct (gently simmer) 1 1/2 teaspoons of slightly crushed fenugreek seeds in one cup of water for ten minutes, and, for a more flavorful taste, add 1 teaspoonful of aniseed to the decoction. Drink three times a day.

Fenugreek combinations:

Combinations of fenugreek seed with other herbs are popular in the US though virtually unknown in Europe. Indeed, specific combinations are so popular that they might as well be called 'traditional American.'

Dosage may vary, depending on the size of the capsule and the quality of the herb. Generally speaking, mothers have to use a higher dosage than is recommended on the package. Start with a low dose and build up until you notice a difference in your milk supply (see general recommendations below). Maintain that dosage to see if your production remains stable. Continue taking the herbs for a few weeks, and then slowly wean from the supplements. Increase the dosage again if your supply drops.

⇨ Combine fenugreek capsules with capsules of one or more of the following medicinals: alfalfa leaves, red clover, marshmallow root, blessed thistle.

⇨ Read up on each of these herbs in their individual sections.

⇨ Like most supplements, capsules of herbal supplements should be taken before a meal.

Fenugreek capsules: Up to 3 capsules, 3 times per day.
Alfalfa leaf capsules: Up to 3 capsules, 3 times a day.
Blessed thistle capsules: Up to 3 capsules, 3 times a day.
Marshmallow capsules: Up to 3 capsules, 3 times a day.
Red Clover: Up to 3 capsules, 3 times a day.

Mothers with persistent low milk supply:

While most mothers use fenugreek for only a short time to give their supply a boost, others depend on fenugreek and fenugreek combinations long-term to keep their supply steady. Some of these mothers find that fenugreek loses its effect with time. The solution is to go off fenugreek and take other galactagogues for a few weeks, to restore fenugreek's effect at a later time.

Flaxseed

See Essential Fatty Acids.

Garlic (Allium sativa)

Garlic is famous for its medical benefits. It is antibacterial, antiviral and antifungal. It is useful in treating inflammation and fungal overgrowth in the intestine. It dilates blood vessels, lowers blood pressure, reduces cholesterol and inhibits the clotting of blood—and so can help prevent heart attacks. It is used in the treatment of circulatory problems, insomnia, colds and flu, arteriosclerosis, arthritis, cancer, heart disorders, liver disease, sinusitis, asthma, and ulcers.

According to Traditional Chinese Medicine (TCM), garlic strengthens a person's *center*, referring to both the digestive system and to the spiritual center of the person. Garlic is therefore considered a strengthening food for mothers in the postpartum.

In Swiss hospitals, nurses and lactation specialists have noticed that women from the Turkish population, whose families bring home-made meals heavily spiced with garlic to the hospital each day, do not have the typical problems of Swiss mothers. The milk of Turkish mothers arrives soon, their babies drink well, and do not cry, or have colic. "There are never problems with mothers from Turkey," one midwife told me.[64] Interestingly, in Native American medicine, ***mothers*** *eat garlic* to heal stomach upset in their babies—through the garlic in their milk. Indeed, garlic has a long history as a galactagogue (see Egyptian Herbal), and one study explained why. In this study, babies were seen to latch on better, suckle more actively, and drink more milk *when the mother had garlic* prior to nursing[65].

Pregnancy: Unfortunately, our culture does not encourage eating garlic, and many people do not tolerate garlic well (or onions, another food which is believed to have a lactogenic effect). For this reason, garlic is not recommended by the American Herbal Product's Association while breastfeeding except under the guidance of a qualified herbalist. However, if you do tolerate garlic and enjoy it in your food, there is no reason that you should not benefit from it. Take garlic in moderation as do women all over the world.

Allergy: Occasional; stomach upset, and rash on contact.

Warning: Garlic can lower blood sugar.

Warning: Do not combine with anticoagulants, as garlic has blood-thinning actions.

Danger: Babies and small children should **never** be given garlic in any form, (whether fresh, dry, powdered or in capsules), to chew, swallow, eat or suck on! Babies should only benefit from the garlic a mother eats, and that passes to him through her milk.

Sources: Grocery stores. Drug stores. Health food stores. Online.

- Dosage and Preparation:
- As medicine: Do not use garlic in therapeutic dosages, unless under the guidance of your healthcare provider.
- As a condiment: If you are not used to garlic, take only 1 – 2 cloves per day. These can be chopped, or pressed through a garlic press into any food after it has finished cooking: vegetables, rice, grains, pulses, salad sauce, spaghetti sauce, or other sauce.

Ginger Root (Zingiber officinal)

Fresh ginger root is a galactagogue. In ancient Ayurvedic medicine, it is described as helping to "cleanse the milk." Any herb that promotes digestion and intestinal health would fit into this category, and ginger is a supreme herb in this respect. Ginger has antibacterial, antiviral and antifungal properties, and has a healing effect on the stomach and intestine. It increases bile flow, helping in the digestion of fat. Ginger also contains high amounts of protease, an enzyme used to digest protein.

As an added benefit, ginger opens the arteries and tiny capillaries, greatly improving and speeding blood circulation throughout the body. It is commonly added to herbal mixtures specifically to speed their transportation throughout the blood system. Ginger is also said to enable other herbs to be better absorbed by the body, and so, indirectly, to enhance their effect. Ginger doubtless increases blood circulation within the breasts as well, promoting the milk ejection reflex and lowering susceptibility to breast infection (see ginger ale and ginger tea on page 203-204).

Ginger has a positive effect on the respiratory system (lungs) and is used in Traditional Chinese Medicine to help prevent and heal depression, which is said in TCM to be linked to the lungs.

Pregnancy: Take small amounts, as a spice.

Allergy: Yes, especially in people who farm and handle the herb.

Warning: TCM warns against using ginger in the early postpartum if there was significant blood loss during birth.

Warning: Do not take ginger immediately after birth due to danger of hemorrhaging.

Warning: Do not use ginger if you have gallstones before consulting your doctor.

Warning: Ginger tends to compound and increase the effects of medication being taken. Talk to your doctor if you are taking medication, especially diabetic, blood-thinning, or heart medicine.

Sources: Grocery stores. Asian stores. Health food stores. Online.

Dosage and Preparation:

- Ginger root can be used fresh or powdered. The fresh root, which tastes like mild pepper, is considered more lactogenic. It can be sliced or grated and added to food, or made into tea.
- A general dosage guideline for powdered ginger is 1 – 3 teaspoons or fresh ginger per day, though some herbalists set the dosage higher, at 1 – 3 tablespoons per day.
- Ginger can be prepared as tea. See page 204 for a recipe.

Ginkgo Biloba (Ginkgo folium)

Ginkgo is not a traditional galactagogue. It has however been observed by lactation consultants to increase milk production. It may work though increasing blood circulation to the breasts.

Ginkgo may be helpful for mothers with syndromes involving poor circulation in the extremities, such as Reynaud's Syndrome.

Allergy: Yes, especially in people who farm and handle the herb.

Side effects: Sometimes, mild gastrointestinal problems.

Rare: Headache, vertigo, dizziness.

Caution: Talk to your doctor before taking Ginkgo if you take anticoagulants or have a blood clotting disorder.

Sources: Drug stores. Health food stores. Online.

Dosage: Follow directions on package. Do not overdose.

Goat's Rue (Galega officinalis)

Goat's rue belongs to the family of the legumes, as do fenugreek, alfalfa, red clover, peanuts[2], chick pea, and lentils—lactogenic herbs and foods.

Many lactation experts believe that goat's rue is especially helpful for mothers with insufficient glandular tissue, in that it helps to build glandular tissue while breastfeeding, and perhaps during pregnancy as well.

Goat's rue balances blood sugar levels, possibly improving insulin sensitivity. If you are diabetic, discuss the use of goat's rue with your doctor. If you have symptoms of hypoglycemia, consult your doctor, and follow the suggestions in this book to stabilize your blood sugar while using this herb.

Pregnancy: Good general safety rating, but no extensive testing. Take goat's rue well beneath therapeutic dosage, for instance, one mild cup of tea a day. Mothers needing the medicinal effects of goat's rue during pregnancy might consider taking metformin instead, under the guidance of their doctor.

Side effect: Can lower blood sugar. Not to be used by diabetics except under the guidance of your doctor.

Warning: The fresh plant is considered to be toxic, but the dried plant is safe to use as tea.

Sources: In bulk as tea, and as tincture, at special herbal stores, online.

Dosage and Preparation:

- Tincture: Take 1 – 2 ml of tincture, or 10 – 15 drops, 3 times a day.
- Tea: Pour 1 cup of boiling water over 1 teaspoonful of the herb, steep 5 –10 minutes. Drink 2 – 3 cups a day.

Hollyhock Root (Alcea rosea)

The huge hollyhock is easy to grow, and it multiplies from year to year. It bears lovely colorful flowers. In early spring, its broad leaves are still eaten as a steamed vegetable in Mediterranean countries today, and its roots are harvested as medicine. Indeed, the hollyhock is the garden variety of the marshmallow plant, and the roots of the two plants share similar medicinal properties: both loosen and draw out congestion from the lungs and sinuses (perfect for a cold or flu), and soothe intestinal inflammation. Both also increase milk supply.

---

[2] Peanuts are not generally advised as a galactagogue due to their being dangerously allergenic for about 1% of all babies. In Asia and Africa, cooked green peanuts are used to build milk supply. It is likely that in this form, they are less allergenic.

In ancient Greece the stem, leaves, and root of hollyhock were decocted to help with milk flow. If you have hollyhock in your garden, you might try this ancient remedy, using the fresh leaf, stem, and root of your plant and simmering them together into a strong brew. Otherwise, use the root of the hollyhock much as you would the marshmallow.

Sources: The garden.

Dosage and Preparation:

- Decoct 1 teaspoon of dried, small pieces of chopped root per cup of water for 10 – 15 minutes. Take three cups a day.
- Hollyhock root tea as beverage: A mild decoction tastes gently sweet. Take 1/4 – 1/2 teaspoon of small chopped pieces of root per cup of water and gently simmer 5 -10 minutes. Sweeten to taste.

Hops (Humulus lupulus)

Hops flowers are used in brewing beer; they provide beer with its color and bitter taste. They are also the source of the relaxing, golden glow that we feel from beer. Hops is highly estrogenic and a strong relaxant. Pillows stuffed with hops flowers have a long tradition of being used to promote sleep. Taken as tea, Hops is extremely bitter.

As a galactagogue, hops may be helpful in triggering the letdown reflex. A cup of hops flower tea is sometimes recommended in the evening, to help a mother relax before bed. However, hops should not be taken by women who are suffering from depression, or who are prone to depression, as it can induce melancholic feelings.

Pregnancy: Hops is strongly hormonal; avoid during pregnancy.

Allergy: Yes, especially in people who farm and handle the herb.

Caution: Some herbalists suggest that hops can increase melancholic feelings, and should not be taken by persons prone to depression.

Caution: Mothers of lethargic babies should avoid large dosages of herbs that have strong sedative effects—such as hops—as these could possibly make their baby even more sleepy and unwilling to drink. Lethargic babies should see their pediatrician as soon as possible.

Sources: Sometimes, health food stores. Herbal stores, online.

Dosage and Preparation:

- Tea: Pour 1 cup of boiling water onto 1 teaspoon of the dried flowers, and steep for 10 – 15 minutes. Take one cup in the late afternoon, evening, or before bedtime.

Lemon Balm (Melissa officinalis)

Balm, also called Lemon Balm, is a tasty tea that grows easily in the garden. It helps relieve nervousness and anxiety, improve sleep, and relieve tension headache and nervous heart palpitations. It eases indigestion, and is useful for intestinal and menstrual cramps. It is reported to be lactogenic in some sources and to be anti-lactogenic in others. It may anti-lactogenic to mothers sensitive to astringent foods. For these mothers, it is probably safe to use as one ingredient in a lactogenic tea mixture.

Pregnancy: It would be wise not to take lemon balm at high dosage during pregnancy.

Warning: People with thyroid problems, such as Grave's disease, should not use lemon balm.

Sources: Sometimes, Health food stores. Herbal stores. Online.

Dosage and Preparation:

- Tea: Pour 1 cup of boiling water onto 1 – 3 teaspoons of the dried leaves, and steep for 5 – 10 minutes. Take one cup in the late afternoon, evening, or before bedtime.
- A light tea is made by steeping 1 teaspoon of the dried herb for one minute in 1 cup of boiling water. Drink up to four cups a day.
- The fresh herb is so potent that 1 – 3 leaves may suffice to flavor a large pot of tea.

Lettuce, Wild (Lactuca Virosa)

Wild and cultivated varieties of lettuce are used in Native American medicine, in ancient Greek medicine, and in Traditional Chinese Medicine to increase milk production and flow. Lettuce contains a milk-like fluid that has sedative properties. It is so powerful that it has been used in traditional medicine as an opium substitute to dull pain during operations, or to relieve pain in rheumatism. (Many sedatives, plant or medical, increase milk production; the body's own chemical opiates also increase milk production). Wild lettuce, like many galactagogues, is an anti-spasmodic, and is helpful for cough, cramps, and colic.

Eating salad made of dark leafy vegetables every day has been reported to support milk supply in some mothers.

Allergy: Rare.

Sources: Herbal stores. Drug stores that carry homeopathy. Online.

Dosage and Preparation:
- Tea: Pour one cup of boiling water onto 1-2 teaspoons of the dried herb, cover and steep for 10 – 15 minutes. Take up to 3 times a day.
- Tincture: 2 – 4 ml (15 – 30 drops), 3 times a day.
- Homeopathy: Lactuca Virosa, X30, combined with Alfalfa, X30. For nervous, tense mothers.

Marjoram, Sweet (Organum majorana)

Sweet marjoram is recorded in German herbals as a galactagogue. Like many better-known galactagogues, it improves digestion, reduces flatulence, encourages sweating, relieves fluid retention, and is anti-spasmodic, useful for bronchial asthma, and menstrual cramps. It is also a mild tranquilizer and mood-lifter.

As a kitchen herb, marjoram is a welcome addition to a lactogenic diet. Slightly bitter, with a sweet aftertaste, it compliments the flavor of many grains, vegetable dishes, and salad dressings. Marjoram is used in Italian cooking, along with basil and oregano. Basil is another lactogenic herb. Oregano, however, is considered anti-lactogenic.

A pinch or two of marjoram, as a dried herb, can be sprinkled directly onto sandwiches, buttered bread, or crackers for a snack.

Pregnancy: Do not take at high dosage; do use as a spice.

Allergy: Rare.

Sources: Spice section of a grocery store, online.

Dosage and Preparation:
- Tea: Add a cup of boiling water to 1 - 2 teaspoons of the dried herb, cover, and steep for 10 - 15 minutes. Take 3 cups a day.
- Mild tea: Steep ½ - 1 teaspoon of the dried herb for 3 minutes.

Marshmallow Root and Leaf (Althea officinalis)

Native Americans use the marshmallow as a galactagogue. The Greeks used the garden variety, hollyhock, to increase milk flow. Marshmallow root is now frequently used by breastfeeding mothers in the US, in combination with fenugreek, red clover, alfalfa, or blessed thistle. Marshmallow contains mucilage, a slimy substance that soothes and calms inflammation in the intestines, stomach, upper respiratory tract, throat, and mouth.

Caution: Marshmallow root may delay the absorption of other drugs that are taken at the same time. May lower blood sugar.

Sources: Sometimes, health food stores. Herbal stores. Online.

Dosage and Preparation:

- Tea: Pour 1 cup of cold water over 1 tablespoon of root powder, and stir frequently while soaking for thirty minutes. Strain, and warm gently before drinking.
- Decoction: Per cup of water, add 1 teaspoonful of the chopped root, and simmer for 10 – 15 minutes. Take three cups a day. Sheila Humphrey recommends that if you are starting a herbal program, you may take higher dosages for a few days to kick-start your milk supply, i.e., take up to one handful of chopped root per cup of water.
- Capsules: 3 capsules, 3 times a day, in combination with other herbs such as fenugreek, blessed thistle, alfalfa, and red clover.

Milk Thistle (Silybum marianum)

Milk thistle has similar benefits to blessed thistle, but it is used for more severe and chronic disease of the liver. Substances in the seed of the milk thistle strengthen the outer layer of the liver's cells, protecting them from the damage of toxins, and prompting the liver to regenerate its tissue. As the tissue regenerates, fat deposits in the liver dissolve, and liver stagnation is relieved. There is also an increased flow of bile from the liver, aiding in the digestion of fat.

Milk thistle is used in India as a galactagogue, and is now commonly used in the US, where it is said by some herbalists to be an even stronger galactagogue than blessed thistle. There is some concern however about a possible release of toxins when the liver's fat melts into the bloodstream. In this case, a mother could feel unwell for a few days until her body cleared out the toxins. These toxins would also enter her milk. Therefore, if a mother has a history of substance abuse such as with alcohol, drugs, or heavy smoking, or if she has many silver-amalgam fillings in her teeth, it may be advisable to wait to take milk thistle until her baby is weaned, or is getting most of her calories from solid foods. At some point, however, milk thistle is just what these mothers need to cleanse and regenerate their livers.

Warning: Use with caution if you have a history of substance abuse, or if you have many amalgam fillings in your teeth.

Dosage and Preparation:

- Tea: Pour a cup of just-boiled water onto 1 teaspoon of the ground seed, cover, and steep for 10 – 15 minutes. Drink 3 times a day.
- Capsule: Take as directed on package. Fresh, whole seeds are more potent than the powdered seeds in capsules.
- Tincture: Take under the direction of your doctor.

Mushrooms:
Reishi (Ganoderma), Shiitake (Lentinus edodes)

The Chinese mushrooms, reishi and shiitake (and others), are two superb immune-boosters. Studies show that these mushrooms contain potent antiviral, antibacterial, and anti-cancer properties. In Traditional Chinese Medicine (TCM), they are known as superb health tonics, greatly increasing the energy that we call *vitality*, and that the Chinese call *qi* or *chi*. These mushrooms were so highly esteemed in ancient China that in wartime they were given only to soldiers and to the King. Today, they are recommended for all those suffering from any condition that compromises the immune system or generates fatigue.

Because they measurably increase the body's immune reaction, *including increasing the immunoglobulin IgA*—the immune substance that prevents large food molecules from passing through the intestine—these mushrooms may be important for breastfeeding mothers of children with colic or allergies.

Mushrooms (all kinds) contain high levels of essential amino acids. This is good news for vegans and vegetarians. The bad news is that mushrooms bind to heavy metals during their growth, so that it is important to buy mushrooms from a source you can trust.

Allergy: Occasional.

Sources: These mushrooms can be found, fresh or dried, in the produce section of many grocery stores and Asian grocery stores, as well as from online sources. If you use the dried mushroom, soak for about twenty minutes. It will be rubbery. Cut into small pieces and chew well, or prepare as you would fresh mushrooms.

Dosage and Preparation:

While these special mushrooms, especially shiitake, can be prepared like other mushrooms and eaten occasionally for a meal, remember that they are potent medicinals. If you decide to use them therapeutically, for instance in the prevention of cancer, it is wise to use *only one half to one whole mushroom* per day, unless otherwise directed by your doctor. Indeed, if you have a compromised immune system, have allergies, feel fatigued, or if you have a serious illness, seek the guidance of a medical doctor for dosage recommendations—if possible, a doctor who has training in TCM. It may be recommended, for instance, to take these mushrooms as supplements on alternating weeks, gradually honing and stabilizing the immune system.

Nettle (Urtica dioica)

Nettle, specifically Stinging Nettle, is one of our most nutritious herbs. Stinging nettle may be prescribed when a person's ability to absorb nutrients is low, as its nutrients are easily absorbable. Its minerals help build blood, explaining its use in the treatment of anemia. It is a good source for calcium and iron, magnesium, manganese, phosphorus, potassium, selenium, sulfur, zinc, copper, chlorophyll, fatty acids, folate, plus vitamins K, B1, B2, B3, B5, C, and E. Nettle has an affinity for the kidneys. It is taken to treat conditions that are associated with weakness in the kidneys such as bladder infections, eczema, bronchial congestion, asthma, arthritis, and rheumatism. It is also a natural antihistamine, and may improve hay fever, allergic asthma, and other allergic conditions.

In different medical traditions, nettle is regarded as appropriate for the first week after birth. Nettle helps the body restore blood that was lost during childbirth. In Asian medicine, the loss of only a few ounces of blood is thought to contribute to postpartum fatigue and depression, as well as to low milk supply. Nettle also contains high levels of chlorophyll, and some lactation experts believe that chlorophyll is particularly conducive to building milk supply after birth. (Dark green leafy vegetables are also rich in chlorophyll.) Finally, stinging nettle does not affect the chemistry of the body and brain as do other lactogenic herbs, (i.e., it is not a sedative, it is not a muscle relaxant, it is not estrogenic) so that it can be taken freely both during the sensitive first week after birth, and long-term in the postpartum.

Allergy: Rare.

Sources: Health food stores. Herbal stores. Online.

Dosage and Preparation:

- Tea: Pour a cup of boiled water onto 1 – 2 teaspoonfuls of the dried herb, cover and steep for 10 minutes. Take 3 cups a day. To kick-start milk production, double this dosage, and take up to 6 cups a day.

- A mild tea is made by steeping one teaspoon of the dried herb for only 1/2 minute in a cup of boiling water. Take three cups a day. (Even the mild tea has a dark-green color and rich taste.)

- Infusion: In a quart jar, add boiling water, cover, and infuse overnight. Use a large handful of nettle. Combine with other lactogenic herbs, such as alfalfa, goat's rue, dandelion leaf, red clover, vervain, and the umbel seeds.

- Tincture: Nettle is frequently an ingredient of specially developed lactation tinctures. Follow the producer's dosage directions.

Nutritional (and Brewer's) Yeast

Mothers frequently find that supplementing with nutritional or brewer's yeast significantly boosts their milk supply. Mothers sometimes say that they feel much more energetic and emotionally balanced while taking yeast. This may signal a lack of essential nutrients in their diet, in particular, chromium, vitamin B complex, including vitamin B12, found in some brands of fortified nutritional yeast. Brewer's and nutritional yeast also contains protein and good levels of phytoestrogen, which doubtless contribute to their lactogenic effect.

Allergy: Persons who are allergic to yeast should avoid these products.

Side-effects: Occasionally, mothers or babies react with flatulence or other stomach problems, more to brewer's yeast than to nutritional yeast. To be on the safe side, start with a small dosage and slowly increase.

Caution: Mothers with fungal infections of the intestine (for instance, who took antibiotics but then didn't take probiotic yogurt or a lactobacilli product to protect their intestinal flora) should avoid taking nutritional or brewer's yeast as it may contribute to their problem.

Sources: Vegetarian stores.

Oats (Avena Sativa)

One of our most nutritious foods, oats contain proteins, vitamins, minerals and trace elements that nourish the nerves, support the metabolism of fats, and uplift the spirit. In traditional medicine, both the seed and the leaf—called oatstraw—are taken. Oats are a *nervine tonic,* used in the treatment of nervous exhaustion—a condition that is all too common in the postpartum. Women traditionally take oats after birth. Oats are widely taken today in the US to increase milk production, both eaten as food and taken as a supplement. Like other galactagogues, oats are antidepressant, antispasmodic, and they increase perspiration.

Allergy: Occasional. Persons sensitive to gluten in wheat are frequently able to tolerate oats.

Dosage and Preparation:

- Taking large dosages of oats is helpful in kick-starting milk production.
- Oatmeal can be taken for breakfast or an afternoon snack.
- Oatstraw is especially rich in minerals. It is available as capsules or as an ingredient in so-called "green-drinks."
- Fluid extract: 3 – 5 ml (15 – 35 drops), three times a day.

Papaya (Green) (Carica papaya)

Green papaya is taken as a galactagogue across Asia. It is a superb source of enzymes, vitamins, and minerals, including vitamin C, A, B, and E. Whereas ripe papaya can be eaten raw, unripe, green papaya, the kind that is traditionally used as a galactagogue, should be cooked. Green papaya can also be taken in supplement form. For a recipe, see page 177.

Allergy: Persons allergic to latex may be allergic to papaya and other fruit.

Warning: Persons taking Warfarin should consult with their doctor before taking papaya supplements.

Red Clover (trifolium pratense)

Red clover is another highly nutritious herb. It has a wide range of usages in traditional medicine, including being used as a poultice to treat cancer, to reduce rheumatic pain, and to soften hardened glands.

Red clover is a blood-cleanser. It is used in the treatment of bacterial infections and to support a weakened immune system. Like many galactagogues, it reduces fluid retention, helps expectorate mucus from the lungs, is antispasmodic, and a sedative, and is useful for cramps and coughs. It is used to treat eczema, especially in children.

Red clover, especially the sprout, is estrogenic; pastured animals that overdose on this plant become infertile—as if taking an estrogen-based birth control pill. This doubtless contributes to its lactogenic effect.

As a galactagogue, red clover is commonly taken as a capsule, together with fenugreek, alfalfa, and blessed thistle. The herb is frequently combined with other lactogenic herbs for a potent infusion. Use red clover with moderation during pregnancy. If you have red clover growing near you, use the fresh flowers in salad.

Pregnancy: Use only in moderate amounts during pregnancy, as one ingredient in an herbal tea mixture, for instance.

Caution: Avoid red clover if you take blood-thinning drugs, aspirin, or hormonal birth control.

Dosage and Preparation:

- Capsules: 2 - 3 capsules, 3 times a day, in combination with other herbs. (See page 280.)
- Tea: Pour 1 cup of boiling water onto 1 – 3 teaspoons of the dried flowers, and steep for 10 – 15 minutes.
- Infusion: Add the herb to a mixture of other lactogenic herbs and infuse for several hours or over night.

Red Raspberry Leaf (Rubus idaeus)

The raspberry vine is native to both America and Europe. The roots, leaves, and berries have long been appreciated for their nutritive value. Native Americans gave raspberry leaves to women and animals during birth to strengthen and speed delivery, and we learned this virtue from them. Today, pregnant women take red raspberry leaf to tone the uterus, and to prevent hemorrhaging during birth.

Red raspberry leaf tea provides an excellent source of minerals and vitamins during pregnancy. As do all highly nutritious lactogenic teas, it is thought that it may help build breast tissue during pregnancy. Humphrey records that it does not appear to contribute to over-supply after birth. Red raspberry leaf is said to bring on the milk and make it richer. However, raspberry leaf tea is astringent (tightens and constricts bodily tissues), and is occasionally anti-lactogenic for women who are sensitive to this effect. For these women, it is probably safe to use red raspberry leaf as one ingredient in a lactation tea mixture.

Pregnancy caution: During pregnancy, red raspberry tea may stimulate the uterus. To be on the safe side, build up dosage slowly, beginning with one cup per day for a week, two cups per day next week, and so on up to four cups per day. Consult your doctor before taking raspberry tea, if you are at risk for miscarriage.

Dosage and Preparation:

Mothers take up a quart of red raspberry leaf tea per day during pregnancy. See above. Red-raspberry tea is said to promote milk production the first week postpartum, though stinging nettle may be the better herb if there is risk of low milk supply.

- Medicinal tea: Pour 1 cup of just-boiled water over 2 teaspoons of the dried leaf and steep for 5 minutes. Sweeten with a natural sweetener to taste. Build up slowly to 4 cups a day during pregnancy

- Do not take the medicinal tea for longer than a few days after birth to avoid a possible anti-lactogenic effect—some mothers however do not see this effect. Experiment with caution.

- Red raspberry leaf as a mild beverage: Steep 1/2 teaspoon of dried leaves in 1 cup of just-boiled water for 1 – 3 minutes. Sweeten with a natural sweetener to taste.

Sesame Seed

Large, black sesame seeds are used to increase milk production across Asia.. Black sesame seeds can be found in Asian food stores. However, they may be difficult for the unaccustomed stomach to digest. Husked, light-colored sesame seeds are also effective, and easier to digest. Look for sesame seeds that have been husked, as substances in the husk prevent the optimal digestion of the seed.

Sesame seeds are an excellent source of calcium. One cup of sesame seed provides a day's requirement. Mothers whose menstrual cycle have begun may find that taking calcium supplements, or foods high in calcium, the latter half of their cycle, evens out their milk supply and prevents the typical slump at that time. The seeds can be taken medicinally, as a galactagogue, as prepared below.

Allergy: Severe, often with a duel allergy to peanut.

Dosage and Preparation:

- Sesame seeds can be taken as food, for instance as sesame-butter, 'tahini,' which can added to hummus, salad dressing, or taken as a spread on bread or cracker, or as 'gomasio,' a salty condiment to sprinkle over grains, vegetables, and salad
- Simmer 1/2 cup of husked sesame seeds for five minutes in 1 cup of water. Chew the seeds well and drink the water. You may wish to add natural sugar, raisons, or chopped, dried fig or date to the seeds while simmering to improve the taste. Take before a meal.
- It may be practical to prepare this medicinal before cooking a meal for your family, so that you can slowly eat the mixture while you cook.

Spirulina

Spirulina is blue-green algae, widely taken because it boosts the immune system. It is farmed in lakes and ponds. As a food source, it is valued for its proteins, enzymes, minerals, vitamins, chlorophyll, and essential fatty acids. Spirulina's nutrients are easily absorbed, even when a person's digestion is not up to par. *It is not wise to rely on spirulina as a source of B12.*

It is important that spirulina be cultivated on a farm that is well tended and protected from insects, and not located in waters that are contaminated, in particular with heavy metals. It is also important not to use spirulina that has been genetically 'improved.' Spirulina and other "green foods" may increase the fat-content of breastmilk.

Dosage: Follow the dosage recommendations on the package. Taken 15 minutes before meals, spirulina improves digestion due to its enzyme content.

Thyme (Thymus vulgaris)

Thyme is used as an expectorant to loosen congestion in the lungs, and to treat a cough or sore throat. Antifungal and antiseptic, it is also used to treat fungal overgrowth of the intestine. Thyme, like many galactagogues, encourages perspiration, and it is mood-lifting. An estrogenic herb, thyme is used to alter menstrual cycles. It is sometimes referred to as a galactagogue in my old, German herbals.

We do not know very much about thyme as a galactagogue. It is possible that large amounts of thyme could be anti-lactogenic in some women, as some lactation consultants recommend taking thyme in combination with rosemary, sage and parsley to mothers who are weaning, to help dry up their milk production.

Perhaps thyme, marjoram, and basil, all lactogenic spices, are best taken as a spice in food, rather than at therapeutic dosage. It is likely that thyme, taken in combination with other lactogenic herbs, may work synergistically as a galactagogue.

Pregnancy: Do not take thyme in large amounts during pregnancy. It is safe to use as a spice.

Warning: Persons with thyroid problems should avoid thyme.

Dosage: Use a moderate amount in a tea mixture, or take as a spice.

Turmeric (Curcuma longa)

Turmeric's use as a galactagogue is not well known in the West. In India, turmeric is viewed as an important herb for mothers after birth – though it is not taken principally as a galactagogue. Rather, turmeric, a potent anti-inflammatory and antioxidant, helps prevent or heal numerous conditions, and is taken to help prevent mastitis.

- One half teaspoon of turmeric a day may help prevent mastitis.

- To help treat mastitis, a paste made of warm water and turmeric powder is applied to the painful area of the breast.

Regarded as a natural antibiotic in India, turmeric is used to treat intestinal disease and digestive disorders, to strengthen the liver, to lower cholesterol, for skin conditions such as eczema or boils, for bacterial, viral and fungal infections, for arthritic conditions, bronchial congestion, asthma and sore throat, among many others. It has shown promising anti-cancer and tumor-reducing abilities in mice, and is being investigated in the treatment of AIDS.

⇨ For allergies, turmeric has been shown to be half as strong as cortisone in its anti-inflammatory effects.

⇨ For arthritis, an extract of turmeric—curcumin—is now commonly used.

⇨ Because turmeric is useful for every kind of intestinal disease, it may help breastfeeding mothers with colicky babies to produce milk with fewer triggers for colic.

⇨ Turmeric may even help us think more clearly—in India it is reported to improve concentration and memory. Recent studies in mice show that turmeric inhibits inflammation and degenerative processes in the brain[66]. In fact, it is thought to be *the* medicinal herb responsible for low incidences of Alzheimer's in curry-loving populations in India. If you feel muddle-minded after birth, you're probably feeling the impact of the hormonal changes that go along with motherhood. But slight inflammation in the brain may also be part of the cause—it's more common than you'd think. Try taking turmeric (and omega 3s) for a few weeks and see if it makes a difference.

Warning: Cancer patients who are *undergoing chemotherapy* should avoid curcumin and turmeric.

Warning: While breastfeeding, it's best to use whole turmeric, as the concentrated extract, *curcumin*, has not yet been tested for breastfeeding.

Warning: Some herbalists say that pregnant women who are not used to taking turmeric should not use a therapeutic dosage if they are at risk for miscarriage.

Warning: Turmeric is considered safe within the recommended dosage. Very high dosages for long periods produced adverse symptoms in rodents.

Dosage and Preparation:

• If you wish to use turmeric therapeutically in preventing or reducing inflammation, it is best to combine it with black pepper. Black pepper contains a chemical, peperine, that researchers at St. John's Medical College in Bangalore, India, have discovered may significantly improve the bio-availability of turmeric.

• Dr. James Duke, botanist and author on medicinal medicine, recommends that we buy a pound of very yellow turmeric powder in an Indian or Asian grocery store, where it costs between $3 - $5 per pound (for those who do not have a local Asian grocery store, check out online sources). Also buy an ounce of black pepper corns. Grind the pepper corns and mix them into the turmeric to make, as Dr.

Duke puts it, "a 10-month supply of anti-inflammatory medicine for around $5."

- **Dosage**: 1/4 teaspoon of turmeric powder or turmeric-pepper powder, 3 times a day. The dosage can be added to soup or veggies. I like to mix turmeric with butter on bread or cracker, and top that with honey. It can also be enjoyed in warm milk with honey, and other spices such as cinnamon or ginger, and sweetened with honey. For those who are brave, it can be stirred into cold water and simply gulped down. As with most supplements, turmeric is best taken before a meal.

Umbel Seeds

Anise, caraway, cumin, dill, fennel, and lovage, (used as a galactagogue in France), grow clusters of small flowers, called umbels. Each tiny flower is linked by a small stem to a central, larger stem. These small groups are linked to a still larger stem, forming larger clusters. In traditional medicine, umbels are said to have an affinity for breasts. The shape of the umbel reminds one of milk glands, connected by milk ducts to the areola; such look-alike factors can play a role in the belief that a plant has certain effects. In the case of umbel seeds, experience shows that they do indeed increase milk production and improve the let-down. In one study, umbel seeds tested on rats generated greater mammary tissue growth than was seen with rats on a control diet.

Umbel flowers produce small, aromatic seeds that are used as digestives, carminatives, and, as galactagogues throughout the world. As spices, these seeds are part of the diets of peoples across Eurasia. However, because some umbel plants and seeds are toxic, wild harvesting is not advisable unless you are very knowledgeable.

Umbel seeds share the following properties: they are estrogenic; they are a slight sedative; they promote digestion, ease colic, and flatulence (may ease a baby's colic through the mother's milk); and because they are anti-spasmodic they aid in the treatment of bronchitis and bronchial asthma.

Pregnancy: Western medicine warns against taking large amounts of anise and caraway during pregnancy. Ayurvedic medicine from India warns against taking large amounts of all umbel seeds during pregnancy.

Allergy: Occasional.

Caution: Traditional Chinese Medicine (TCM) says that "warming" herbs, such as the umbel seeds, should not be taken in large amounts by mothers who tend to develop breast infections. According to TCM, these mothers typically have dry skin and hair, and tend to get rash or eczema.

Caution: In Germany, a lactation tea has been produced for decades by Weleda containing equal amounts of stinging nettle, fennel, anise, and caraway seeds. The producers warn that taking more than three cups a day can lead to loose stools in the mother and baby.

Caution: Mothers of lethargic babies should avoid large dosages of herbs that have sedative effects—such as hops and umbel seeds—as these could possibly make their baby sleepier. Lethargic babies should see their pediatrician as soon as possible.

Dosage and Preparation:

- Umbel seeds can be taken individually, together, or combined with other herbs to make a lactation tea. They can be infused overnight in cold or hot water, can be decocted, or steeped as tea.

- Umbel seed tea: Gently crush 1-2 teaspoons of the seeds, and add one cup of boiling water. Cover and steep for between 5 - 20 minutes. Longer steeping produces a more potent tea. Sweeten to taste.

- Umbel seeds as a beverage: Steep 1 – 3 minutes for a milder taste and effect.

- Infusion: In Eastern Europe, umbel seeds such as anise, given to breastfeeding mothers to promote milk production, are covered with boiling water and infused for four hours.

- In India, umbel seeds are placed in cold water and soaked overnight. The liquid is strained and gently warmed before drinking. This way, none of the volatile, medicinal oil is lost to steam.

- The usual recommended dosage is 3 cups a day. To increase milk production, take up to 6 cups a day initially, as necessary, observing your reaction, and your baby's reaction. If you or your baby get loose stools or become gassy, reduce the dosage or try other galactagogues.

- To treat flatulence, drink umbel seed tea slowly before meals, or take it in sips throughout the day.

Valerian (Valeriana officinalis)

Valerian root is not a galactagogue, but because it can be useful to mothers suffering from sleep deprivation, it is included here. Valerian has been shown to improve sleep quality—though it does not reduce waking times during the night[67]. In this study, best results were achieved after four weeks of taking an extract of *the whole valerian root*. Other studies, based on commercial brand products, did not show significant benefits.

Mothers who are sleep-deprived because their baby frequently wakes during the night may find relief with valerian tincture. Even when waking to feed her baby, a mother will remain physically and emotionally relaxed and will easily slip back into deep sleep. If she takes the "right-for-her" dosage, she will not feel drugged or lethargic, but rather, relaxed and refreshed.

⇨ If you are suffering from lack of sleep or stress, it may be wise to take a vitamin-mineral supplement, and an additional vitamin B-complex, vitamin C, magnesium, and zinc supplement. The body depends on these nutrients during times of stress and they become depleted.

Pregnancy: Do not use valerian during pregnancy except under the guidance of your health care provider.

Warning: Valerian should not be taken by persons who also drink alcohol, or take sedatives, or antidepressants.

Caution: Mothers of lethargic babies should avoid large dosages of herb that have sedative effects—such as hops, valerian, and umbel seeds—as these could possibly make their baby even more sleepy and unwilling to drink. Lethargic babies should see their pediatrician as soon as possible.

Caution: A review of studies has shown that valerian is a potent but *safe* sedative that does *not* lead to addiction. Like all sedatives, however, it should used cautiously while caring for a baby. Sedatives tend to sink the inhibition threshold, and mothers on sedatives are more prone to shake or spank their babies. If a mother notices any violent urges toward her baby, she should speak to her healthcare provider immediately.

Caution: As with all sedatives or antidepressants, be extra careful when driving or using machinery.

Dosage:

- Discover your individual dosage. Taking too large a dosage can lead to a drug-like sleep, with the mother feeling as though she has a hang-over next day.

- With herbal tinctures, the dosage can be fine-tuned. Although 30 – 40 drops of valerian before sleep is the recommended dosage, 3 – 10 drops may be sufficient for mothers who respond more sensitively to medicinals.

- Take valerian before going to bed if you are taking it specifically to help you sleep more deeply. Take it in small dosages during the day if you are using it to help calm your nerves.

- If you co-sleep with your baby, make sure to arrange your sleeping positions so that there is no danger of your baby suffocating in bed.

- It may take up to four weeks for the herb to unfold its full effect.

Verbena (Verbena – various species)

Verbena, also called vervain, or lemon verbena, was a holy herb of women in ancient days. It is an estrogenic herb, a liver tonic, and a digestive. It is calming, mood-lifting, and is said to prevent depression from developing. It is particularly useful after a viral infection, such as a cold or flu to prevent exhaustion from lingering, and to restore a person's strength. Because verbena fortifies the nerves while relieving tension, it is a nervine tonic. Also an antispasmodic, verbena helps relieve tension headaches, menstrual cramps, and asthma.

⇨   Verbena extract is taken to balance the thyroid, both when it under- and over-functions.

All species of verbena are said to promote milk production.

Pregnancy: Verbena's effect on the uterus is not understood; experts suggest avoiding it during pregnancy.
Warning: Verbena may interfere in the action of medication for blood pressure or hormone therapy.
Warning: Although traditionally a galactagogue, Traditional Chinese Medicine sees verbena as having a drying property, so that when over-used regularly it may decrease supply. Verbena should therefore be alternated with other teas or beverages.

Dosage and Preparation:
- Medicinal tea: Pour 1 cup of boiling water onto 1 – 3 teaspoonfuls of the dried herb and steep for 10 – 15 minutes. Drink three times a day.
- Tincture: 2 - 4 ml of tincture (10 – 30 drops), three times a day.
- Verbena tea as a beverage: Verbena has a delightful taste. A light tea is made by steeping 1/2 – 1 teaspoon of dried herb for 1 – 3 minutes in a cup of boiled water. Add stevia or other natural sweetener to taste.

Contact Information

For bookstores, "Mother Food for Breastfeeding Mothers" is available through Ingrams, or Baker and Taylor.

For individual sales, "Mother Food for Breastfeeding Mothers" can be ordered through BarnesandNoble.com, Amazon.com, and other online bookstores.

To contact Hilary Jacobson, please write to one of the following email addresses:

Persons with information on lactogenic traditions should write to: **galactagogue@mother-food.com**.

Comments on food sensitivity should be sent to: **foodsensitivity@mother-food.com**.

Comments on colic or GERD: **colic@mother-food.com**, or **gerd@mother-food.com**.

Requests for personal Mother Food Questionnaire Evaluations: **consult@mother-food.com**

Visit www.mother-food.com to read contributions from parents, and for updates, articles, artwork, and links.

Endnotes

1. Bingel AS, Farnsworth NR. Higher plants as potential sources of galactagogues. *Econ Med Plant Res* 1994; 6:1–54 [review].

2. U. Renzenbrink, "Mit Kindern Leben, Chapter 2, Ernährungsfragen", (1979) Stuttgart: Verlag Freies Geistesleben GmbH

3. A.M. Siega-Riz, "Frequency of Eating in Second Trimester Helps Predict Risk of Premature Delivery." *Am J Epidemiol* 2001;153:647-652.

4. Uvnas-Moberg, Kerstin. "Role of efferent and afferent vagal nerve activity during reproduction: integrating function of oxytocin on metabolism and behaviour." *Psychoneuroendocrinology* 1994; Vol. 19, Nos. 5-7, 687-695

5. L. B. Dusdieker et al., "Effect of supplemental fluids on human milk production." *Pediatr* 106:207, 1991

6. D. E. Larson-Meyer, "Effect of Postpartum Exercise on Mothers and their Offspring: A Review of the Literature." *Obes Res* 2002 Aug;10(8):841-53. Review.

7. Information kindly provided by Christiane Husi-Simonis, holistic lactation consultant, yoga teacher and certified nutritionist in TCM.

8. A. Wright et al., "Cultural interpretations and intracultural variability in Navajo beliefs about breastfeeding." *American Ethnologist* 1993. 20(4)781-796

9. U. Ravnskov, "The questionable role of saturated and polyunsaturated fatty acids in cardiovascular disease." *J Clin Epidemiol* 1998 Jun;51(6):443-60.

10. Developed by Linsey McLean
http://abcnews.go.com/sections/business/PatentlyWeird/patent_990113.html

11. K. Fischer et al., "Cognitive performance and its relationship with postprandial metabolic changes after ingestion of different macronutrients in the morning. " *Br J Nutr* 2001 Mar;85(3):393-405.

12. P. M. Kris-Etherton et al. "The effects of nuts on coronary heart disease risk." *Nutr Rev* 2001 Apr;59(4):103-11.; R. Lopez Ledesma, et al., "Monounsaturated fatty acid (avocado) rich diet for mild hypercholesterolemia." *Arch Med Res* 1996 Winter;27(4):519-23.

13. H. Kawagishi et al., "Liver injury suppressing compounds from avocado (Persea americana)." *J Agric Food Chem* 2001 May;49(5):2215-21

14. H. Isensee, "Differential effects of various oil diets on the risk of cardiac arrhythmias in rats." *J Cardiovasc Risk* 1994 Dec;1(4):353-9. (As example for study with hydrogenated saturated fat.)

15. J. Riedler et al., "Exposure to farming in early life and development of asthma and allergy: a cross-sectional survey." *Lancet* 2001 Oct 6;358(9288):1129-33.

16. S. Rautava et al., "Probiotics during pregnancy and breast-feeding might confer immunomodulatory protection against atopic disease in the infant." *J Allergy Clin Immunol* 2002 Jan;109(1):119-21.

17. T. Dunder et al., "Diet, serum fatty acids, and atopic diseases in childhood." *Allergy* 2001 May;56(5):425-8.

18. N. M. de Roos et al., "Replacement of dietary saturated fatty acids by trans-fatty acids lowers serum HDL cholesterol and impairs endothelial function in healthy men and women." *Arterioscler Thromb Vasc Biol* 2001 Jul;21(7):1233-7. C.M. Oomen et al., "Association between trans-fatty acid intake and 10-year risk of coronary heart disease in the Zutphen Elderly Study: a prospective population-based study." *Lancet* 2001 Mar 10;357(9258):746-51. (Netherlands). R.N. Lemaitre et al. "Cell membrane trans-fatty acids and the risk of primary cardiac arrest." *Circulation* 2002 Feb 12;105(6):697-701. (USA).

19. Ginsberg et al., "Increases in dietary cholesterol are associated with modest increases in both LDL and HDL cholesterol in healthy young women." *Arterioscler. Thromb. Vasc. Biol.* 15:169-178.

20. D. F. Horrobin, "Essential fatty acid metabolism and its modification in atopic eczema." *Am J Clin Nutr* 2000 Jan;71(1 Suppl):367S-72S; S. Wright, C. Bolton, " Breast milk fatty acids in mothers of children with atopic eczema." *Br J Nutr* 1989 Nov;62(3):693-7; R.G. Jensen et al,

"Possible alleviation of atopic eczema in a breastfed infant by maternal supplementation with a fish oil concentrate." *J Pediatr Gastroenterol Nutr* 1992 May;14(4):474-5;

21.   J. R. Hibbeln, "Seafood consumption, the DHA content of mothers' milk and prevalence rates of postpartum depression: a cross-national, ecological analysis." *J Affect Disord* 2002 May;69(1-3):15-29

22.   C. L. Jensen et al., "Effect of docosahexaenoic acid supplementation of lactating women on the fatty acid composition of breast milk lipids and maternal and infant plasma phospholipids." *Am J Clin Nutr* 2000 Jan;71(1 Suppl):292S-9S

23.   Dosage limitation from Dr. Jack Newman, *The Ultimate Breastfeeding Book of Answers* (2000) pg 132

24.   A. Cant et al., "The effect of maternal supplementation with linoleic and gamma-linolenic acids on the fat composition and content of human milk: a placebo-controlled trial." *J Nutr Sci Vitaminol* (Tokyo) 1991 Dec;37(6):573-9

25.   Graduate student study, under the direction of BB Teter at the University of Maryland.

26.   S.K. Weiland et al., "Intake of trans fatty acids and prevalence of childhood asthma and allergies in Europe." *The Lancet* 1999; 353 (9169): 2040-2041.

27.   B. Teter et al., "Milk Fat Depression in Mice Consuming Partially Hydrogenated Fat." *Journal of Nutrition*, 1990, 120:818-824

28.   Zwillich, T. US Panel Finds No Safe Level of Dietary Trans Fatty Acids Reuters Health Information 2002. © 2002 Reuters Ltd. available at http://www.medscape.com/viewarticle/438341

29.   S.B. and D. Kritchevsky, "Egg consumption and coronary heart disease: an epidemiologic overview." *J Am Coll Nutr* 2000 Oct;19(5 Suppl):549S-555S.

30.   F. Kern, "Effects of dietary cholesterol on cholesterol and bile acid homeostasis in patients with cholesterol gallstones." *J. Clin. Invest.* 93:1186-1194.

31.   E.N. Smit, et al. "Effect of supplementation of arachidonic acid (AA) or a combination of AA plus docosahexaenoic acid on breastmilk fatty acid composition." *Prostaglandins Leukot Essent Fatty Acids* 2000 Jun;62(6):335-40

32.   S.H. Zeisel, "Choline: needed for normal development of memory." *J Am Coll Nutr* 2000 Oct;19(5 Suppl):528S-531S

33.   J.M. Hopkinson, et al., "Milk production by mothers of premature infants: influence of cigarette smoking." *Pediatrics* 1992 Dec;90(6):934-8

34.   B. Koletzko, F. Lehner. "Beer and breastfeeding." *Adv Exp Med* Biol 2000;478:23-8

35.   B. Koletzko, F. Lehner. "Beer and breastfeeding." *Adv Exp Med* Biol 2000;478:23-8

36.   R. Pols, D. Hawks, "Is there a safe level of daily consumption of alcohol for men and women. Recommendations regarding responsible drinking behaviour." NH¬MRC pamphlet, Canberra.

37.   K.M. Jarvinen et al., "Does low IgA in human milk predispose the infant to development of cow's milk allergy?" *Pediatr Res* 2000 Oct;48(4):457-62

38.   See Sally Fallon's, "Nourishing Traditions."

39.   This testimonial was sent to me directly, but it also appears on a website. I have been unable to locate the author as her email address has changed in the interim.

40.   S.D. Holladay, "Prenatal immunotoxicant exposure and postnatal autoimmune disease." *Environ Health Perspect* 1999 Oct;107 Suppl 5:687-91

41.   R. Nakagawa et al., "Maternal body burden of organochlorine pesticides and dioxins." *J AOAC Int* 1999 May-Jun;82(3):716-24

42.   W. Karmaus, "Does the sibling effect have its origin in utero? Investigating birth order, cord blood immunoglobulin E concentration, and allergic sensitization at age 4 years." *Am J Epidemiol* 2001 Nov 15;154(10):909-15

43.   J. Hergenrather et al., "Pollutants in Breast Milk of Vegetarians," *New England Journal of Medicine* 304:792, 1981; P.C. Dagnelie et al. "Nutrients and contaminants in human milk from mothers on macrobiotic and omnivorous diets." *Eur J Clin Nutr* 1992; 46: 355-366.

44.   " PERSISTENT ORGANIC POLLUTANTS AND HUMAN HEALTH—Dioxins in Breastmilk " Based on the materials of the seminar "Women's Role in Addressing Problems of Persistent Organic Pollutants" " Moscow, May 15-16, 2001 © Eco-Accord Centre http://accord.cis.lead.org/cooperation/sem-engl/yufit.htm

303

45. D.O. Carpenter, "Effects of metals on the nervous system of humans and animals." *Int J Occup Med Environ Health* 2001;14(3):209-18; A.F. Castoldi, "Neurotoxicity and molecular effects of methylmercury." *Brain Res Bull* 2001 May 15;55(2):197-203

46. D. Klinghardt, P. Kane, "Schwermetalle und ihre Wirking auf die Gesundheit", video-recorded lecture from Oct. 31,2001. (2001) Paracelsus Apoltheke CH-8840 Einsiedeln, Switzerland

47. R.L. Siblerud et al., "Psychometric evidence that mercury from silver dental fillings may be an etiological factor in depression, excessive anger, and anxiety." *Psychol Rep* 1994 Feb;74(1):67-80

48. G.A. Ulmer. "Heilende Oele." Günter Albert Ulmer Verlag: Tuningen

49. As I wrote this section, I thought it was original. Now I believe I may have read something similar, but do not know where. I am sorry that I cannot provide a source, but will gladly do so in future editions if contacted about it.

50. A.W. Shiell et al., "High-meat, low-carbohydrate diet in pregnancy: relation to adult blood pressure in the offspring." *Hypertension* 2001 Dec 1;38(6):1282-8.

51. T.R. Mikuls et al., "Coffee, tea, and caffeine consumption and risk of rheumatoid arthritis: results from the Iowa Women's Health Study." *Arthritis Rheum* 2002 Jan;46(1):83-91

52. A.L. Craigmill et al., "Pathological changes in the mammary gland and biochemical changes in milk of the goat following oral dosing with leaf of the avocado (Persea americana)." *Aust Vet J* 1989 Jul;66(7):206-11

53. G.E. Fraser et al., "Effect on body weight of a free 76 Kilojoule (320 calorie) daily supplement of almonds for six months." *J Am Coll Nutr* 2002 Jun;21(3):275-83

54. L.H. Kushi et al., "Health implications of Mediterranean diets in light of contemporary knowledge. 1. Plant foods and dairy products." *Am J Clin Nutr* 1995 Jun;61(6 Suppl):1407S-1415S

55. "Just a mouthful of whale meat is toxic." *New Scientist*, Friday, June 7, 2002

56. M. BURROS,"EATING WELL—F.D.A. Cautions Against Eating Certain Fish During Pregnancy" *The New York Times* May 9, 2001

57. http://www.drjaygordon.com/nutrition/goodfood/danger07.htm

58. L. Marasco et al., "Polycystic ovary syndrome: a connection to insufficient milk supply?" *J Hum Lact* 2000 May;16(2):143-8

59. This insight is found at IBCLC Lisa Marasco's interview at Obgyn.net: http://www.obgyn.net/displayarticle.asp?page=/pcos/articles/childers-chats

60. James Braly, M.D. *see* bibliography.

61. F. Batmanghelidj, M. D. *see* bibliography.

62. K. Bone, "Clinical Applications of Ayurvedic and Chinese Herbs." Warwick, Australia, *Phytotherapy Press.*

63. P.G. Merz et al. "Prolaktinsekretion und Verträglichkeit under der Behandlung mit einem Agus-castus-Spezialextrakt (BP1095E1). Erste Ergebnisse zum Einfluss auf die Prolaktinsekretion."

64. *hytopharmaka in Forschung und Klinischer Anwendung*, ed. D. Loew und N. Rietbrock, Darmstadt, Skein Kopff.

65. Personal interviews.

66. J.A. Mennella et al., "The effects of repeated exposure to garlic-flavored milk on the nursling's behavior." *Pediatr Res* 1993;34:805–8.

67. G.P. Limet al., "The curry spice curcumin reduces oxidative damage and amyloid pathology in an Alzheimer transgenic mouse." *J Neurosci* 2001 Nov 1;21(21):8370-7; S.A. Frautschy et al., "Phenolic anti-inflammatory antioxidant reversal of Abeta-induced cognitive deficits and neuropathology." *Neurobiol Aging* 2001 Nov-Dec;22(6):993-1005

68. PD. Leathwood, et al. " Aqueous extract of valerian root (Valeriana officinalis L.) improves sleep quality in man." *Pharmacol Biochem Behav* 1982 Jul;17(1):65-71

Selected Bibliography

Balch, Ph. A., and Balch, J. F. *Prescription for Nutritional Healing*, 3rd ed. New York: Penguin Putnam Inc., 2000.

Bateson-Koch, C. *Allergies, Disease in Disguise*. Burnaby BC, Canada: alive books. 1994.

Batmanghelidj, F. *Your Body's Many Cries For Water*. Norwich, Great Britan: The Tagman Press, 2000.

Blumenthal, Mark et al. *THE COMPLETE GERMAN COMMISSION E MONOGRAPHS*. Computer CD. *Austin, Texas: American Botanical Council 1999*

Braly, J. *Dr. Braly's Food Allergy & Nutrition Revolution*. New Canann, Connecticut: Keats, 1992

Brostoff, J., Gamlin, L. *Food Allergies and Food Intolerance – The complete guide to their identification and treatment*. Rochester, Vermont: Healing Arts Press, 2000.

Cabot, S. *The Liver Cleansing Diet*. Scottsdale, AZ: S.C.B. International, 1996

Crook, W.G. *The Yeast Connection Handbook*. Jackson, Tennessee: Professional Books, INC., 2000.

Culpeper, N. *Complete Herbal & English Physician Enlarged*. Glenwood, Illinois: Mayerbooks, 1990.

Dalton, K. *Depression after Childbirth*. Oxford: Oxford University Press, 1989.

DesMaisons, K. *Potatoes not Prozac*. New York, NY: Fireside, Simon & Schuster, 1999.

Duke, J. A. *The Green Pharmacy*. New York, NY: St. Martin's Press, 1997.

Duke, J.A. *Handbook of Medicinal Herbs*. Boca Raton, Florida: CRC Press LLC, 2001.

Enig, M. G. Know Your Fats: The Complete Primer for Understanding the Nutrition of Fats, Oils, and Cholesterol. Silverspring, MD: Bethesda Press, 2000.

Fallon, S. Enig, M. G. *NOURISHING TRADITIONS*. Washington, DC: NewTrends Publishing, 1999

Flaws, B., Wolfe, H. *Prince Wen Hui's Cook: Chinese Dietary Therapy*. Paradigm Pubns, 1985.

Galland, L. *Superimmunity for Kids – What to Feed Your children to Keep Them Healthy Now—and Prevent Disease in Their Future*. New York, NY: Copestone Press, Dell Trade Paperback, 1988.

Gladstar, Rosemary. *Herbal Healing for Women*. New York: A Fireside Book, 1993.

Gunter, R. T. *The Greek Herbal of Dioscorides*. New York, 1959.

Harris, C. Carey, A. *PCOS A woman's guide to dealing with polycystic ovary syndrome*. London: Thorsons, 2000.

Hoffman, D. *An Elders' Herbal*. Rochester, Vermont: Healing Arts Press, 1993.

Hudson, T. *Women's Enycyclopedia of Natural Medicine*. Los Angeles: Keats Publishing, 1999.

Huggins, K. *The Nursing Mother's Companion*. Boston, Massachusetts: The Harvard Common Press, 1999.

Humphrey, Sheila. *The Nursing Mother's Herbal*. Minneapolis, Minnesota: Fairview Press, 2003.

Jain, S.K., R.A. DeFilipps. *Medicinal Plants of India*. Vol. 2. Algonac, Michigan: Reference Publications, Inc., 1991.

Joneja, J. *DIETARY MANAGEMENT OF FOOD ALLERGIES & INTOLERANCES – A Comprehensive Guide*. Burnaby, British Columbia: J.A. Hall Publications, 1998.

Kranowitz, Carol Stock. *The Out-of-Sync Child*. New York, NY. 1998

Kühne, P. *Säuglings-Ernährung*. Bad Liebenzell: Arbeitskreis für Ernährungsforschung e.V. 1988.

Laderman, C. *Wives and Midwives: Childbirth and nutrition in rural Malaysia*. Berkeley: University of California Press, 1984.

La Leche League International. *The Womanly Art of Breastfeeding*.

Lawrence, R.A. *Breastfeeding 4th ed. A guide for the medical profession*. St. Louis, Missouris: Mosby-Year Book, Inc., 1994

Leung, A., Foster, S. *Encyclopedia of common natural ingredients used in food, drugs, and cosmetics*. 2nd ed. New York: John Wiley & Sons. 1996.

Lim, Robin. *After the Baby's Birth – A Complete Guide for Postpartum Women*. Berkeley, CA: Celestial Arts, 1991.

306

Longsdorf, N., MD, Butler, V., MD, Brown, M., Ph.D. *A Woman's Best Medicine.* Los Angeles: Tarcher/Putnam, 1993.

Luetjohann, S. *The Healing Power of Black Cumin.* Twin Lakes, WI: Lotus Light Shangri-la, 1998.

McGuffin, M. et all. (1997). *American Herbal Products Association's Botanical Safety Handbook.* Boca Raton, Florida: CRC Press LLC

McIntyre, Anne. *The Complete Woman's Herbal, A Manual of Healing Herbs and Nutrition for Personal Well-being and Family Care.* New York: Henry Holt and Company, Inc., 1995.

Minchin, M. *Breastfeeding Matters.* St.Kilda, Vic: ALMA Publications, 1998

Molony, D. *The American Association of Oriental Medicine's Complete Guide to Chinese Herbal Medicine.* New York, NY: Berkley Books, 1998.

Morgan, B. Audio-book. *Reading Your Baby's Body Language. San Jose, CA: Milky Way Press, 1998.*

Mutter, J. *Amalgam – Risiko für die Menschheit.* Weil der Stadt: NaturaViva Verlag GmbH, 2001

Newman, J., Pitman, T. *The Ultimate Breastfeeding Book of Answers.* Roseville, CA: Prima Publishing, 2000.

Northrup, Ch. *Women's Bodies Women's Wisdom – Creating Physical and emotional Health and Healing.* New York, NY: Bantam Books, 1998

Northrup, Ch. Audio-book. *Your Diet, Your Health.* Chicago, IL: Heitz/Wilson, Inc., 1999.

Odent, Michel. *The Nature of Birth and Breastfeeding.* Westport, Connecticut, London: Bergin & Garvey.

Palmer, L.F. *Baby Matters – What Your Doctor May Not Tell You About Caring For Your Baby.* Lancaster, Ohio: Lucky Press, 2001.

Pedersen, M. *Nutritional Herbology.* Warsaw, IN: Wendell W. Whitman Company, 1998.

Pierce, A. *The American Pharmaceutical Associations Practical Guide to Natural Medicines.* New York, NY: Stonesong Press, William Morrow and Company, Inc., 1999.

Price, W. A. *Nutrition and Physical Degeneration*. La Mesa, CA: The price-pottenger Nutrition Foundation, Inc., 2000.

Raphael, D., Davis, F. *Only Mothers Know: Patterns of Infant Feeding in Traditional Cultures*. Westport, CT: Greenwood Press, 1985.

Rapp, D. *Is This Your Child? Discovering and Treating Unrecognized Allergies in Children and Adults*. New York, NY: Quill, William Morrow, 1991.

Rapp, D. Audio-book. *Infant Food Allergies*.

Ranade, Subhash, Ph.D. (1994). *Ayurveda: Wesen und Methodik*. Heidelberg: Karl F. Haug Verlag

Renfrew, M., Fisher, Ch., Arms, S. *The New Bestfeeding – Getting Breastfeeding Right for You*. Berkeley, CA: Celestial Arts, 2000.

Renzenbrink, U. *Die Ernährung des Säugling*. Aus: Verein für ein erweitertes Heilwesen. *Mit Kindern leben: zur Praxis der körperlichen und seelischen Gesundheitspflege*. Stuttgart: Verlag Freies Geistesleben, 1979.

Riddle, J. M. *Contraception and Abortion from the Ancient World to the Renaissance*. Cambridge, Massachusetts, London, England: Harvard University Press: 1994.

Rotblatt, M., Ziment, I. *Evidence-Based Herbal Medicine*. Philadelphia: Hanley & Belfus, 2002.

Tamaro, J. *So that's what they're for!* Holbrook, MA: Adams Media Corporation, 1996.

Tricky, R. *Women, Hormones & The Menstrual Cycle – herbal & medical solutions from adolescence to menopause*. St. Leonards NSW Australia: Allen & Unwin

Teeguarden, R. *Radiant Health – The Ancient Wisdom of the Chinese Tonic Herbs*. New York, NY: Warner Books, 1998.

Weed, S. S. *Herbal Childbearing Year*. Woodstock, NY: Ash Tree Publishing, 1986.

Willfort, Richard. *Gesundheit durch Heilkräuter*. Linz: Austria: Rudolf Trauner Verlag, 1959.

Herbs Index

ANTI-LACTOGENIC:

Parsley, **123-24**. Can be anti-lactogenic if taken frequently; can promote milk production if taken sparsely. 23,81,104, 197,294. Allergenic.
Do not take at high dosage during pregnancy.

Peppermint, **123-24**, Can be anti-lactogenic if taken frequently; the essential oil, also as flavoring, is anti-lactogenic. 164,188. **Do not take at high dosage during pregnancy.** Allergenic

Rosemary, **123-124**,194. Possibly anti-lactogenic if taken frequently.
Do not take at high dosage during pregnancy. Allergenic

Sage, **123-24**,188,294. Strongly anti-lactogenic. **Do not take at high dosage during pregnancy**

Thyme,: **294**. Can possibly be anti-lactogenic if taken in combination with other anti-lactogenic herbs; otherwise, can promote milk production.
Do not take at high dosage during pregnancy

LACTOGENIC:

Alfalfa Leaf, **261**,279. Nutritious; vitamin K; supports pituitary gland, i.e., prolactin. Allergenic Contraindication: Persons with Lupus should avoid alfalfa.

Anise Seed, **262**. Digestive, estrogenic, relaxing. Allergenic
Do not take at high dosage during pregnancy.

Asparagus racemosus, see Shatavari.

Astragalus Root, **263**. Tonic, immune booster, IgA. Contraindication: Do not take during a cold or flu.

Barley, Seed and Grass, **197**. Tonic, immune booster, intestine, liver, bronchial. Caution: Too much barley may be anti-lactogenic, especially barley-sprout.

Basil, **264**. Estrogenic, anti-microbial, relaxant.
Do not take at high dosage during pregnancy.

Black Pepper, **264**.

Black Seed (Nigella Sativa), **264-65**. Digestive, tonic, bronchial dilator, immune booster.

Do not take at high dosage during pregnancy.

Black Tea, **265**.

Blessed Thistle, **266**,279. Liver, gall-bladder, intestine, appetite. Allergenic **Avoid during pregnancy.**

Borage, **267**. Euphoric, stress reducer. Counterindication: do not take at therapeutic dosage.

Caraway, **267**. Digestive, estrogenic, relaxing. Allergenic
Do not take at high dosage during pregnancy.

Chasteberry, **268**. Hormone-balancer. Counterindication: Take only under the guidance of your healthcare provider.
Do not take during pregnancy, except the last two weeks.

Cumin, **271**. Digestive, estrogenic, relaxing. Allergenic
Do not take at high dosage during pregnancy.

Dandelion, **271-73**. Liver-herb, gall-bladder, diuretic, nutritious. Allergenic Counterindication: gall-bladder blockage.

Dill Seed, and Leaf: **273-74**. Digestive, estrogenic, relaxing. Allergenic
Do not take at high dosage during pregnancy.

Dong Quai, **274-75**. Blood tonic, women's herb, immune booster.
Do not take during pregnancy.
Counterindication: Do not combine with blood-thinning medication.

Elder Flowers (and Berries), **276**. Promotes sweating and fever when treating a cold or flu. Antiviral.

Fennel seed, **277**. Digestive, estrogenic, relaxing. Allergenic
Do not take at high dosage during pregnancy.

Fenugreek seed*, **278-80**. Promotes sweating and fever; digestive, estrogenic. 30,53,106,111,159 Allergenic
Do not take during pregnancy.
Caution: diabetes or hypoglycemia; use under doctor's guidance.

Garlic, **281-82**. Strengthens digestion. Antibacterial, antiviral, anti-fungal. Counterindication: Do not combine with blood-thinning medication. 67,82,85,111, 126,128,165,166,176,177, 195,197,215, 221-3,236-242,253,273 Allergenic

Ginger*, **282-83**. Improves circulation. Drying. Antimicrobial. Digestive.

---

* Herbs that are cautioned against during pregnancy are marked with an asterix "*".

Food Index

Food Index

Dill, 14,67,68,91,121,161,163,164,167,
169,171,172,204,215,218,221,222,
223,237,240,241,256,260,273,274
see Herbs Index for Counterindication.
Dong Quai, 29,51,176,253,260,263,274
allergy, 249
anemia, 99,174,187
Egg, 39,40,43,45,47,49,50,51,52,53,69,71,
144,150,151,196,203,**217,06,213,214,**
221,222,227,229
and cholesterol,49,50
Egg Dressing, for salad,240
Essential Fatty Acids (EFAs), *see* Subject
Index.
Evening primrose oil, 46-48,111,252
Fennel seed, 3,23,51,68,91,101,111,121,122,
124,128,142,158,160,161,163,166,167,
169,170,172,175,187,191,192,193,195,
196,200,204,209,224,225,232,233,234,
235,239,242,248,246,264,**277**
Fennel, vegetable, 3,101,111,122,128,142,163,
187,195,196, 224-5,232,234,235,239,248,
277
Fenugreek, 30,53,106,111,159,162,170,171,
173,186,192,194,204,208,209,258,256,
260,266,272,276,278-80
Fig, 3,101,120,121,130,160,161,178,193,
198,202,215,216,226,244,
in barley-water, 193
fig-ginger topping, 244
fig-wine, 161
Fish, 118,146-148
Fish oil, *see* Subject Index.
Flaxseed, *see* Subject Index.
Flaxseed oil, *see* Subject Index.
Fruit, 29,30,31,69,71,73,82,108,109,120,125,
127,129,130,145,151,156,198,203,
206,207,210,216,218,224,243
Fruit, dried,27,70,87,102,120,210,227,245
Fruit-Nut Shake, 203
Garbanzo, *see* Chickpea
Garlic, 3,5,51,68,82,85,111,126,128,165,166,
176,177,195,197,215,221,222,223,
236-242,253,273, **281-82**
Baked Garlic Spread, 223
Ginger, 68,82,130,167,169,170,172,175,177,
192,199,200,202,203,204,215,224,
242,248,250,253,256,260,**282-83**
Counterindication: anemia; blood loss.
Ginger ale, for let-down, milk flow, 203
Ginger tea, 204, **282-283**
Ginkgo biloba, 283
Goat's rue, 106,159,166,186,276, 283-84

and mammary development, 186
Gomasio, 131,152,154,178,221,294
Grain-drinks, 190-193
Grains and legumes, 82, 143,144,145,
146,151,152,174,252
preparation, 136,145,**228-31**
Granola, 122
Green-bean, 81,109,111,119,122,128,129,134,
154,232,233,234,235
Green-drink, green-juice, 159,195-98
Green soup, 81
Halvah, 218,244
Hollyhock root, 161-2,204,260,284
Hops, 262,285
Hummus, 222
Jerusalem artichoke, 111,122,128,166
Juice, 24,27,81,82,123,126,152,156,190,195,
196,197,198
combinations, 195
green, with blender, 196
Kale, 103,122,128,152,196-7,233
Kefir, 139,142,200-201
Leftovers, 227
Lemon Balm, 123,204,**286,** *see* Herbs Index.
Legumes, *see* Grains and legumes,
Malt, **59,**70,86,102,136,151,159,166,192,199,
202,205,206,209,**244,**260
Marjoram, 23,30,67,121,192,217,221,223,233,
236,238,240,241,264,**287,**295
Marshmallow root and leaf, 14,162,248,260,
272,279,284,**287**
Marzipan, 244
Mayonnaise, 220
Meat, 30,32,35,38,39,40,48,49,74,75,78,100,
104-5,110,128,129,143-5,150-1,153,
155,156,177,190,222,229,237,238
lactogenic, 118,144
Milk, spiced milk, 199
substitute, 121 *see* almond-milk, rice-
milk, coconut-milk.
Milk Thistle, 83,249,253,256,288
Millet, 3,23,30,108,109,119,134,137,174,178,
187,**191,**192,209,210,212,**229,230,**241
millet-flake tea, 191
Miso, 70,134,221
Molasses, blackstrap, 87,102104,114,120,152,
199,202,203,209,221,258
molasses coffee, 114,202
Moshi (pounded rice-cakes), 120
Muffins, basic recipe, 214-215
Mung bean, 119,134,**170,**208,212,231,239,
split mung bean soup, 242
sprouts, 239

312

Subject Index

D

E

Subject Index

sesame seed oil, 42,46,48,53,121,**132**
trans-fats, *see* Trans-fatty acids.
    vegetable oil, polyunsaturated,
        37,40,43,**52**,133,220
    processed, 35,38,40
    sunflower, safflower, 133
    Omega 3 and omega 6, *see* Essential
        Fatty Acids
Oral defensiveness, 20
Orthomolecular medicine, 157
Osteoporosis, 56,141
Over-active milk-ejection reflex, and low
    milk supply, 188, *see also* Milk
    ejection reflex and Milk flow.
    and scissors hold,189
Overweight, 34,36,104,143,195,228
Oxytocin, 8,924-5,110,184
    oxytocin-spray, 9
    and digestion, 24-5,110
    and let-down, 8,9,203, *see also* Milk
    ejection reflex.

P

Pain, *see* Breast.
Palate, high 19
PCOS (polycystic ovarian syndrome),
    104,183-186
    and breast hypoplasia, 183-4
    and insulin resistance, 104
    and low milk supply, 183-4
    overproduction of milk, 188
    overactive milk ejection reflex, 187-9
    and overweight, 104
    see also, Glandular breast tissue,
    development of.
Palmer, Linda Folden, 71,72,78,138
Peanut, 3,52,63,68,69,70,71,120,139,250,
    280,283
Phosphorus, 151,261,271,290
Pitocin, 181
Potassium, 271,272,290
    lack of, 99,261,
    and calcium depletion, 125
Phytates, 226
Phytic acid and enzyme inhibitors, 136,
    210,213,
Phytoestrogen, (plant-estrogen) 129,135,
    208,209,215,239,261,262,264,265,
    270,271,274,278,283,285,290,292,
    294,297,299
Placenta, and delayed milk production, 6
Plugged milk ducts, 8,15,16,177,189,255
    lecithin, 255
Polysaccharides, 59,135,191

Postpartum health problems, 99-105
Pregnancy, preparation for
    breastfeeding, 184-186
Premature birth, 83
Prenatal vitamins, supplements, 155,156
Probiotics, *see* Lactobacillus Acidophilus.
Progesterone, natural, oral micronized, 184
Prolactin receptors, 187
Prostaglandins, 39,50
Protein, 29,36,57,61,62,63,66,67,69,70,71,
    75,83,84,85,90,100,104,105,109,110,
    111,116,131,133,134,137,138,140,
    143,146,150,159,184,185,191,196,
    197,200,205,216,219,221,222,225,
    231,242,250, 282,290,291,293
    amount needed, 144
    animal, 143
    and calcium depletion, 141,151
    complete plant, 134,231
    and low milk supply, 144
Pumping, 6,7,8,9,10,11,15,18,19,20,21,
    22,25,47,57,86,88,98,103,111,117,
    182,184,187,188,197,203,222,248
    frequency, 9
    hand-express, 7,10
    Pumps, types, 7

Q

"Qi" energy, 171,173,289

R

Ravnskov, Uffe, 35
Raw food, 30
Raw milk, 35,36,37,38,63,104,142,
Refusal to breastfeed, 6,20,87,56,88,255
Reglan™, *see* Medication, to boost milk
    supply.
Relactation, **21**,164,165
Riddle, John M., 4
Rapp, Doris, 31,60,72,74,93,94

S

Saponins, 129,135,191,208,215,
Saracoglu, Iclal, 166
Saturated fat, *see* Oils and Fats
Screaming baby, 74,84,92
Sensory integration dysfunction, 19,93
Serotonin, 110,111
    and carbohydrate cravings, 110,116
    milk production, 111,129,130
    serotonin-rich foods, 110-11
Sesame oil, 38,52,53,54,132,152,169,176,
    195,217,239
SIDS (Sudden Infant Death Syndrome),

Printed in the United States
213900BV00002B/32/A

9 780979 599507